CULTURE AND HEALING
IN ASIAN SOCIETIES

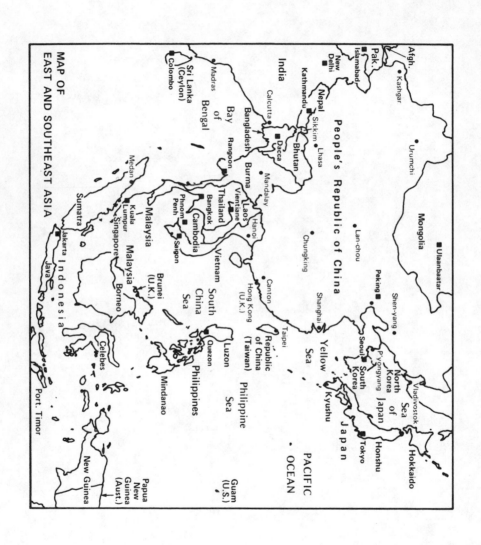

MAP OF
EAST AND SOUTHEAST ASIA

CULTURE AND HEALING IN ASIAN SOCIETIES

Anthropological, Psychiatric and Public Health Studies

Edited by

Arthur Kleinman
Peter Kunstadter
E. Russell Alexander
James L. Gate

G.K. HALL & CO.
70 LINCOLN STREET, BOSTON, MASS.

SCHENKMAN PUBLISHING COMPANY
Cambridge, Mass.

Library of Congress Cataloging in Publication Data
Main entry under title:
Culture and healing in Asian societies.

    Includes index.
    1. Medicine, Oriental.   2. Medicine, Chinese.   3. Medical
anthropology — Asia.   4. Medical anthropology.
I. Kleinman, Arthur. [DNLM: 1. Anthropology — Asia.
2. Cross-cultural comparison.   3. Delivery of health care —
Asia.   4. Medicine, Oriental.   5. Socioeconomic factors.
WB50 JA1 09]
R602.C845   362.1'095   78-16401
ISBN 0-8161-8248-5

This publication is printed on permanent/durable acid-free paper
MANUFACTURED IN THE UNITED STATES OF AMERICA

CONTENTS

Part B: Other Asian Societies

SECTION II: CROSS-CULTURAL PSYCHIATRIC AND PUBLIC HEALTH STUDIES

SECTION III: THEORY AND METHODS

LIST OF CONTRIBUTORS

EMILY M. AHERN, Ph.D., Department of Anthropology, Johns Hopkins University.

E. RUSSELL ALEXANDER, M.D., Department of Epidemiology and International Health, School of Public Health and Community Medicine, University of Washington.

E. N. ANDERSON, JR., Ph.D., Department of Anthropology, University of California, Riverside.

FREDERICK L. DUNN, M.D., Ph.D., Department of International Health, University of California, San Francisco.

JAMES L. GALE, M.D., Department of Epidemiology and International Health, School of Public Health and Community Medicine, University of Washington.

BERNARD GALLIN, Ph.D., Department of Anthropology, Michigan State University.

H. JACK GEIGER, M.D., Department of Community Medicine, State University of New York, Stony Brook.

KATHERINE GOULD-MARTIN, Ph.D., Department of Community Medicine and Public Health, University of Southern California School of Medicine.

JOHN KAREFA-SMART, M.D., Harvard Medical School.

ARTHUR KLEINMAN, M.D., M.A., Division of Social and Cross-Cultural Psychiatry, Department of Psychiatry, and Department of Anthropology, University of Washington.

PETER KUNSTADTER, Ph.D., East-West Population Institute, East-West Center, and Department of Anthropology, University of Hawaii.

RANCE P. L. LEE, Ph.D., Social Research Center, Chinese University of Hongkong.

CHARLES LESLIE, Ph.D., Department of Anthropology, University of Delaware.

EVERETT MENDELSOHN, Ph.D., Department of History of Science, Harvard University.

GANANATH OBEYESEKERE, Ph.D., Department of Anthropology, University of California, San Diego.

JOHN C. PELZEL, Ph.D., Department of Anthropology and Harvard-Yenching Institute, Harvard University.

MELFORD E. SPIRO, Ph.D., Department of Anthropology, University of California, San Diego.

MARJORIE TOPLEY, Ph.D., Center for Asian Studies, University of Hongkong.

WEN-SHING TSENG, M.D., Department of Psychiatry, University of Hawaii.

PREFACE

This book has been assembled to meet the desire for a single source of readings in both medical anthropology and cross-cultural medical studies which can be used by anthropology students, medical students, residents in psychiatry and other clinical fields, and students of international health. Its chapters were written by anthropologists, a medical sociologist, clinicians, epidemiologists, and several experts in international health and community (or social) medicine, all of whom participated in an international conference on the "Comparative Study of Traditional and Modern Medicine in Chinese Societies," sponsored by the University of Washington and the Fogarty International Center, National Institutes of Health, which was held in Seattle, Washington, February 4-6, 1974. That conference dealt with two interrelated topics: medicine in Chinese and other Asian societies and interdisciplinary comparative cross-cultural research approaches to the study of health care. Most of the chapters which follow were originally part of a much larger work, *Medicine in Chinese Cultures: Comparative Studies of Health Care in Chinese and Other Societies*, edited by the same editors as this volume. That volume, published by the U.S. Government Printing Office for the Fogarty International Center, National Institutes of Health, contained the entire proceedings of the conference. The present volume consists of reports of empirical investigations (anthropological, epidemiological, and clinical), comments on various aspects of health care in Asian societies, and several chapters on general theory and methods in medical anthropological and cross-cultural medical research. Several of the chapters below have been expanded (Chapters 8 and 12). One (Chapter 21) has been abridged. Chapter 17 was prepared specially for this volume as was the *Introduction*.

Although the focus of the empirical and commentary chapters is medicine in Chinese and other Asian societies, this book speaks to more general questions in medical anthropology and cross-cultural medicine. The chapters illustrate problem- and solution–frameworks that are basic to most studies in these two closely related fields, independent of cultural setting. It will be seen from these studies that social scientists and medical people engaged in cross-cultural research on health care are studying very much the same subject matter, but from often quite distinct perspectives and, of course, with different purposes in mind. By presenting work from both fields, we hope to help advance each and also to lay the groundwork for interdisciplinary research and teaching.

Because most of the cultures under study are associated with large-scale, post-traditional societies, including several with sophisticated literate healing traditions, this book represents a new direction when compared with previous works focused on small-scale, preliterate groups. Unlike the latter, from which much of past medical anthropological and cross-cultural medical research and theory has emanated, the Asian societies examined here contain highly organized and even modernizing indigenous medical systems. Like Western societies, their systems of health care are pluralistic. Interaction between these medical systems and Western medicine occurs in more complex ways than in small-scale, preliterate societies; and, not surprisingly, comparisons with Western cultures are closer and more relevant.

We believe the book can be profitably used in courses in several fields: medical anthropology, cross-cultural psychiatry, social medicine and social science in medicine, and international health. Advanced students and even researchers should also find useful the data and concepts discussed in the chapters that follow.

the Editors

CHAPTER 1

INTRODUCTION

Arthur Kleinman and Peter Kunstadter

Healing systems are found in all known cultures, but their variety is enormous. This variety accounts for the desire of both social scientists and medical personnel to examine medicine in different cultures. Healing systems, as cultural universals, are of intrinsic interest to anthropologists who want to document and understand the distribution and determine the general features of these complex forms of behavior. We have come to understand that healing systems are more or less well integrated parts of sociocultural systems, and as such they contain social organizational and cognitive aspects as well as the technological features upon which there is so much concentration in Western societies. Thus in studying healing systems in Asia, one of our tasks is to describe the social organization, thought processes, behaviors, and techniques related to healing in various sociocultural settings. The primary interest of Western-oriented medical personnel in Asian medicine has been the technology of healing, as they have sought to transfer items such as acupuncture or improved training of paramedical personnel from one medical system and sociocultural setting to another. Using an interdisciplinary (medical science and social science) and cross-cultural comparative (Chinese and other Asian societies) approach we intend this book to help explain the utility of broadening their perspective. We also wish to explore what anthropological and medical studies of the cultural context of healing in Asia can tell us about the relationship between culture and healing generally.

Beyond this, as medical and social scientists concerned with the improvement of health, we want to use the comparative method to learn about fundamental processes at work in health and healing. Comparisons of medical systems which have developed in different traditions raise and help to answer questions such as the definition and classification of sickness, and the role of society in setting priorities and criteria for evaluating healing.

In this *Introduction* we describe the main features of each chapter, identify some major issues in the study of medical systems in society, and suggest some of the disputes with respect to these issues. The book is organized in three sections. The first contains anthropological case studies

1

describing and interpreting health care patterns in Chinese populations of Taiwan, Hongkong, and Malaysia and non-Chinese groups in Thailand, Burma, India, Sri Lanka, and Japan. These chapters raise questions about the form of accommodation which takes place when Asian and Western medical systems come into contact. Section II includes studies combining applied medical and social science perspectives in Taiwan, Hongkong, the People's Republic of China (PRC), other developing countries, and the United States. The underlying questions in these chapters are the outcome of the application of contemporary Western medicine in Chinese societies, its interaction with indigenous Chinese healing traditions, and the possible use of contemporary forms of health care from the People's Republic of China in other societies. The final section deals with general problems in anthropological and comparative cross-cultural research on medical systems in different sociocultural settings, and the theoretical and practical applications of such studies.

By including several empirical studies from each of several Chinese populations, we illustrate the range of healing systems within a major cultural tradition as well as perspectives from anthropological, clinical, and public health disciplines. Thus, the reader can compare several different pictures of rural and urban health care systems within distinct Chinese settings (Taiwan, Hongkong, Malaysia), before comparing these systems with those found in other countries.

The reader will not find a unified set of concepts and methods, or even agreement on several important issues. This diversity represents the state of the art in a field of inquiry which is both theoretical and applied, contemporary and historical—a field which studies questions that are biological and psychological, social and cultural, and which deals with rapid changes in all these dimensions. We have not developed an integrated theory in this *Introduction*. We have presented our favorite candidates in the final section of this book, but we feel that there is as yet no single set of concepts that successfully integrates either medical or anthropological views of healing systems in society. Nor have we yet developed an overriding interdisciplinary framework for medical anthropology and cross-cultural medical and psychiatric studies. There is a parallel lack of common methodology. Some of the empirical descriptions and all the more theoretically oriented chapters offer alternate frameworks for conceptualizing and studying shared problems, and Chapters 20 and 21 suggest ways in which discipline-bound approaches might be better organized.

The material in this book stresses the social anthropological aspects of medical anthropology and the cultural and behavioral aspects of clinical and public health research. Thus, the book is not intended as a comprehensive survey of medical anthropology, which would also contain studies of culture and biology, the cultural context of stress, and many other issues. The focus of the book is clarified in the following summary of the chapter contents.

The first part of the book contains seven anthropological studies of medicine in contemporary Chinese settings. Ahern (Chapter 2) and Gould-Martin (Chapter 3) have drawn ethnological pictures of the symbolic worlds in which shamans and other folk-healers, patients and their families exist in rural Taiwan. They describe the expectations of the patients who seek healing from shamans, and show the relationship between these expectations and the culturally sanctioned systems of meaning and support which the shamans manipulate. Gould-Martin considers all the resources available in the local health care system, including traditional Taiwanese healing and Chinese-style and Western-style professional medical practice, and shows how they are related to one another and to their clients. Both Ahern and Gould-Martin try to determine how the patients use and evaluate these co-existing systems.

The Andersons have done comparative ethnography of folk and popular medicine in two quite different Chinese communities, in Hongkong and Malaysia (Chapter 4). They focus on the self- and family-based diagnosis and treatment of illness relating to herbal and dietary therapies. These are probably the most common Chinese forms of health care, and are all too often overlooked by Western-biased observers. After reviewing symbolic and instrumental uses of diet, they suggest why dietary therapy continues to flourish in the Hongkong community, but seems to be dying out in the community in Malaysia. They also describe the thought patterns which support dietary therapy (as does Topley in Chapter 6), and use their case studies to comment on the generally deleterious impact of modernization and technological change on diet in Southeast Asia. They convincingly show the need to broaden social anthropological perspectives to look at diet and the symbolic systems maintaining diet as a determinant of health.

Ahern's study of the interaction of traditional and modern medical systems in a rural Taiwan community (Chapter 5) was planned in conjunction with Gale's research (Chapter 14). Gale's major interest was in comparing the health-related attitudes of Chinese-style and Western-style practitioners and their patients in Taipei. The methodological effect of the collaboration between anthropologist and epidemiologist is shown in Ahern's use of some quantitative measures of attitudes and behavior. Gale, taking a cue from anthropologists, used participant observation and attempted, in a manner more sophisticated than the usual epidemiological inquiry, to understand attitudes and beliefs underlying the behavior of the doctors and patients he observed.

Topley (Chapter 6) describes historical, political, and cultural determinants of Hongkong's complex mixture of traditional and modern health care. She outlines the cognitive and behavioral features of the clients and describes the institutional organization of the system and its internal conflicts. Topley shows how the symbolic universe of Chinese culture incorporates professional, secular folk, and religious Chinese medical traditions, and she looks at various combinations of Chinese and Western medical practices currently functioning in Hongkong. Her chapter should be compared with Lee's (Chapter 15) survey research on the health system of a rapidly modernizing satellite town of Hongkong. Working with. different methods they paint different pictures of the interactions between traditional and modern medicine in Hongkong, representing the ethnographic and sociological-epidemiological poles in research methodology, but also reflecting quite different assessments of the political-historical context (e.g., whether or not it is imperialistic).

Dunn (Chapter 7) outlines the Chinese medical system in Malaysia. He proposes an elegant model implying that medical systems must be understood as a part of the ecological adaptation of the population which uses them. Dunn suggests that a differential epidemiology is associated with the particular social and ecological characteristics of the Chinese minority in Malaysia as compared with the other segments of the population. This ecological orientation is developed further by Kunstadter (Chapter 20) and Kleinman (Chapter 21) in their discussions of general theories.

In Chapter 8 Gallin reviews the work of Ahern, Gould-Martin, the Andersons, Topley, Tseng, and Lee, and bases his comments on material from his own long-term field research in rural and urban Taiwan. He looks critically at the general problems which field studies of Chinese populations raise for the comparative anthropology of medicine. He comments particularly on the tendency of the researchers to fall into "reverse ethnocentrism." These studies have lauded traditional healing and have been highly critical of modern health care for failing to fit into traditional cultural patterns, while neglecting to consider the relative effectiveness of the two systems or the choices made by their patrons. Obeyesekere (Chapter 12) makes the same point in his comments on Sri Lanka.

Viewed as a whole, chapters 2 through 8 demonstrate the richness and local variations of health care systems in Chinese societies, and the cultural continuities which run through them despite large geographical, social, and political differences. The studies disclose a lack of agreement on definitions, terminology, and methods within the anthropology of medicine, and thus suggest some of the difficulties confronting efforts to integrate research findings or to plan comparative and interdisciplinary work. These points are further illustrated in the second part of section I, which contains five anthropological accounts of medicine in non-Chinese Asian societies.

In Chapter 9 Kunstadter proposes a general model of choice in medical behavior and applies the model to choices made within the plural medical systems found in the ethnic mosaic of northwestern Thailand. He questions the hypothesis that people strive for cognitive consistency and suggests that choice of entry into a medical system and action within it relate to social ranking and boundaries, to economic and geographical factors, and to perceptions of effectiveness, as well as to cultural traditions. Spiro (Chapter 10) examines the folk medical tradition of Burmese in Mandalay, emphasizing the importance of their beliefs in supernatural causes of illness and the treatments organized around these indigenous diagnoses of sickness.

Leslie (Chapter 11) describes the recent history of Ayurvedic medicine in India, and contrasts this with attempts to integrate elements of traditional Chinese medicine in the contemporary official medical system of the People's Republic of China. Using examples from Sri Lanka (Ceylon), Obeyesekere in Chapter 12 points to the continued contemporary importance and potential for survival of Ayurvedic medical concepts. This is in marked contrast with Leslie's negative prognosis for Ayurvedic practice in India. Although he agrees with Leslie's analysis of professionalization of Ayurvedic medicine, Obeyesekere argues that the articulation of illness as a cultural experience links that experience with the larger societal system of cultural values and world view, which in turn makes "cultural diseases" more real and meaningful for people than biomedically defined disorders. This, he believes, will insure the survival of traditional medicine. Obeyesekere also uses data from his Sri Lanka field work to argue several fundamental theoretical points. He implies that the ethno-scientific method of analyzing indigenous medical *beliefs* is in error when it ignores the practical *uses* to which traditional medicine is put. He reasons that the diagnosis of illness in traditional cultural terms provides the culturally accepted logic for the choice, use, and evaluation of indigenous treatments. He characterizes as *pragmatic* the orientation of members of traditional societies who select indigenous or modern scientific systems of medicine based on their rational calculation of the practical and symbolic strengths and costs of each. And he concludes that Western medicine and indigenous healing traditions are in fact *effective for different kinds of problems:* the former for biomedically defined diseases; the latter for the psychosocial problems associated with those diseases as well as for "cultural diseases."

Pelzel (Chapter 13) compares the development of modern medicine in China and Japan and discusses general questions of the response of these societies to contact with the West.

Carrying these themes further, the second section of the book contains six chapters focused specifically on cross-cultural problems in health care. Gale (Chapter 14) and Lee (Chapter 15) look at practitioner and patient attitudes and behaviors where traditional Chinese and modern Western medicine coexist in Taipei and Hongkong. Gale's research used the epidemiological technique of defining the study population as consisting of doctors of the different types and their patients, and then considered similarities and differences between these groups. Lee used a survey of the total population. Despite the different approaches there is considerable similarity in the results of these studies, though comparability could have been improved by starting with a common list of questions.

Tseng (Chapter 16) compares several types of Chinese folk healing and modern psychotherapy as practiced in Taiwan. He identifies both culturally variable and universal elements of therapy and explains the place of these varied treatment forms in the overall picture of health care in Taiwan. Tseng theorizes that both traditional and modern forms of psychotherapy provide a system of reference which is essential in giving meaning to sickness. He raises the basic clinical question of effectiveness of the traditional healing practices in comparison with modern procedures for treatment of disorders such as psychoses. He calls attention to the limitations and negative aspects of the traditional practices, as well as their successes.

In Chapter 17, Kleinman compares the interaction of doctors and patients in different traditional and modern settings in Taiwan. He extrapolates from these comparisons a more general understanding of the cultural construction of clinical reality and explanatory model transactions in health care relationships, and carries these theoretical notions further in Chapter 21.

Two distinguished health care experts, Karefa-Smart (Chapter 18) and Geiger (Chapter 19), examine developments of health care in the PRC in a search for lessons to be applied in developing countries and in the U.S. The overlap and tension between academic and applied interests is highlighted by these chapters. Results of academic research on the place of medical systems in society and the mutability of their cultural aspects are brought to bear directly on the problem of designing better health systems and improving the health of the population.

The final section of the book presents three theoretical perspectives. Kunstadter (Chapter 20) considers anthropology to be a comparative and integrative science of man as a biological and cultural species. He shows that studies of health care systems fit with a series of traditional anthropological concerns, including the ecological adaptation of societies to their natural settings, the persistence and change of cultural traditions, and the relationship of ethnic identity to behavior. He views medical anthropology not as the handmaiden of medicine, but as a part of the broader anthropology of culturally-mediated adaptation.

Kleinman (Chapter 21) outlines some of the chief theoretical problems in the relationship between culture and medicine, and discusses a variety of conceptual models from different disciplines. He suggests what the future of comparative cross-cultural studies of medicine and psychiatry might be if cultural, clinical, and health care system perspectives are integrated. Both Kunstadter and Kleinman offer definitions of health care systems. They raise questions about their components, their cultural context, measurement of their effects, and the appropriate tasks for social and medical scientists studying them.

In Chapter 22, Mendelsohn stresses the importance of the historical understanding of medicine and science as creations of particular social and historical settings. He argues that evidence from the development of Western science and medicine shows that decisions were made to limit these fields to inquiry and practice which were appropriate to those settings. The cultural and social origins of science and modern scientific medicine, he argues, must be considered in their cross-cultural transfer and propagation in non-Western societies. The same would also apply in transfer from Asian to Western societies. Anthropologists and medical scientists studying various aspects of contemporary health care in Asian societies can and should place these in proper social historical and cultural perspective by using the historical documents from these literate civilizations. Such studies can contribute both to the development of a general theory of interaction between societies and their medical systems, and to the solution of practical problems of transfer of medical social organizations, thought patterns, values, and technology from one society to another.

Some of the common issues expressed or implied in the series of comparative case studies and attempts at theoretical generalization have already been mentioned. (Table I gives an issue-by-issue grouping of the chapters.) First is the need to *define the subject* in a way which corresponds both to the realities of the particular case and to the common features generally existing wherever the phenomenon is found. As Pelzel suggests, we have alluded to the importance of the problem, but we have not solved it. There is a need to work toward common methodologies and conceptual schemes even if we cannot achieve a unified theory. In fact, this is a suggestion for an approach to unified theory to the extent to which theory grows both out of the nature of the phenomena being observed and from the tools available for observation and interpretation.

An important aspect of the definition of our subject concerns definitions of *medical systems*. To begin with, most current anthropological and cross-cultural medical models of medicine in society view medicine as a

TABLE I

A Reader's Guide to the Contents of the Chapters

1. Empirical descriptions of, or commentary on, medical systems:
   a. in Chinese societies: Chapters 2, 3, 4, 5, 6, 7, 8.
   b. in non-Chinese societies: Thailand, Chapter 9; Burma, Chapter 10; India, Chapter 11; Sri Lanka, Chapter 12; Japan, Chapter 13; non-Asian developing societies, Chapter 18; United States, Chapter 19.
2. Discussions of problems of comparative analysis of these systems, including explanations of similarities and differences: Chapters 4, 6, 7, 8, 11, 12, 13, 15, 20, 21.
3. Actual and potential applications of this knowledge: Chapters 18, 19, 20, 21.
4. Examination of the relationship between anthropological and medical sciences in research, teaching, and practice: Chapters 8, 20, 21, 22.
5. Discussion of specific theoretical and practical issues emerging from the empirical studies:
   a. Development of theoretical models of culture, society, and healing: Chapters 7, 9, 20, 21.
   b. Methods and techniques for the comparative study of culture and healing: Chapters 5, 7, 8, 9, 14, 15, 16, 17, 20, 21.
   c. Pluralism in medical systems: Chapters 3, 5, 6, 7, 9, 11, 12.
   d. Implications of culture and society for healing—clinical models: Chapters 16 and 17.
   e. Implications of culture and society for healing—public health models: Chapters 14, 18, 19.
   f. Relationship of culture to illness: Chapters 2, 3, 4, 5, 6, 7, 10, 12, 20, 21.
   g. The cultural context of biomedical science as a problem for the comparative science of illness and care: Chapters 21 and 22.

system. That is, beliefs about sickness, illness behavior, health care decisions, patterns of use of health care facilities, patient-practitioner relationships, and medical institutions are viewed not as isolated phenomena, but as part of systematic societal organization of health, illness, and health care. Questions begin with this appreciation of medical systems: how are such systems to be construed? Here, the book accurately reflects the various major orientations to medical systems. Ahern (Chapter 2), Gould-Martin (Chapter 3), and Kleinman (Chapters 17 and 21) all center on medical systems as cultural systems. They also consider medical systems to be local systems. Lee (Chapter 15), Leslie (Chapter 11), and Topley (Chapter 6) tend to view medical systems principally as social systems. They alternate between local and macro-social definitions of these systems. While taking into account both of these aspects of medical systems, Dunn (Chapter 7) and Kunstadter (Chapter 9) regard medical systems as adaptive systems. They are concerned with the environmental and epidemiological context of local medical systems. In Chapters 20 and 21, Kunstadter and Kleinman develop broad, integrative models of medical systems as ecological systems, which try to incorporate these other models.

From the last perspective, it is insufficient to study medicine in society *solely* as a system of beliefs, norms, and values (the cultural system model). Beliefs, norms, and values must be seen as attached not only to distinct cultures but also to particular social structural postions and social roles (the social system model), which are engaged in processes of modernization, indigenization, and institutional change (the social change model: see Leslie, Chapter 11; Obeyesekere, Chapter 12; and Pelzel, Chapter 13). These changes produce, in the systems undergoing them, adaptive, and maladaptive, effects. They need to be studied in relation to environmental influences and stress (the adaptive and ecological models).

Clinical, public health, and social science interests pull the models in different directions. One of the tasks for interdisciplinary collaboration is to figure out ways to integrate these models, and the interests that stand behind them, so that they can be used as a framework for carrying out more sophisticated medical ethnography and systematic cross-cultural comparisons. Even though such a single unified framework does not emerge from this book, the fact that some chapters make explicit the models they use is a real advance over most studies in medical anthropology and cross-cultural medicine and psychiatry, which, like other chapters in this volume, fail to specify the models they tacitly employ. Moreover, Chapters 7, 9, 20, and 21 suggest hypotheses, based on their models, which can be disconfirmed when tested against existing data, or supported when tested in future field studies. This is one of the gains to be derived from directly confronting the question of how to define medical systems.

Additionally important definitional problems are the different ways the concepts of *culture* and *society* are used in the contexts of illness and healing. Western clinical and public health research is only beginning to integrate the concept of shared, learned, organized, symbolically meaningful behavior as a crucial explanatory principle or as a criterion for selection of problems and evaluation of their solutions. The practical importance of the application of sociocultural principles to problems of health care seems far better understood (though without much evidence of self-conscious systematic research on the topic) in the PRC. Inattention to these concepts has made many of the non-technological aspects of contemporary medicine in the PRC unintelligible to many Western observers, for example, the use (or lack of use) of scientific research and statistical data in the setting of health policy and the evaluation of health programs. This inattention has also helped create major problems for health care in Western societies and in developing societies into which Western medicine has been introduced.

The systematic translation between social science and health science perspectives remains an objective for future work. The recent development in anthropology of methods to study symbolic aspects of culture has not been systematically applied in medicine, where it should prove useful in understanding the meaning of illness to patient and family, and thus should be a helpful therapeutic device in primary care. Nor has the concept of culture been operationalized in health care research in anything like the precision and detail with which it is treated in anthropology. Conversely, research on the anthropology of health has not made use of recent medical, psychiatric, and public health concepts, techniques, and results, including those of epidemiology which imply the need to document and understand differential responses within a population. Also frequently overlooked by medical anthropologists are clinically relevant questions that require them to understand and apply biomedical nosology, along with their understanding of indigenous illness categories. Similarly, anthropologists have made only very limited use of stress theory and findings.

The case studies illustrate the need to *specify the perspective of the actors* under which various components of the medical system are being used and evaluated. This caveat has two aspects: first, we must ask what level of common understanding must exist between practitioner and clientele in order that the medical system as a whole, or any particular diagnostic or therapeutic act, be judged effective; second, we must ask what is the cognitive basis for, and what are the effects of, the common occurrence of considerable variety and choice of medical agencies or health behaviors for individuals in the societies we have examined.

In which contexts is cognitive consistency important? This remains an unresolved issue for investigation. The chapters illustrate contrasting positions. On the one hand, it can be argued that understanding is an essential feature of illness, diagnosis and treatment, that there must be some common understanding for curer and patient to come together in the first place, and that common understanding and cognitive consistency are essential for the diagnosis to be accepted and for the therapy to "work." On the other hand, it can be reasoned that common understanding is unlikely to exist in a pluralistic society, in a situation where curers have special knowledge not enjoyed by their patients, where there is inherently a great deal of uncertainty, and where a service (curing) is being purchased. To the extent that some aspects of healing are purely technological, the buyer no more needs to know how the cure works than a truck driver needs to know thermodynamics in order to operate a truck. To the extent that much of healing, however, involves therapeutic communication and the provision of personal and social meaning for sickness and its treatment (Kleinman, Chapter 17), it is necessary that patient and practitioner share cultural explanatory systems. The difference in these approaches is most clearly seen by comparing Ahern (Chapter 2), Gould-Martin (Chapter 3), and Kleinman (Chapter 17) with Kunstadter (Chapter 9).

What are the effects of systematic differences or alternatives in the medical systems? Because the case studies were written primarily by anthropologists and were based largely on observation of the people directly involved in healing, these chapters tend to emphasize the views of the people as participants (patients, relatives, healers) rather than taking an official, legal, professional, or biomedical science position. These views may vary significantly with respect to what they see as the goals of healing activities. None of the chapters shows how the efficacy of medical systems is to be evaluated. This is a key question for future comparisons of medical systems, which must include assessment of the impact of specified differences in their structure and functions.

A major theme which recurs in these chapters is the importance of *variation within a given society.* The variation has at least two sources: sustained contact between people with different cultural traditions, and the effects of modernization on traditional medical systems. The case studies give examples of the definition of one or a few traditions as official or orthodox, the effects of government sponsorship or support for one or a few out of many available traditions, the persistence of non-orthodox theories and practices in the face of empirical evidence and official opposition, the indigenization of Western medical institutions, and the association of distinct forms of medical practice with different segments of society. We are repeatedly presented with evidence that there is no single uniform Chinese (or Burmese, Indian, or Thai) medical system, but there are many systems brought into play under different circumstances (Kunstadter, Chapter 9). With the exception of Chapter 17 (Kleinman), none of the case studies presents direct evidence on the extent to which the patients (or healers) actually are aware of inconsistencies among the multiple theories of disease cause and cure, and if they do see inconsistencies, the ways in which this awareness affects their behavior. An investigation of this question could contribute both to a general understanding of processes of perception, "rationality", logic, and innovation, and to an understanding of how people choose among multiple alternatives in a complex medical system. But such an investigation, as Kleinman shows in Chapter 17, requires a conceptual framework that will support comparisons of biomedical and professional clinical forms of rationality, on the one hand, with folk and popular medical rationality, on the other. We do not yet possess such a framework for comparing forms of medical rationality, and to construct it will mean developing a comparative cross-cultural science of illness and healing in which biomedicine is but one component, not the standard for comparison. Here is further reason for the value of an autonomous anthropology of suffering and healing, not dominated by the paradigm of biomedicine, which can give an independent account of professional, folk, and lay arenas of health care, including their plural beliefs and logics.

Leslie's case study of an Ayurvedic medical institution in India illustrates the need for caution in assuming that plural medical traditions are always compatible. He suggests that even with the best of intentions, and even where there is some political support, the practical superiority of modern scientific (cosmopolitan) medicine eventually becomes evident to the practitioners and teachers of the traditional system. Obeyesekere, writing from observations of patients in Sri Lanka, suggests, on the contrary, that beliefs in the traditional theories of disease cause are so deeply embedded in the thought patterns of the population that Ayurvedic medicine will persist there for many years. Kunstadter, Ahern, and Gould-Martin seem to support this conclusion with evidence from other Asian societies. Their work shows that the demonstration of the practical superiority of modern scientific medicine is problematic as is the counter demonstration of the failure of traditional medicine. Moreover, as Kleinman shows in Chapter 17, there is a complementary process of indigenization, whereby modern scientific medicine is modified when it is incorporated in differing cultural environments, making this question even more complex.

All of the case studies suggest the importance of *pluralism* of medical systems in Asian societies, and describe a range of responses to plural traditions, from attempts at exclusivity to active competition, or to mutual co-existence or incorporation of diverse traditions into the official legitimate national medical system. Various official rationalizations are offered for this latter policy, including necessity due to lack of scientific personnel, lower cost, appropriateness to the local scene, or nationalism and the rejection of the universalistic pre-eminence of Westernism, even in scientific medicine, especially as it has been associated with colonialism. These phenomena are clearly exemplified in both Chinese and non-Chinese case studies which have been described in the first section of this book. They provoke us to rethink what the relationship should be between traditional and modern scientific medicine in different societies.

The examples of Chinese populations in non-Chinese societies (Chapters 4 and 7) suggest the practical therapeutic relevance of pluralism in medical systems by pointing to the cultural variability of theories of diagnosis, disease cause and cure which are culturally Chinese (as contrasted with the cultures of the dominant segment of the societies within which the Chinese minorities exist). Beyond the possibilities of cultural misunderstandings or "conflict," Dunn's paper suggests, as we have noted, that differential epidemiology is associated with the particular demographic, social, and ecological characteristics of the Chinese minority.

Each of the case studies contains examples of *changes* in medical forms as a response to the widespread diffusion of the external features of Western medicine, what Pelzel has called the "hardware." Leslie and Obeyesekere, in discussing Ayurvedic medicine, also indicate *changes in the organization* of the traditional medical professions in response to modernization of the societies in which they are found. Such changes do not always take place in the medical systems within which there was no traditional professional organization (formal training, licensing, examination, disciplining of the members, etc.). Traditional curing in Burma and northwestern Thailand is still carried out by individuals who are not members of professional organizations, though they may have served more or less formal apprenticeships. There are officially recognized schools and licensing procedures for practitioners of traditional medicine in Thailand but these have had no effect on the practice of traditional medicine in the area of northwestern Thailand described in Chapter 9. We do not yet know in general the social conditions under which traditional medicine becomes professionalized.

Questions of *modernization of theories* of disease and healing are equally important but harder to study because evidence of the thought patterns of consumers is difficult to gather. Kleinman attempts to examine this difficult problem in Chapters 17 and 21, where he argues that this should become a central focus of medical anthropological studies. At least in some situations it appears that behavior can change or alternatives can be added without requiring that traditional theories or practices be abandoned (Kunstadter, Chapter 9), while in others, both indigenous and Western medical concepts seem to be undergoing active interaction and change (Kleinman, Chapter 17).

The descriptive chapters give numerous examples of the importance in determining the individual and societal response to medical systems of beliefs concerning .the nature of illness, curing, and the position of the patient in the social system, as well as the nature of the society and its commonly held objectives. Neither the commonly held beliefs about illness nor more general cultural beliefs and values can be ignored as important topics for applied medical research. Likewise, neither the distribution of diseases within and between populations, nor the physiological nature of these diseases can be neglected in understanding how health care systems work.

This book should give its readers a sense of the scope and purposes of both medical anthropological and cross-cultural medical studies as well as an understanding of their utility in the study and promotion of healing. We believe that the best way to learn these interrelated subjects is by simultaneous immersion in empirical details and theoretical arguments from both fields. This should help to dissolve disciplinary blinders, and to illustrate the shared questions underlying both these fields. We believe in the importance of informing medical anthropology with ideas and research results from clinical practice and public health, and vice versa. The cross-cultural study of medical systems also provides a valuable opportunity for progress in theory and application of social science (particularly anthropology and historical sociology).

After reading this book, students of anthropology should come away questioning what is or should be important and distinctive about anthropological studies of health care in society: how these studies should be conducted, what hypotheses they might test, how they might contribute to the cumulative building of theory, and what relationship they should have with medical science studies of the same problem areas. Hopefully, students of cross-cultural medicine and psychiatry and international health will be provoked to ask similar questions about their disciplines. In particular we hope medical and public health students and advocates of change in health care systems will come to recognize that medical and public health practices are sociocultural as well as applied scientific activities. We believe this recognition can be achieved by using teaching materials both from our own and other societies to illustrate how specific cultural factors and social settings (in addition to "pure" biomedical science) influence their daily clinical and health planning and promoting activities. We hope that as a result they will begin to work out new methods for studying the impact of culture on health care, and will recognize the necessity for including the cultural dimension in medical education and public health planning.

Perhaps the most significant effect this book could have is to increase the awareness among medical and public health workers of the fundamental means by which culture affects the way they and their patients think about and respond to sickness. That awareness should enable them to see medicine as a cultural system. This same insight should lead anthropologists to a further exploration of what this cultural system is, how it works, and how it varies in different cultural and social settings.

Studies which make implicit or explicit comparisons of health care systems across cultural boundaries, or within pluralistic societies, can contribute to a general understanding of human behavior, and to the practical solution of some universal problems of human existence. For these purposes a book such as this should bring into question the conventional dichotomies between pure and applied science, between hard and soft science, and between biological and cultural or behavioral science. Similarly, it should make us think hard about interdisciplinary work, and the different interests that stand behind and guide it.

Because the editors believe that science grows by arguments over specific contradictions and the testing of individual hypotheses, as well as by new descriptive discoveries, and because we also believe that medical anthropology and cross-cultural medicine are at present weakest in the former areas, we have called attention to key issues, developing controversies, and alternative models contained in the chapters which follow. If these chapters are to contribute to the advancement of medical anthropology and cross-cultural medical and psychiatric studies, then readers must confront these issues, sharpen and refine the contradictions, dig out and test specific hypotheses, explore and further develop alternative models, and, in sum, continue the interdisciplinary dialectic begun in these chapters.

SECTION I
ANTHROPOLOGICAL STUDIES

Part A
Chinese Studies

CHAPTER 2

SACRED AND SECULAR MEDICINE IN A TAIWAN VILLAGE: A STUDY OF COSMOLOGICAL DISORDERS

EMILY M. AHERN

Chinese villagers, like people anywhere else in the world, must confront sickness and pain as well as the threat of death. Like other people also, they have ways of conceptualizing what the causes of bodily sickness are and ways of acting to prevent or to stop its course once it has begun. In this essay I explore some of the basic concepts that play a part in Chinese villagers' understanding of bodily health or sickness.[1] First I introduce two idioms that are used to describe the health of the body: The balance between hot and cold elements in the body and the relation between the *yang* body that exists in the world of the living and the *yin* body that exists in the world of the dead. Then I show that these two idioms are also used when discussing processes that occur beyond the human body—in human society as a whole or subgroups within it. That is, analogous vocabularies are called into play to describe procedures at two levels—the human body and human social groups. Comparison of the way these two idioms are applied to the body and to social groups will reveal not only analogies and congruencies but also fundamental dissimilarities and incongruencies. In the last part of the paper it is shown how people utilize these dissimilarities in a practical way when they seek causes and cures for illness.

Hot and Cold, Yin and Yang in the Body and in Society

References to hot or cold substances and their effect on the body are made very frequently in the course of everyday conversations. When I grew faint with the heat I was told to drink some bamboo-shoot soup because it was "cold" (*lièng*).[2] When my landlady served some eggs she announced that they were not "hot" (*zuâg*) because they had been boiled in tea, which was "cold." Intricately associated with hot and cold are two other substances described as "clean" and "poison." They, too, are mentioned very often. For example, when I happened upon a woman who was bathing a sore on her lip in a solution of brown sugar and water, she explained that the sugar was "clean" (*chieng-khi*) and would take out the "poison" (*tôk*) in the sore. A full discussion of the intricacies of this vocabulary would be extremely long and complex; in this context I have chosen to simplify the presentation, discussing only some of the most basic properties and uses of hot and cold, clean and poison substances.[3]

17

To understand how hot and cold substances function one must realize that the body requires them both. Exactly how much of each a person requires is determined by the time of year (one tries to take in fewer hot substances in the summer and fewer cold substances in the winter), the individual's particular constitution (some people can tolerate more hot substances than others), and the stage of the life cycle (old people must be more careful to maintain a proper balance than young people who can eat "carelessly" and not fall sick).

When the body is out of balance, a lack of one substance, say hot, can be overcome by ingestion of that substance; a surfeit of one substance, hot or cold, can be counteracted by an addition of the opposite substance. The body is believed to lack hot substances, for example, when it has lost blood. Consequently, women customarily consume an extremely hot mixture for a month after giving birth to help them replace the blood lost in childbirth. A soup made up of hot ingredients—chicken, wine, and sesame oil—is prepared for the mother to eat practically to the exclusion of any other food. This soup is one of a class of foods known as tonics or, literally, "patching medicines" (pô-iôuq), taken whenever the body lacks hot substances or needs strength. A person who has lost blood in an accident or an operation will take tonics; a child who is too thin and is not growing at a normal rate will be given tonics; boys and girls are both given a special kind of hot tonic when they reach puberty to help them successfully complete the physical change; everyone customarily takes another kind of hot tonic during the twelfth lunar month to better endure the cold weather. The hot substances in tonics build strength, help the body undergo necessary growth and replace the loss of vital blood.

Sometimes, however, the body can become too hot. Signs of too much heat in the body are certain kinds of overflow out of body orifices. Whereas loss of blood in an accident or childbirth means the body has a deficit of hot substances that should be made up by taking tonics, a nose bleed is thought to be a sign that the body has too much heat, too much blood, so that it is forced to overflow spontaneously. For this condition one takes honey mixed with water (a cold substance) to counteract the excess of hot. Similarly, the vomiting associated with sunstroke is a sign of an excess of hot in the body and is cured by taking cold bamboo-shoot soup.

Maladies closely associated with too much heat are caused by the presence of poison in the body. Like excess heat, poison exudes across body boundaries, most often in the form of skin sores like those associated with skin diseases or with measles. To eliminate poison in the body, one avoids eating hot substances and makes a special effort to take in clean substances. Some examples of clean substances are golden needle soup, pig's-blood soup and certain herbal teas. Their functions are various, but all involve cleansing: they can stop the poison in sores, clean the body of foreign matter such as lint that collects in the lungs of textile workers, and eliminate the contamination that results from contact with ritually defiling substances like menstrual blood.

Certain substances, such as pearl powder, winter melon soup, and some herbs, are considered to be both cold *and* clean. These are used when there is an obstruction somewhere in the body so that the blood and *ch'i* (vital force) cannot flow freely through the body as they should. One informant compared the body to a plant: "A plant kept in a small pot will be small and poor because the roots are bound up and are not able to spread out. Another plant kept in a large pot will spread out its roots and be healthy. So if a person is healthy his body will be entirely unencumbered. If there is a fault or obstruction somewhere, blood and other things cannot get through and his health will be bad." Swelling is often taken as a sign of an obstruction in the body caused by a collection of *hông* (wind) at the swollen spot. For example, the place where a bone is broken often swells because of an accumulation of *hông*. The remedy is to ingest or apply cold-and-clean substances that will disperse the *hông,* remove the obstruction and allow the blood and *ch'i* to flow freely again.

Each of these substances, then, produces a different effect: hot substances build up a deficit in strength or blood; cold substances reduce an excess of hot elements and allow them to flow out of the body; clean substances draw out harmful matter that exudes from the body or prevent it from building up in the body; and cold-and-clean substances disperse obstructions and make the blood and *ch'i* flow freely. These functions fit remarkably well with the actual physical characteristics of the things that are classified as hot, cold or clean. Hot things tend to be oily, sticky, or made of animal matter (considered to be the most nutritious food). Examples are sesame oil, fried foods, glutinous rice, chicken and duck. Cold, clean and cold-and-clean things tend to be soupy, watery or made of vegetable matter (considered to be less nutritious than animal foods). Examples are golden needle soup, herbal teas of various sorts, and honey dissolved in water (honey is considered vegetable matter because bees make it from the pollen of plants). It is fitting that hot things, eaten to build and add to the body's resources, are viscous, oily, sticky and, it is believed, full of nutrition. They are taken in to stay. On the other hand, cold, clean, and cold-and-clean things are ingested to remove or disperse harmful substances; they are watery, free-flowing, and not considered particularly nutritious. The physical characteristics of these substances are appropriate to the tasks it is hoped they will perform (Anderson and Anderson 1969:113–14; and Anderson in this volume, Chapter 4).

Beyond hot and cold, there is another vocabulary that people use to talk about sickness or discomfort, a vocabulary that involves the relationship between one part of the body, visible and palpable to the living people in this (*yang*) world, and another part of the body that exists in the (*yin*) underworld, strangely enough, in the shape of a house and tree. The underworld is the realm of the dead to which one soul of each deceased person travels after death. It is there, too, that the dead are punished or rewarded according to the merit of their past lives. Although the living have no regular access to knowledge of the activities of their deceased ancestors in the underworld, on certain occasions they are able to get a glimpse of what is happening there. In Ch'inan, when a particular shaman* (tang-ki) visited village, he often read certain incantations that enabled villagers to enter a trance state and thereby travel to the underworld. People explained this by saying that the soul of the living person is sent down to the underworld to look around (kuan-louq-îm).[4] Once there, the traveller may seek out deceased relatives of his own or of others present at the session, or he may travel about, reporting on the interesting sights in the underworld where people live, work and play much as they do in the yang world.

Travellers to the underworld also almost inevitably visit a certain region where there are trees and houses linked with the bodies of living men and women. Each living person has a house and a tree (a flowering tree for females) in the underworld that correspond to the various parts of his or her body—the roof of the house is linked to the head, the walls of the house to the skin, the flowers on a woman's tree to her reproductive organs, and similarly other parts of the house and tree correspond to other parts of the body. A person who is in pain or discomfort may send the traveller to visit his or her tree and house, look them over, and describe their condition. The traveller may announce that the root system of the tree is damaged or eaten by bugs (meaning that there is something wrong with the person's feet) or that the roof has missing tiles (meaning that something is wrong with the person's head). After describing the condition of the house, the traveller is usually asked to arrange for repairs by hiring workmen in the underworld to do the necessary work. When this is done, it is hoped that the corresponding part of the yang body will be fixed as well.

The villagers were reluctant to say whether trouble originates in the yin world and spreads to the yang body or vice versa. The only relevant fact seemed to them to be the yin body is in exactly the same condition as the yang body. There are several different ways one might describe the relationship between these two entities. One could simply call them two different bodies and leave it at that. However, this way of speaking may tempt us to miss the extent to which the two bodies are interdependent—whatever happens to one happens to the other. Somewhat differently one could speak of the yin body as a symbolic representation of the yang body. But this seems to imply that the yin body is causally dependent on the yang body such that the yang body's condition initiates changes in it. As we have seen, the villagers were unwilling to agree with this proposition. One fruitful way of describing the relationship between the two entities is to speak of two parts of the same body—

---

*Editors' Note: In this volume the Taiwanese word for shaman is romanized variously as tang-ki by Ahern, Gould-Martin, and Gallin, as dang-gi by Tseng, and as tâng-ki by Kleinman.

yang and *yin*—rather than either of the two alternatives above. If this is the way people see the relationship between the *yang* and *yin* components of the body they would be likely to believe that both the *yang* portion of the body and the *yin* house and tree must be in good repair in order for good health to prevail. This is in fact one thing that motivates people to take trips to look at underworld houses and trees. If simpler efforts fail to restore health, one can travel to a part of the body that is more directly alterable than the *yang* half; alteration of that part of the body is believed to entail alteration of the *yang* half of the body.

Although the two vocabularies I have discussed—hot, cold, clean, and poison and *yin* and *yang*—are commonly used to describe health in the human body, they are also frequently applied in contexts which involve the wider society. In what follows I first stress the analogies between the use of these vocabularies at the level of the body on the one hand and the level of the larger human society on the other. Secondly, I point out some basic dissimilarities between their use at the two levels.

Hot food substances play a vital role on certain social occasions, in particular those on which a group is growing, expanding and increasing in prosperity. Just as hot things are given to the body when it needs to grow or add to its resources, so hot foods are prepared and consumed when groups of people see their numbers enlarging or their prosperity increasing. For example, on the occasion of an engagement, the members of the husband's family look forward to acquisition of a new worker (the wife) and more importantly, the sons and daughters the wife will bear who will ensure their posterity. Fittingly, at engagements the ceremonial foods are composed of hot substances. Engagement cakes, given out to the boy's and girl's friends and relatives are made of a very short pastry filled with bits of pork fat and coated with sesame seeds—all items that are considered hot. In addition, a soup composed of small balls of ground glutinous rice floating in syrupy sugar solution is made. The gooey glutinous rice in its sticky broth epitomizes the viscous nature of hot substances. When the eagerly anticipated birth of the couple's first child occurs, more hot substances are prepared. Large quantities of "oily rice" *(iu-png)* are made by stir-frying glutinous rice in oil and adding bits of pork and pork fat; this hot dish is distributed to relatives, neighbors, the go-between for the couple and sometimes the natal family of the bride.

Occasions on which the gods are worshipped with the hope of increasing the prosperity, peace and happiness of a group—a family, a village or even a township—are also occasions for preparing hot foods. Glutinous rice, the stickiest, gooiest substance in Taiwanese cuisine plays a large part on all such occasions. At New Years, when all the highest gods are beseeched for peace and plenty, a very large, sweet, steamed cake is made of ground glutinous rice. At other worship ceremonies *(pài-păi)* at which the gods are worshipped, smaller molded cakes of glutinous rice *(āng-kû)* are often made. People like to praise the cook for making the cakes so sticky and gooey (*liám*); the more glutinous they are, the better they taste. In this respect the uses of hot foods when the body is growing and when social groups are growing seem directly analogous. Viscous, adhesive substances are taken in to help add to the resources of the unit concerned—the body or the larger social group.

There is also an analogy between the body and social groups in the use of clean substances to counteract poisonous substances: just as clean substances can eradicate poison in the body, so can clean substances eliminate harmful elements in society. At the beginning of the fifth lunar month numerous measures are taken to banish dangerous spirits of the dead (ghosts or *kui*) from among the living. Some people say this is also an occasion for banishing the "five poisonous things"—wall lizards, toads, centipedes, spiders and snakes. One essential procedure is the hanging of several clean herbs from each doorway. Doolittle (1865) more than 100 years ago described this custom for Amoy.

> On the morning of the first day of the fifth Chinese month every heathen family nails up on each side of the front doors and windows of its house a few leaves of the sweet-flag—and of the artemisia. The leaves of the sweet-flag are long and slender, tapering to a point, resembling the general shape of the sword. When used as above, they represent swords. It is said that evil spirits, on coming near the house and seeing these leaves nailed up, will take them for swords, and run off as fast as they can!

Just as sweet-flag or artemisia, both clean herbs, can be used to wash bodily sores in order to draw out the poison, so they can be used to eliminate harmful spirits from among social groups of the living.

Given that hot and clean substances function for social groups not unlike the way they function in the body, one might also expect parallels between the *yin* and *yang* parts of the body and the *yin* and *yang* parts of society. One parallel is that the *yin* world replicates the *yang* world in many ways just as the *yin* body replicates the *yang* body. People say that the *yin* world is very much like the *yang* world: there are villages there precisely like the ones here; there are townships and countries there which are replicas of the ones in the *yang* world, all located directly below their earthly counterparts. Many of the same things happen in both worlds as well: rice planting takes place at the same time and people utilize the same amusements—movie houses, beautiful gardens and even houses of prostitution.

Beyond this, the *yin* world resembles the *yin* part of the body in that both are associated with trouble, discomfort and pain. Just as one can go to the *yin* part of the body to see what is causing problems with one's *yang* body, so one can look to the *yin* world to find the source of trouble and discomfort in the *yang* world. The *yin* world is the usual residence for ghosts, who, however, are all too often able to find an entrance into the *yang* world. When they do so, they are liable to bring sickness, discord or even death to those who encounter them. Sometimes people act foolishly and make it easy for ghosts to cause trouble. For example, if a child urinates near a grave, ghosts, who frequent such places, find it possible to "follow" the child causing him to be ill and fretful. At other times, people quite inadvertently run into ghosts, with consequences equally as bad. One story was told of an incident on the eve of a "ghost marriage" in which a man and a woman were to be posthumously married so that their souls would rest satisfied in the underworld. As the story was told to me,

> On the night before the wedding, at about midnight, a girl appeared in a beauty parlor in the market town asking to have her hair washed and set. All the assistants had gone home, but the owner was still there, and he agreed to set her hair. While doing so, he remarked that she was terribly cold. She said, "Oh, it's just the damp weather." He also remarked on her arriving so late at night. She said, "Oh, I'm getting married in the morning." He asked where, and she replied, "In the town of Cheng-fu." When he finished, she gave him some money and left. In the morning his wife asked him for some money so that she could buy vegetables. He told her to look in the pocket of the jacket he had worn the night before where he put the money given to him by the late customer. In a little while, his wife came back, very puzzled. The money she had found in the pocket was im-cuá, money which is burned for the dead to spend in the underworld. At this discovery, they were both terribly frightened. The man remembered that she said she was getting married in Cheng-fu, so they went there to see if any weddings were taking place. When they found out that a ghost marriage was scheduled to occur, all their worst fears were realized. After this the man's business failed utterly.

Aside from causing sickness and the decline of one's livelihood, ghosts can also bring about discord in the family. Faced with any of these troubles, people usually seek the help of powerful gods, residents of the *yang* world, in driving away the offending ghosts.

As I have shown, it is quite possible to point out parallels between the functioning of hot, cold, clean, poison, *yin* and *yang* at the level of the body and of larger social groups. It is also possible to find places where their functioning is not analogous. With regard to the hot-cold idiom, there is one major dissimilarity: Whereas in the body hot and cold should ideally be in balance, in society there is no corresponding ideal balance of hot and cold occasions. For each festival at which hot foods are prepared, there is not a corresponding festival at which cold foods are prepared. Instead of attempting to achieve a delicate balance between hot and cold, people's effort seems to be to increase the occasions on which hot foods are prepared because they are positively valued. The more engagements, births, and *pai-pais* one has in the course of a year, the better off one is. There is no feeling that happy occasions must be offset by an equal number of sad ones, and when sad ones such as funerals occur they are not marked by the serving of cold food. In fact, at sad events, the classification hot/cold seems quite irrelevant; people may happen to serve hot or cold foods, but there is no stress on one or the other as being particularly important.

Far from trying to achieve a balance between hot social occasions and cold ones, excessive amounts of hot substances are sometimes used in order to drive out unwanted elements, a procedure that would be very dangerous within the body, because the excess of hot elements could cause death. In Ch'inan an extreme measure used to banish a ghost from among the living is the application of hot substances directly to the ghost. It is hoped that the power associated with the hot substance can be used in this instance to drive something out rather than to bring about growth and increase. In one attempt to exorcise a ghost from a small boy, the ghost finally departed the boy's body, only to enter the body of a pig. In a final effort, the god aiding in the exorcism displaced the ghost from the pig into a pot of boiling oil (a hot substance). This destroyed it, leaving only a single black bone. Similarly, Jordan describes the use of oil, wine and sesame seeds (all hot substances) to exorcise ghosts from a village in southern Taiwan (1972: 55–56, 59, 123–25, 127–28, 131).

Whereas within the body a delicate balance of hot and cold is sought, outside the body there is instead a struggle between antagonists (for example gods versus ghosts) in which hot elements can be used to drive out damaging *yin* elements in an attempt to increase people's measures of health, peace and life.[5]

Further dissimilarities between the body and society can be discovered by comparing their *yin* and *yang* components. Within the body, both *yin* and *yang* parts must be in good repair before good health can prevail. But order in the *yang* world is not dependent on a corresponding order in the *yin* world. On the contrary, order in the *yang* world is achieved by banishing evil, dangerous elements to the *yin* world. The *yin* world is the repository of agents who cause harm in the *yang* world.

If the relationship between the *yang* and *yin* worlds does not parallel the relationship between the *yang* and *yin* parts of the body, perhaps it parallels the relationship between hot and cold in the body. In a sense it does, for the *yang* and *yin* worlds both exist at the same time within the wider cosmos, just as the elements hot and cold coexist within the body. But there is a crucial difference between the two cases. Hot and cold coexist within the same entity, the body, all of whose parts are interdependent. But the *yin* world and the *yang* world are in many ways independent of each other; events happen in the *yang* world which do not affect the *yin* world and vice versa. One could say that the two worlds are nonetheless parts of the same cosmos, but they are divided in a way that hot and cold in the body are not. A *tang-ki* told me that the *yin* and *yang* worlds are divided by a line as thin as a piece of paper and that because of his special abilities he could often see ghosts fading in and out across the line. Yet, thin and permeable as it may be, the line of division between the two worlds exists.

One consequence of these dissimilarities between the operation of hot and cold, *yin* and *yang* in the body and outside is that they allow forceful action to be taken against certain kinds of dangerous and evil agents: evil agents can be separated from the world of the living and relegated to a distinctly separate realm. If the *yang* and *yin* worlds were related in the same manner as the *yin* and *yang* parts of the body then it would be impossible to eradicate evil elements from the *yang* world by sending them to the *yin* world, since in that case the two would be exact reflections of each other. Or if the two worlds were related in the fashion of hot and cold in the body, it would be equally impossible to separate the undesired elements out; they would have to coexist in balance within the same entity, presumably the world of the living. As it is, however, the line of separation between the two worlds allows certain agents to be banished from the world of the living. This separation is clearly expressed in the language of exorcism. When a man was being followed by a particularly tenacious ghost, the god called in to help said that the victim must "*yang*" the ghost, that is, assert the presence of the *yang* world around it in order to force it to the *yin* world. This consisted, among other things, of setting loose a paper boat on the river which would carry the ghost back to the underworld.

The other dissimilarity, between hot and cold substances in the body (where they must be in balance) and hot and cold substances outside the body, can be put to a different use: an excess of hot elements such as boiling oil can help in the exorcism of dangerous *yin* agents abroad in society.

Knowing the Cause of an Illness

The foregoing discussion of Taiwanese ideas about bodies and the rest of the cosmos can be given a concrete grounding in the actions people take to find cures for illnesses that plague them. The notions of hot/cold and *yin/yang* in the body and outside it provide a way for people to handle illness by searching for ever more serious causes, which are in turn treated by ever more complex methods. In extreme cases, the division between the *yin* and *yang* worlds is brought into play as the gods are requested to carry out an exorcism. In the following, I present some of the basic elements of disease treatment among these Taiwanese villagers, trying to show how a seemingly abstract cosmology is in fact a powerful tool that allows those stricken by distressing sickness to understand what afflicts them, cope with it and ultimately to prevail over it.

One element in the villagers' attempt to find cures for illness is their concern about finding the *cause* of the illness. Anecdotal evidence of this is plentiful. One man who had been to several practitioners in an unsuccessful attempt to find relief from severe stomach pain exclaimed to me, "I can't stand it. Unless I can find out what the cause of this illness is, I don't know what cure to use. I'm completely at a loss." In an effort to find out whether the importance this man gave to knowing the cause of an illness was widespread, I asked several questions to this point on a questionnaire administered informally to about 40 villagers.[6] In one question 46 informants were asked to indicate which of eight factors they felt was most important in choosing a doctor. Sixteen (35 percent) chose the answer, "He explains the cause of an illness clearly." No other single answer came close to this percentage.[7] Another question was phrased as follows: "Suppose there are two doctors in the same town. It is equally convenient for you to go to either of them. One explains to you the cause of your sickness whereas the other just gives medicine with no explanation. Would you think it important to visit the one who gives explanations?" Forty of the 43 (93 percent of those responding to this question) gave a positive answer. Thirty-two of these 40 (80 percent) gave an emphatic answer such as, "It's very important to visit the doctor who gives explanations." These answers indicate that many people regard finding out the cause of an illness as an important part of the process of seeing a doctor.

But this is not the whole story, for the kind of illness one has determines the range of causes that might possibly be relevant, and, in turn, the kind of practitioner one should seek out. People commonly distinguished between two kinds of illness. The first, called *phuà-pi:*, refers to trouble that arises from within the body; the phrase used to describe this kind of illness, *sīn-thè în-khì*, translates literally "arising from within the body." The symptoms of this kind of illness are extremely diverse, but the term is usually not applied unless the discomfort is rather serious, with the person incapacitated and forced to lie in bed. In this event the effort to find the cause of the trouble is taken very seriously. Minor ailments like colds also arise from within the body, but are not called *phuà-pi*; people do not feel compelled to find the cause of a simple, uncomplicated cold the way they do an illness called *phuà-pi*. They merely say, "Colds just happen. No one knows why."

The second kind of illness is commonly called *chiōng-tiouq,* which means being bumped into or hit by something. As one might guess, the thing most often blamed for "hitting" someone is a ghost, whether encountered at a grave, a funeral, or elsewhere. At times, potentially malevolent spirits such as those which reside in the ground or in various objects around the house can also hit out at someone, causing him or her to fall sick. With a few exceptions the symptoms characteristic of *phuà-pī* and *chiong-tiouq* can be precisely the same. The classification is not made on the basis of different kinds of discomfort and pain, but on the basis of different kinds of initiating causes. Apropos of this point, one informant told me about an illness in which one half of the body becomes numb and without feeling. He said there are two very different kinds of illness that manifest themselves in exactly this way; one, brought about from within the body, is very hard to heal because medicine does no good. The other is caused when a person is hit by a ghost and can readily be cured through proper use of a charm to banish the ghost. Thus, when a person becomes sick with something regarded as more serious than a simple cold, the focus of people's activities is to ascertain whether the illness is caused by something within the body, or by something external to the body; once the answer is known, an appropriate cure is chosen and it is hoped that the ultimate goal of fully alleviating the painful symptoms will be achieved.

Which kind of practitioner one seeks out depends on which kind of illness one suspects is involved. In general, illnesses caused from within the body are believed to be best treated by Western or Chinese-style doctors.[8] Western-style doctors, many of whom are available near Ch'inan, diagnose with the help of a stethoscope, blood pressure readings and various tests on urine and blood. They treat by administering medicine— antibiotics, vitamins, etc.—in the form of orally-taken powders or injections. Chinese-style doctors, also available to the Ch'inan villagers, diagnose with the help of feeling the pulse or studying the color of the complexion. They treat by administering herbs or other natural substances and by warning the patient away from certain foods, measures often designed to correct an imbalance of hot and cold. Although their methods are very different, both kinds of doctors are seen as being able to cure disease that arises from within the body.[9]

Illness that is caused by a spirit "hitting" a person is best cured by the gods, however, for it is they who have the ability to handle the responsible ghosts or malevolent spirits. Using different words, many people explained this basic division of labor to me. One old woman told me: "The way gods and men cure illness is not at all the same. Men use stethoscopes or feel the pulse, but the god just looks at you and can tell that way. Gods are only better at healing if the illness is caused by a ghost or some other spirit hitting into you." Similarly, another informant said that you need both men and the gods. "If you have appendicitis, you have to go to the hospital and have your appendix taken out; the god has no way to help you. But if your illness is caused by a ghost, medicine is of no benefit and only the god can help." Of course, some medical practitioners are willing to accept these propositions and others are not. By and large, those who speak for the gods or act as intermediaries between them and men are quite willing to accept this division of labor, whereas Western- and Chinese-style doctors are less willing to do so. A woman known as a *Siān-sī:-mà,* who enlists the aid of the gods to cure a disease in which a child's soul is dislodged from his body, said, "I have no way to treat any illness 'within the body'. For that you need a doctor. If two children came to see me and one had lost his soul, but the other had a cold, I could only help the one who had lost his soul. People need both my skills and those of the doctors."

This notion that an illness with one set of symptoms can have different causes at different times means that people always have in mind the possibility that the first practitioner they choose to heal an illness may not be the correct one. If the cure he administers fails to get results, they will be likely to switch to another practitioner of the same type or to a practitioner of a different type entirely. The important premise seems to be that there are specific cures attached to specific causes. Given that, if the cause is correctly ascertained, the cure appropriate to that cause will work. If the cure does not work, then the cause was incorrectly ascertained. Reasoning based on this premise was particularly transparent in one case in which a young woman had been taken to the hospital with abdominal pain. As her mother told me: "The doctors there told us she had 'stones in her abdomen.' When we got her home, we gave her a kind of herb called 'stone grass' but nothing happened. If the sickness had really been 'stones in the abdomen,' the herb would have made the stones come out in the stool, without a doubt." At this point, the family was preparing to take the girl back to the hospital again. It also follows from this line of thinking that if a cure works, the cause associated with it must necessarily have been the correct one. Consequently, if people are going through a whole sequence of practitioners to find a cure, the one who happened to administer the treatment followed by ˚amelioration of the condition will be said to have found the correct cure. A young doctor in a small market center near Ch'inan expressed it this way: "People usually go on a round of searching for help, from one doctor to another. Whichever one they happen to be at when they begin to feel better is the one they credit with helping them."

The Escalating Process of Finding a Cure

At this point I move from the general considerations above into a preliminary analysis of the things that motivate people to make decisions about seeking cures. According to my general impressions, if initial attempts to seek a cure for a malady first classified as *phuà-pi:* ("arising within the body") fail, the patient moves toward the assumption that the illness is *chiōng-tiouq* (caused by a harmful spirit "hitting" him). Recourse to the gods who alone are able to cure such an illness gives the patient access to techniques specifically suited to reveal the cause of the illness, namely, the ability of the gods to "see" what is wrong with him. If the course of treatment is carried to its ultimate and most extreme conclusion, it is possible for the gods to make use of the separation between the *yang* and *yin* worlds so that they can banish the evil spirit finally and irrevocably from within the world of the living.

Since most people assume at the onset of an illness that it is caused from within the body, they consequently seek out a Western- or Chinese-style doctor if they wish for the help of a specialist.[10] An informant said, "We only go to see a *tang-ki* who can enlist the aid of a god if a doctor's medicine or shot has been tried and failed. If the patient just doesn't get well or if the sickness comes back too quickly, people assume that medicine is not going to work." In seeking a doctor's help, people have two primary goals. They want, of course, relief from symptoms, but as was shown above, they also desire an explanation of what is causing the illness. However, in many cases, whether or not doctors provide relief from symptoms, they do not satisfy the patient's desire to understand what is wrong with him. In the course of having assistants transcribe doctor-patient interactions in the offices of nine doctors to whom people in Ch'inan regularly have access, I noticed that in many instances a patient's direct request for some explanation of the illness went unanswered or was shunted aside. In one case a 35-year-old woman sought help from a Western-style doctor. The dialogue went as follows:

> Doctor: "Do you feel pain here?" (The doctor touched the patient's abdomen.)
>
> Patient: "No, I don't."
>
> (The doctor took the patient's pulse.)
>
> Patient: "I was told that it is nephritis. Is that true?"
>
> Doctor: "Let me see." (The doctor listened with a stethoscope.)
>
> Doctor: "You feel pain here don't you?" (He touched another part of the abdomen.)
>
> Patient: Yes. When I lie down I always feel pain."
>
> (The doctor asked the patient to give him a urine sample. Afterward, the dialogue resumed.)
>
> Patient: "It was diagnosed as nephritis before. Is that true? Now I have chest pain and feel cold."
>
> Doctor: "Your symptoms are not like those of nephritis."
>
> Patient: "I don't dare eat any kind of pork."
>
> Doctor: "You can eat just as a normal person does. Now take this drug and come back again tomorrow." [11]
>
> (The patient nodded and left.)

In another example, after an exchange in which the Western-style doctor recommended that a mother feed her baby less concentrated milk, the mother asked: "Why are his feces blackish?" The doctor replied: "Because you gave him some medicine." The mother retorted "But they were black before I gave him the medicine." The doctor gave no response to this, and the mother did not ask again.

I am unable to say how often the request for an explanation of an illness is met with the kind of lack of response evident in the two incidents described above. Though it is not uncommon in the transcripts of doctor-patient interactions I have, the sample of doctors is not extensive enough to draw any definitive conclusions. However, the attitudes of doctors themselves also indicate that people are often unable to find out what the doctor thinks is wrong. In an informal interview both Western- and Chinese-style doctors were asked: "If a patient describes his symptoms and offers his own explanation of what his sickness is, do you correct, ignore or accept it?" In answering, four of the doctors mentioned how stubborn patients are and how difficult it is to convince them of anything. Three said that they would simply ignore whatever the patient said and only two said that they would explain the difference between the patient's diagnosis and their own. Again, in response to the question "Does it help a patient to get well if he understands what is wrong with him," three doctors said no, two said yes, provided the patient has sufficient education, and only four gave an unqualified yes. One Western-style doctor expressed his feeling as: "I hardly ever tell patients what I think is wrong with them. What I say might disagree with other doctors' opinions and besides, knowing what is wrong won't help them get well at all. I think most doctors feel the same way."

It is perhaps safe to say that if a patient's discomfort is alleviated by the treatment a doctor gives him and if his symptoms do not recur, he will consider himself cured, and will not seek further medical help whether or not he has been given a satisfying explanation of the disease. Not *every* illness must be explained; colds, stomach aches, skin sores and other minor complaints "just happen" and as long as the doctor can provide relief, no further action need be taken.

The more unfortunate, though for our purposes the more interesting, case arises when the doctor first sought out for help fails to provide what the patient perceives as a satisfactory cure. If the trouble persists, becomes more serious or recurs with any frequency, people often begin to suspect that the illness requires the special abilities of a god. One woman put it very clearly: "People usually try doctors before asking a god for help. This is because, if none of the doctors can heal the illness, the god can tell you what the real cause of the illness is. Gods are better able to know this than others. Unless you know what the cause of the illness is, you don't know what method to use in healing the illness." When people decide that doctors are unable to provide a cure, finding out the correct cause of the illness becomes of vital importance, the more so because in many cases patients will not have been given any kind of explanation from the doctors they consulted. Gods are consulted because they are regarded as those eminently able to ferret out the cause of an illness. One woman told me that there are two kinds of tang-ki (shamans). One kind can ask the god questions about any subject at all while the other has the specialized talent of finding out through the inspiration of the god, "what kind of an illness you have (e-thâng ka lî kòng sîm-mîq pī:)." The same attitude apparently exists toward consulting the tang-ki in Singapore described by Elliott (1955: 91): "The consultant will leave the diagnosis as well as the treatment to the dang-ki, demanding a sufficiently plausible reason for the trouble as well as the prescription of a remedy."

In similar fashion, a young mother who had just decided to take her child to see the Sian-si:-ma explained that she was seeking the aid of this specialist because she would be able to find out "all about what kind of illness the child has—whether it's soul loss, or something else." Unlike doctors, who often disregard a patient's request for an explanation, gods and their assistants are sought out specifically because they are able to tell the patient what is wrong.

I cannot discuss the dramatic methods used in healing sessions presided over by the gods in any detail here. Suffice it to note that after various kinds of examination of the patient they build to a climax in which the god or his assistant reveals what the cause of the illness is. When a child is taken to see the *Sian-si:-ma,* for example, she prepares a heaping bowl of raw rice over which she wraps tightly a piece of the child's clothing. Then she rubs this all over the child's body for several minutes while she calls on the help of the god. After repeating this process, she finally moves to the light of the doorway, stands erect, unveils the bowl of rice, examines it carefully and announces with great effect that the child is sick because it lost its soul when it was dropped, or when it was bathed in hot water, or alternatively that it was hit by a ghost, and so on. The prescribing of cures, which in any event are familiar and specific for each kind of ailment, seems to come as a definite dénouement of the part of the performance in which the cause of the illness is announced.

Determining the cause of an illness is often described in terms of "seeing" what the illness is. This is a talent which ordinary doctors have and the common phrase used to mean diagnosis—*k'an-ping*—literally translates "to look at the sickness." But ordinary doctors are forced to rely on other techniques besides just looking at the patient: feeling the pulse or listening through a stethoscope. Some people were quite scornful of doctors who used stethoscopes because their reliance on an instrument clearly indicated they had less native ability to diagnose the illness. Gods, however, need only look, and require no other techniques. As the above-quoted said: "The god just *looks* at you and can tell that way." The looking that gods do is of a different quality than that of which men are capable, however. They do not require eyes in the ordinary sense, because the *tang-ki* whose bodies they possess are often blindfolded. In addition, they are capable of feats that men would find impossible. In one session in which a god was diagnosing an illness after midnight on a moonless night, the *tang-ki* ran out into the dark several times with no lantern or flashlight and was able to find numerous rare medicinal herbs.

The ability of gods to "see" the cause of the illness is especially important when the patient has been "hit" by some evil spirit. When this happens, they do not just act as especially skillful doctors, they utilize abilities that doctors do not have. One *tang-ki* told me that when a god is diagnosing an illness, he makes the agent which is at fault "drop in" (*toù-laí*) to the room where the patient is. If the spirit of the door lintel is angry, for example, the part of the house in which the angry spirit lives will "drop in." Then the *tang-ki* and the god look it over and determine what the trouble is. Alternatively, if the sickness is caused by a ghost, the ghost itself may appear. The god looks the ghost over and may communicate with it to find out what offerings will appease it.

Likewise, on a trip to the underworld, the gods are said to accompany those who travel there, enabling them to make the transition to the other world and to see things when they arrive. The image of seeing is carried over here, too. Trips to the underworld are literally called "looking around the underworld"; visits to the underworld house and tree consist of the traveller simply looking carefully at all parts of these objects, to *see* whether or not anything is wrong. Those who help the gods diagnose for men—*tang-ki*—or even those who travel to the underworld, often themselves possess special abilities to "see" what causes illness. This is sometimes expressed by saying that these people have "low" eight characters, or a horoscope that gives them in some sense a close affinity with the *yin* world. These are the people who are able to enter a trance and visit the underworld; it is said that other people can enter a trance, but when they arrive in the underworld, they cannot "see" anything. These people can also see ghosts and other *yin* beings who are invisible to most humans. On one occasion a *tang-ki* who often visited in the village announced to his hosts that he could see a female ghost sitting on the door mantel of their living room. He helped them make a wooden charm to keep the ghost away.

The special abilities of the gods and those who can travel to the underworld allow *yin* causes of illness to be made patently observable. Seeing and describing the cause of an illness provides a way, the correct way, of dealing with that illness. Otherwise, people are left in the state of the despairing man quoted above as saying "Unless I can find out what the cause of this illness is, I don't know what cure to use. I'm completely at a loss." As Victor Turner (1967) has put it: "To reveal or portray is to expose, and exposure of the 'true character' of a disease ... is half the therapeutic battle, for the known is not nearly so dangerous as the hidden and unknown. Action can be taken against something visible and classified in terms of traditional thought and belief, and positive action, as has often been said, reduces anxiety and promotes confidence."

One might surmise that the wonderfully accurate ability of the gods to "see" the cause of illnesses would allow them to offer a kind of court of last appeals in which all illnesses could be diagnosed and cured. Unfortunately, the course of healing is not always so simple. If the cause of illness is indeed a *yin* agent, the gods will attempt to handle it themselves and will not suggest recourse to other practitioners. But sometimes the god consulted determines that the illness is caused from within the body of the sick person. In this event, some gods, who possess knowledge of how to heal these illnesses, will prescribe a dose of herbal medicine. Others will refuse to act themselves and will instead refer the patient to a Western-style or Chinese-style doctor, sometimes specifying the place at which the proper doctor is to be found. This understandably brings on a certain amount of dread. If the cause of the illness lies within the *yin* world, then the gods' superior abilities can be called into play. But if the cause lies within the body of the patient, then the gods' abilities may not be of any use and it becomes far from certain that a cure can ever be found. One woman who suffered from goiter persisted in consulting the gods time and again only to be told repeatedly that her illness was caused from within the body and that the gods could be of no help. The family of an elderly man who seemed to be failing rapidly told me that the old man's plight was now hopeless. The gods had insisted that the disease was caused from within his body and none of the doctors they had consulted had been able to provide a cure. At least part of their hopelessness seemed to derive from their acceptance of the fact that only a limited number of measures were now relevant to the old man's cure and that some of the most powerful cures possessed by the gods were not applicable.[12]

If, in contrast, the gods do decide that the illness is a result of some spirit "hitting" the sick person, the full range of exorcising techniques can be utilized. In the first stages, the goal is simply to dislodge the harmful agent from the body of the sick person. This is done by making certain offerings to the spirit to appease it and coax it to leave the patient alone. If the ghost is a kinsman and is causing sickness in order to force his descendants into providing some service for him such as repairing his grave or worshipping him more often, then this demand will be met. In either case, the ghost is merely separated from the body of the patient; it is not banished from the world of the living or destroyed.

In an extreme case, when an especially fierce ghost is not deterred by these measures, then the kind of exorcism described earlier can be called into play. Hot substances and special ritual procedures can be utilized not merely to detach the ghost from the patient, but to banish it from the world of the living entirely. The cosmological belief that the *yang* and *yin* worlds are independent of each other and that *yin* agents can be kept separate from the *yang* world when the correct procedures are used is here given a practical use. It allows the gods and the *tang-ki* who help them to relegate the ghost to another realm.[13]

In the process of exorcism, the images used are appropriate to the goal. In his description of Sinhalese curing rituals, Nur Yalman (1964: 117) states that the rituals are designed to deal with opposed categories such as pollution and purity, sickness and health; the object of the rituals is to "turn one side of the opposed category into the other," thus increasing the quantity of desired elements in the world. The symbols used in Sinhalese rituals clearly express the idea of exchange between two elements. But in the Taiwanese case, the symbols used in exorcising rituals seem to express not the idea of exchange but the idea of removal, detachment, and departure. In many ceremonies paper boats are placed on the river to float downstream, carrying the malign spirits away with them to the underworld. Alternatively, powerful hot elements are applied to the ghost or the person possessed to literally blast out the offending spirit. Rather than the idea of exchange, here there is the idea of separating the world of the *yang* from the world of the *yin* by isolating the living who ideally possess health, life and plenty from the spirits of the dead who can bring sickness, death and destitution.

Conclusions

In the study of cosmologies, it has become well established that there are analogies between different levels of experience such as the human body and wider society. Griaule and Dieterlen (1954: 81–110), Levi-Strauss (1966: 168–69), and Douglas (1970) provide striking analyses of such homologous patterns. Douglas puts the point most forcefully: "Just as the experience of cognitive dissonance is disturbing, so the experience of consonance in layer after layer of experience and context after context is satisfying . . . The human body is always treated as an image of society" (1970: 70). In this examination of Taiwanese beliefs I have shown that despite the existence of many homologies between the organization of the human body and of the world outside it, there are also basic disagreements between the two levels. Consonance among different levels may be, as Mary Douglas holds, intrinsically satisfying, but the ability to make short work of evil spirits by separating them out from the *yang* world, an ability which depends on dissimilarities between the way *yin* and *yang,* hot and cold function in the body and in society, must surely bring satisfactions of its own. It is at least a possibility that a search for incongruencies among the more noticeable homologous patterns in the cosmologies of other peoples will yield similar insights into the role of what might be called cosmological disorder.

But this kind of disorder is only perceptible when a cosmology is viewed from a distance so that all its parts can be set alongside each other at once. As these beliefs are used in the process of healing, they seem to bring about renewed order. Levi-Strauss (1963) has given us a striking illustration of how a shaman can imbue the disordering, fear-inspiring experience of difficult childbirth with order by giving the woman a mythological description of what is happening within her body. The Taiwanese material shows us another way that the same goal can be achieved. When the pain and discomfort that accompany illness are not alleviated by initial efforts to remove them, the patient seeks a way of understanding what is wrong by consulting a god who will assign a cause to the illness. Knowing the cause of the illness limits the number and scope of possible threats to the body the patient need consider, and at the same time provides a rationale for him to act in a specified manner to stop the pain. The same applies to the patient's kinsmen and neighbors, who, if he is too young or becomes incapacitated, will seek a cure on his behalf. In this case the disordering fear created by the illness may be derived both from people's dread over the possible loss of a loved kinsman or friend and from their vicarious fear of experiencing pain and death. Whether the sick person himself acts or whether action is taken on his behalf, one of the most important effects of seeking a cure is that the patient and those around him are given a language with which to describe and understand the illness. Whether or not the treatment succeeds in curing the illness itself, it will have succeeded for a time in affecting people's *experience* of the illness, a result scarcely less vital than achieving a final bodily cure.

NOTES

1. Fieldwork for this paper was supported by the General Research grant (N.I.H.) through the Department of Epidemiology and International Health, The University of Washington, during the summer of 1973. I am especially grateful to E. Russell Alexander and Peter Kunstadter for their help in arranging this grant. Nearly all of the material was gathered in the village of Ch'inan, Taiwan, where I had done a year's work in 1969–70, and in a nearby market town. The beliefs about illness and health outlined are those of villagers— farmers, coal miners, or small merchants—unless I specifically indicate otherwise. I will not address the important but enormous question of how these beliefs fit with those of trained practitioners such as Western- or Chinese-style doctors.

I owe many thanks to the two assistants who aided in this research: Chou Pi-se and Liu Hsiou-yüan. Their persistence and imaginativeness in interviewing doctors and patients were genuinely indispensable. I would also like to express my appreciation to James L. Gale of the University of Washington, who took time from his research in Taipei to offer support, suggestions and invaluable medical information.

2. Taiwanese words are spelled according to the system outlined in Nicholas C. Bodman's *Spoken Amoy Hokkien* (1955). Mandarin is used for place names and for words that commonly appear in their Mandarin forms.

3. Hereafter the quotation marks around the words hot, cold, clean and poison are omitted. They are subsequently used consistently in the special sense introduced here.

See Ahern (1973: 228-35) for an extended description of one such trip. See Gould-Martin in this volume (Chapter 3) for an extensive account of shamanism in Taiwan.

5. This is not to imply of course that ideas of balance function nowhere in Chinese society. I am singling out only the idiom of hot and cold food stuffs for consideration. In fact, in another time and place in China the vocabulary of hot and cold was used to express regular alternation between opposed states. Skinner (1964: 21) reported that in Szechwan "hot" market days were said to alternate with the "cold" days in between.

6. The sample was selected to include males and females in several categories: those with more than a grade school education and those with less; those in three stages of the life cycle: (1) unmarried, (2) married but still living with parents or parents of spouse, (3) married and living in independent households.

7. Answers in the order of frequency with which they were chosen are as follows:

	No. Choosing	%
He explains the cause of an illness clearly	16	34.8
He is available at all times	9	19.6
He is understanding and takes a personal interest in the patient	8	17.4
He is well known over a wide area	7	15.2
He is a registered doctor. (Some doctors have the requisite medical training to be certified by the government. others who do not can still set up an office, diagnose illness and dispense medicine.)	3	6.5
He is well known through long residence in the community	2	4.3
You have *yüan-fen* (relationship by fate) with him. (It is believed that some individuals who are not kinsmen are fated to develop a close relationship. This applies equally to friends of about the same age and to the doctor-patient relationship.)	1	2.2
His treatment is inexpensive	0	0.0
	46	100.0

8. The terms "Western-style" and "Chinese-style" doctors are direct translations of the commonly used Taiwanese terms: *Sē-siêng* and *Tiōng-ī-siêng*.

9. In lumping Chinese- and Western-style doctors together this way I naturally gloss over important differences between them, not only in the kinds of treatment they use but in the attitudes people have toward them. See my other chapter (5) in this volume for a discussion of this.

10. Of course, some people first use home remedies based on their impressive knowledge of the uses of herbs and other plants; still others purchase patent medicine without consulting a doctor at all. If these remedies do not work, however, most people eventually consult a doctor.

11. This reference to eating restrictions is related to the belief that certain hot or cold foods are incompatible with certain illnesses. This patient, like most laymen and many Chinese-style doctors, places great emphasis on these practices and so is fearful that she will eat the wrong thing. Western-style doctors like this one more often than not disregard such habits and encourage people to eat normally.

12. It is at this point that people are likely to have their underworld house and tree viewed, if a *tang-ki* who knows the proper incantations is available. Because the opportunity to visit the underworld arises infrequently, people cannot count on regular trips as a way of

treating illnesses when they first begin and are still assumed to be caused from "within the body." But since alteration of the underworld house and tree is considered an appropriate treatment only for such illnesses and not for *chiōng-tiouq,* it tends to be used for chronic complaints that are not serious enough to be treated by the gods or that the gods have declared to be caused from "within the body."

13. In Ch'inan I came on no instance in which the gods professed inability to exorcise ghosts completely (Elliott 1955: 95). People did say, however, that when ghosts are very fierce several gods must be consulted and several exorcisms must be attempted. If the patient does not seek treatment soon enough, the ghost may kill him before the exorcism is complete.

REFERENCES

AHERN, E. M.
   1973   The Cult of the Dead in a Chinese Village. Stanford: Stanford
          University Press.

ANDERSON, E. N. and M. ANDERSON
   1969   Cantonese Ethnohoptology. Ethnos: 107–117.

BODMAN, N. C.
   1955   Spoken Amoy Hokkien. Kuala Lumpur: Charles Grenier and
          Son, Ltd.

DIAMOND, N.
   1969   K'un Shen, A Taiwan Village. New York: Holt, Rinehart and
          Winston.

DOOLITTLE, REV. J.
   1865   Social Life of the Chinese: with some account of their Reli-
          gious, Governmental, Educational, and Business Customs and
          Opinions. New York: Harper and Bros.

DOUGLAS, M.
   1970   Natural Symbols: Explorations in Cosmology. New York:
          Random House.

DURKHEIM, E.
   1915   The Elementary Forms of the Religious Life. London: George
          Allen and Unwin Ltd.

ELLIOTT, A. J. A.
   1955   Chinese Spirit Mediums: Cults in Singapore. London: Royal
          Anthropological Institute.

GRIAULE, M. and G. DIETERLEN
   1954   The Dogon of the French Sudan. In African Worlds, Daryll
          Forde, ed. London: Oxford University Press.

JORDAN, D. K.
   1972   Gods, Ghosts and Ancestors. Berkeley: University of Califor-
          nia Press.

LEVI-STRAUSS, C.
   1963   The effectiveness of symbols. In Structural Anthropology.
          New York: Basic Books.
   1966   The Savage Mind. Chicago: The University of Chicago Press.

SASO, M. R.
   1972   Taoism and the Rite of Cosmic Renewal. Washington State
          University Press.

SKINNER, G. W.
   1964   Marketing and Social Structure in Rural China, Part 1. Journal
          of Asian Studies 24: 3–43.

TURNER, V.
   1967   Lunda medicine and the treatment of disease. *In* The Forest
          of Symbols. Ithaca: Cornell University Press.
YALMAN, N.
   1964   The Structure of Sinhalese Healing Rituals. Journal of Asian
          Studies 23: 115–150.

CHAPTER 3

ONG-IA-KONG :

THE PLAGUE GOD AS MODERN PHYSICIAN

KATHERINE GOULD-MARTIN

Traditional religious methods of treating disease seem to have been replaced by secular ones on the Chinese mainland, but the religious methods coexist with the modern ones on Taiwan. They exist behind, beyond, and under the modern system; they fill in its gaps.

In order to understand the total health care system of the area of rural Taiwan (that is being industrialized) where I did field work in 1972–73,[1] it is important to understand the cult of their plague god, *Ong-ia-kong** [2]— the diagnoses and prescriptions given by his shaman and the community life that goes on around him. The *Ong-ia-kong* cult is one of hundreds throughout Taiwan. Though it is only part of a rather comprehensive Chinese and Western medical-resource system, it has major health care significance. First, it is concerned with a specialized area of medicine, that is, it treats matters perceived as health-related that most of the other available facilities do not. It also treats untreated aspects of matters that are treated by the others. Second, the kind of treatment it offers differs markedly from that of the non-religious health care resources in its response to the personal and social needs of the patient.

In this paper I will first describe the setting and background of the *Ong-ia-kong* cult and an evening's session there (1). Then I will discuss the kinds of ailments treated and the kinds of treatments (2). Finally, I will return to the comments I just made, emphasizing the features that distinguish medical practices associated with *Ong-ia-kong* from the rest of the health care available (3).

There are three types of available health care, which I have chosen to call Chinese sacred medicine, Chinese secular medicine, and Western-style medicine. *Ong-ia-kong* is one of many cults in the Chinese sacred medical system, which refers to a part of Chinese religion which I have systematically separated out as specifically health-related. Chinese secular medicine (usually called traditional Chinese medicine) shares its pharmacopoeia and much of its theory with the *Ong-ia-kong* cult, but in manner and setting it resembles Western-style medicine far more closely. "Western" or "Western-style" medicine in this paper refers to that practiced by Taiwanese doctors who have been trained in Taiwan in the principles and practices of a medical system similar to that prevalent

*Asterisks occurring in this chapter denote that the Chinese-Taiwanese phrase is to be found in the Glossary appearing at the end of the chapter.

41

in the United States. Some of the differences, particularly in psychiatry, are due to the fact that Taiwanese Western medicine was originally taught by Japanese doctors who had studied German medicine. Others are due to Taiwan being a developing country and to the ancient establishment of the "proper" medical role and behavior by doctors of traditional Chinese medicine (See Croizier, 1968).

1. Setting and Background of the Ong-ia-kong Cult

The trip from the village where *Ong-ia-kong* resides to Taipei, Taiwan's largest city, takes less than an hour by modern transportation. Taipei has numerous hospitals: municipal and missionary, the National Taiwan University Hospital, the National Defense Medical Center, and innumerable smaller private hospitals and clinics. Taipei is where people go for treatment for diphtheria, premature births, tuberculosis, or any major or mysterious disease. The University hospital is the usual referral goal of the local doctors and hospitals. Both in terms of Western medicine and Chinese secular medicine, Taipei is the recognized capital; not so, however, for religion or the Chinese sacred medical system.

The market town, about one-half hour by train, bus, or taxi from Taipei, is well-provided with Western-style doctors and clinics. There are three hospitals with beds: the surgery hospital (sixty beds), the labor insurance hospital (fifty beds), and the lying-in hospital (five beds). Some of the ten "doctors" at the first two hospitals are probably pharmacists or paramedical assistants. There are an additional six Western-style doctors, two of whom also practice at the University hospital in Taipei. There are 19 Western-style druggists, although doctors dispense most of the drugs they prescribe. There are four miscellaneous Western-style clinics, seven dentists, and three midwives. The public health office has a part-time doctor, two midwives (who do check-ups but not deliveries), and two nurses. The midwives and nurses spend more than half their time in community public health work, particularly vaccinations and immunizations. The market town also has a man we call "Wang the Examiner" who runs a small laboratory to do tests on blood, urine, and stool either for the patients of local doctors or for individuals who come on their own. Some factories have full or part-time medical staff and facilities. In short, Western medicine as we know it, or as we knew it only a few years ago, is fully available and much used.

Chinese secular medicine is also available. There are five bone-setters, seven doctors who work in their own drugstores, three druggists who do not consider themselves doctors, and four stores selling Chinese herbs. Most of the Chinese doctors claim to have mastered acupuncture, though none practices it. They explain, "There is no demand for it." There are also itinerant peddlers who claim to cure everything, particularly boils, eye disease, and lack of virility. Their evening displays resemble medicine shows and include sleight-of-hand tricks.

This medical inventory needs a brief description of the religious facilities where Chinese sacred medicine, i.e., the treatment of illness, fright, bad luck, and bad fate through soul covering, patching the fate, crossing a gate, calling the soul, magic, and numerous other means, is available (see Ahern's Chapter 2 in this volume). The market town has two large temples, one of them quite new, which may loosely be deemed Taoist as each has a full-time resident Taoist priest. There are numerous smaller temples, but only one commonly resorted to by people from *Ong-ia-kong's* village. Two large temples further up the river in San Hsia* and Pai Chi*, a Matsu* temple across the river, and two of the temples in Taipei, the Lung Shan temple and the Min Chuan Road Kuan-Kung* temple, were also frequented. There is a geomancer in town, an old woman who cures fright in children, and two or more fortune tellers who treat simple ritual problems. There are also three Buddhist temples on the mountainside to the northwest of town but, though most of the nuns are Taiwanese, the higher priests are of Mainland origin and I am under the impression that the temple clientele are generally Mainlanders and/or upper-class. Thus these temples are here barely relevant (see Ahern's Chapter 2 in this volume).

To complete the picture of the town, I should add that there are one Catholic and two Protestant churches, three nursery schools, two primary schools, one lower-middle school, and one private upper-middle school. There is a train station, post office, town office, police station, a credit-cooperative bank, a large Farmers' Association building with auditorium and library, and two movie theatres. About five factories employ from 200 to 2000 workers each (in textiles, electronics, concrete, medicine, and wine industries), and many more smaller factories employ workers and send out piecework. The population of the market town and its adjacent villages amounts to more than 43,000 people *(Taiwan Demographic Fact Book,* 1970) of whom only about 200 or 0.66 percent are Christian. (Wang, 1972.)

The administrative district or li* where we lived, at the far end of town, is a rapidly industrializing rural area. Most of the remaining farmers are over 50 years of age and most have sons and daughters in factories. At the furthest point from the town within the area of the li is the nucleus of the old village—a densely clustered multi-surname area where the *Ong-ia-kong* resides.

The house in which the *Ong-ia-kong* resides differs slightly from those that surround it. The family members whose house it is are unusually sweet and thoughtful. The family consists of an old lady, her two grown sons, and the wife and three children of the elder son. The entire family is capable of kindly and relaxed hospitality every night of the week from seven to midnight and all night long on many occasions. They provide drinking water, cigarettes, toilet paper, and other necessities. They converse with the supplicants, help them in their worship, take an active interest in their cases, and take care that they are provided with the equipment both for prior sacrifices and for initial treatment. The house differs from those of the neighbors in having a plastic shelter over the courtyard to protect the god's birthday party from rain, and in having a large outdoor incense pot donated by two Taipei business-men. Both of these acquisitions appeared while I was living in the village. This house is more old-fashioned than many of the neighboring homes: it still has an outdoor pump instead of running water, and a pit toilet among the unused pig pens instead of the flush toilets that have gained favor in newer houses.

Inside the house the arrangement of the ancestor hall is an elaboration of the usual one. On the back wall, in front of the two ordinary scrolls of the three happinesses (wealth, sons, long life*) and the five gods which are hung in almost every house, are not only the usual tablets, divination blocks, candles, wine cups, incense pots, and so forth, but also the statue of the *Ong-ia-kong* flanked by his two guardian gods, each with an incense pot. During the year I spent there, two other god-statues moved in, each of them with its incense pot. The left-hand wall of the central room is also devoted to the cult. There is a table to store, display, and sell the spirit money, firecrackers, candles, and incense needed for worship, and also a board where hang the *chhiam** or fortune papers. There are two square tables, instead of the usual one, in front of the high altar table. On the tables are candles, vases of flowers, dishes of fruit, a money box, the seal of the god, and the *poe** or divination blocks for getting yes and no answers to simple questions such as "Have you (the god) finished eating?" The other paraphernalia needed for sessions with *Ong-ia-kong* are kept in the drawers of these tables. There are assorted chairs, stools, benches, and a couch in the room. In summer, the benches are moved outside and people go out to chat and to avoid the thick incense smoke inside the room.

Ong-ia-kong with the surname of *Hêng* was once a man on the Mainland. There is little knowledge of or interest in that phase of his existence among his devotees in modern Taiwan. What is known and related is that his statue was brought over around the time that the god Koxinga (modelled after the man Koxinga) came to Taiwan, i.e., about 200 years ago. By once stopping the procession of another god, this *Ong-ia-kong* made its efficacy known to those who had neglected it. It was set up more than 100 years ago in the area in which I worked. Though the statue has frequently moved from house to house and even resided in a community across the river, it is now located in the older part of the village.

The statue is mute but *Ong-ia-kong* is not. There are two ways for the god to make his wishes known. The primary way is through a *tang-ki,* variously translated as "shaman" or "spirit medium." The *tang-ki* is, in this case, a man of 40 who is nightly possessed by the god and speaks in his voice. Secondly, lacking a *tang-ki* as *Ong-ia-kong* did after the retirement of the previous one, *Ong-ia-kong* can make his *kīo-á** or divination chair write in the dust. The characters are deciphered by a *khīa-toh-thâu** or assistant who is literate and who chants and writes for the *tang-ki,* when there is one.

The former *tang-ki* involuntarily entered that profession at age 18 and continued to go regularly into trance for *Ong-ia-kong* until he was more than 60. When he retired, there was no one to take his place. At the birthday of the god, the present *tang-ki,* who had simply taken his children to watch the firewalk, suddenly went into trance.[3] His wife claimed that it was punishment from the god for appearing without first washing. But the arm of the divination chair wrote in the dust that *Ong-ia-kong* had chosen this man for his new *tang-ki.*

The present *tang-ki* is an energetic, somewhat nervous man of 40 who lives with his mother, wife and four children. Though he did not choose to become *tang-ki,* he met the two requirements set by the god— that he be illiterate and that he be willing to go into trance whenever earnestly entreated to do so. The assistant is a man in his sixties who is related by blood and adoption to the former assistant. He is a cheerful, stocky man who is retired from work and lives with his adult sons. He learned the business of assisting from the former assistant, who chose him in preference to his own two sons. Assisting requires considerable literacy and some study. Although it is not physically exhausting, as trancing is, the assistant devotes from 3 to 6 hours a day to it.

In the evenings, most villagers come home from work by bicycle, motorcycle, or on foot. They bathe before eating supper. If they are not going out again, they usually watch television or sit outside or at stores and neighbors' houses to chat. Those who are going to see *Ong-ia-kong* gather at his house. Some come by just to worship the god, either regularly or for favors granted. The worship consists most simply of bowing and offering incense or, more elaborately, of purchasing spirit money, candles, incense, and firecrackers and burning all of them. Sometimes fruits, cookies, or candies are offered as well, and taken home after a throw of the divination blocks indicates that the god has partaken of them. People who are going to ask the god about some problem always buy the spirit money, incense, and candles to burn. The members of the host household are unfailingly friendly to the supplicants. The old mother talks to both men and women; the daughter-in-law sells the incense and spirit money and usually sits with her baby on her lap talking to the other young mothers with children; the household head, a man in his early thirties, sits outside smoking with the men and burning firecrackers for those who don't like the explosion.

The assistant arrives from the market town on his bicycle. He chats a bit and then goes inside to prepare for the ceremony. The supplicants follow him inside to tell him the name of the patient (or of the patient's father if it is a child), the birthdate and time, the address, and the problem. People often come to ask for help for others—their children, spouse, parents, friends, or grandchildren. The assistant writes the necessary data on the back of a piece of blank spirit money. The family members make sure there is enough incense, that candles are lit, that boiled water is prepared, and that all the supplies for the session—red envelopes, the god's seal, the ink stone, and other ritual and practical objects are readily available.

About this time the *tang-ki* usually arrives. He lives only two doors down, but he works as a laborer in a suburb of Taipei some distance away. He comes home to bathe and eat before trancing. If there are not many people yet, he may wait and smoke and chat with the others until more patients arrive. Otherwise, he will just straighten the god's robes, perhaps speak to him, light a cigarette for him (which is placed in an ashtray in front of the statue by the god's incense pot), and stand to say his prayers. The assistant starts to burn wads of the folded spirit money and begins a chant which starts slowly but picks up speed and rhythmic intensity as it goes on.

During the chant the *tang-ki* first stands praying, hands folded. Then he sits on a stool, facing the god, with his hands on his knees. His eyes close. After a while he begins to tremble, then shake. His hands start to beat on his knees. Then in a half-crouch he begins jumping, his feet hitting the floor as his hands hit his knees, his head down, almost hitting the table in front of him. As he starts to jump, someone removes the stool behind him. He jumps for about a minute, then comes down hard on the table—his forehead hitting the table, his hands clasped together and trembling rhythmically over his head, his legs stiff, his feet apart, one slightly behind the other.

Once the *tang-ki's* head comes down, the assistant stops chanting and begins to read off the first case: "believing man or woman"*, name, birthdate, address, problem. During the reading the *tang-ki* starts to make sounds in a strange falsetto. He continues for some time. This is considered to be the god speaking in his native dialect, i.e., that which was spoken in his area of the Chinese mainland in the T'ang Dynasty. No one can understand those sounds. The actual advice is given in Taiwanese in a voice similar to the *tang-ki's* normal speaking voice, but deeper, more forceful, and more inflected. The sentences of advice are often followed by, "Did you understand that?" They are interspersed with the falsetto noises. Often there is some discussion. The patient asks the god or the *tang-ki's* helper a question. The god speaking through the *tang-ki* may reply or, if it is simple or the god seems annoyed, then the helper or even another patient or listener may answer the question. The god does not like to repeat himself and will be annoyed at that, but he will answer further questions. At the end the god, speaking through the *tang-ki,* says, "next case" and lapses into soft falsetto while the data of the next case are read to him.

During the session people listen, walk around the room, smoke, and chat. New people come in to worship or to tell the assistant their problems. It is, in fact, new patients trying to get the assistant to write down their problems that usually causes the original patient to ask the god to repeat. *Ong-ia-kong* speaking through his medium may shout with annoyance at that, but the listeners just giggle at his anger, though they attempt not to annoy him again. People often comment on the patient's case, offering supplementary advice on the basis of their own experience. The atmosphere is quite casual.

The *tang-ki* may spend the entire evening, up to 4 hours, in the same position bent over the table. He occasionally lifts his head and disengages his hands in order to scribble the magic character or *hû-á** with brush and ink on spirit paper. (He claims to be unable to write this or anything else when not in trance.)[4] There is only one case for which he changes position. This is when a patient, most often a child, is judged to have a *im** thing in him which must be exorcised. Then the *tang-ki* first writes the *hû-á* on spirit money while the patient, or mother with patient on her lap, sits on a stool facing the door with her back to the *tang-ki* and altar. She uncovers the afflicted area, most often the baby's belly. After the *tang-ki* writes the magic character, the assistant burns it, and drops the burning paper into a glass of boiled water. The *tang-ki* fills his mouth with this, walks stiffly around until he is facing the patient, writes the magic character with brush on the afflicted part, and then suddenly stamps and spits the mouthful of water on the same place.

When all the patients have been diagnosed and prescribed for, the assistant begins to chant and burns one more wad of spirit money. At this the *tang-ki* stirs, groans, slowly raises his head and rubs his neck with a look of obvious discomfort on his face. He goes outside to wash his hands and face at the basin the host family has prepared for him. The remaining men, the host, the assistant, the *tang-ki,* and any other adult males still there, talk a bit, smoke a bit, and divide up the money. Some is given to the *tang-ki,* some to the assistant, some to the host household, and some is left in the large money box which is the fund for the *Ong-ia-kong* birthday and for the temple they will eventually build.[5]

This area of Taiwan is, as we noted, well-provided with public health, environmental health and preventive medical facilities and personnel for Western-style medical treatment. The area has enjoyed rapid and widespread economic improvement, and mortality has declined rapidly. On the other hand, we have the *Ong-ia-kong* cult, which is in type quite common throughout Taiwan. It also is doing well, judging from the number of hours it operates each week, the numbers of people in attendance, and the gifts to the cult. The *tang-ki* is asked to go into trance almost every evening of the week. Some evenings only three or four people show up and he may not go into trance until 8:30 or 9:00 and come out again by 10:30. Other evenings he begins by 7:30 and is not done until after midnight. This occurs despite the fact that doctors' offices are open in the evenings, people have television to watch at home, and the nearby market town has movie theaters and a very colorful and lively evening market. Furthermore, the people who come to see the *Ong-ia-kong* are not just those from the village. Every evening they come from the market town, and frequently even from Taipei and other more distant cities and market towns.[6]

The success of the *Ong-ia-kong* cult must be seen as part of the prospering of Taiwan's economy and the flourishing of many aspects of Taiwanese religion. This flourishing of religion is partially due to the fact that Taiwanese people are accustomed to directing their resources and energies in ritualistic ways. Excess money is usually put into religious ritual, family ceremonies (such as weddings and funerals), education, and investments (land, factories). But prosperity alone does not explain the existence or continuance of *Ong-ia-kong* as physician. For this we must look at his medical practice.

2. Ailments and Methods of Ong-ia-kong Treatment

Constructing a classification of the matters treated by *Ong-ia-kong* is exceedingly difficult. What would be recognized by a Western-style doctor as a single disease, such as hepatitis, might be perceived by the patient in a variety of ways, only some of which would make sense to the doctor. Since I did not work on native taxonomy, I can only present two amateur classifications: one loosely "Western" (relying on myself as informant); the other loosely "Taiwanese old-fashioned" (my reorganization of informants' views). The types of conditions listed below under one classification do not necessarily correspond to the conditions given the same numerical designation under the other classification.

MATTERS TREATED BY ONG-IA-KONG

(A)	(B)
Western	*Taiwanese Old-Fashioned*
(1) trivial, self-limiting (some psychosomatic) ailments	(1) non-serious physical ailments
(2) non-trivial, easily curable illness	(2) disease from the body
(3) non-trivial, difficult to cure illness	(3) disease from supernatural problems, especially offenses
(4) serious, incurable disease	(4) fate
(5) social, mental, other semi-medical problems	(5) choice of time and site
(6) non-medical, e.g., business matters	(6) social, financial, and career problems

Western doctors are best with (A2) non-trivial, easily curable ailments. When they treat (A1), (A3), and (A4) (Western classification), patients often perceive them as fallible and themselves uncured. The right-hand listing covers the same range of problems. I have called it "old-fashioned" as Taiwanese classify according to at least some of the left-hand chart as well.

(A1) The so-called trivial and self-limiting diseases make up most of those we suffer from. These are ailments which Western-style medicine treats but has limited effect on. They occur particularly in children and include some fevers, diarrhea, colic, the common cold, the mysterious "virus," and rashes. They usually go away after a few days with Western medical treatment; they usually go away after a few days with *Ong-ia-kong's* treatment. A mother's choice of which treatment to use, since the price is roughly the same, probably has mainly to do with where she lives and what her mother, mother-in-law, and neighbors say. Going or not going to *Ong-ia-kong* for a trivial complaint may express solidarity with a significant person. It may allow a wife to revisit her natal home or to show her allegiance to her conjugal home and neighborhood. Furthermore, some of the prescribed herbs are the natural forms of certain common medicines. For instance, *kam chháu** (*Glycyrrhiza glabra*), prescribed by *Ong-ia-kong* for coughs and colds, is found in many Western and Chinese cough medicines.[7]

(A2)(Non-trivial, easily curable illness.) Since most people go to a Western doctor before seeing *Ong-ia-kong* in the case of an illness which they view as serious, the class of illnesses which are non-trivial but easily curable are usually cured by Western doctors. Therefore they rarely appear at *Ong-ia-kong*. I imagine simple pneumonia, syphilis, appendicitis, and many others would fall into this category.

(A3)(Non-trivial, difficult to cure.) However, there are often cases of disease where the sickness has been defined by the patient as one which should be treated by Western medicine, but either the disease has continued longer than expected, another disease has taken the place of the original one, or another member of the family has become ill. Since the disease does not follow the patient's expectations of Western medical treatment, the patient or family begins to think that a supernatural being is trying to tell them something. If they ask *Ong-ia-kong,* they might find, for instance, that the sick child's father's brother, who died in childhood, is wanting an heir. If they appoint this child his heir, to worship him as a father, then their problems will be solved. The disease will be cured or at least will revert to one that can be handled successfully by Western medicine.

(A4)(Serious, incurable disease.) Some illnesses cannot be cured by the Western medicine available to these people. In old people, I suspect that such problems would include liver damage, gynecological problems, cancers, lung damage, and various weaknesses due to excessive child-bearing, hard physical labor, poor diet, life-long anemia, chronic respiratory infections, asthma, tuberculosis, exposure to toxic agents, and so on. The next generation will be more free of these ailments, but there is little to be done for people in their sixties and over. Two of the more sympathetic Western-style doctors in the market town said they prescribe or recommend Chinese medicine for these ailments, particularly cancer, as they feel it will do no harm, and it is better for the patient and his family to maintain hope. For example, the following case: A man from a small town to the south came to ask about his father-in-law. The father-in-law had a tumor, as yet not clearly diagnosed as malignant or benign, despite the family having spent in excess of 1000 U.S. dollars on his care in the Armed Forces Hospital and other places in

Taipei. Having given up hope in Taiwan's sophisticated Western medicine, they had come to *Ong-ia-kong* for herbs and ritual.

Among children there are also problems Western medicine cannot solve. A child who has recovered from polio or a severe meningitis infection will be "disease free" but partially crippled. Maybe *Ong-ia-kong* can help, at least to tell the parents why, when they tried their best, this child must suffer. Another case illustrates this: A 3-year-old girl is brought in because she cannot walk well. *Ong-ia-kong* forbids several fruits, prescribes water with a *hû-á* for washing the feet, herbs for drinking, and tells the mother, "Early in the morning put the baby on the floor to make her take in the earth flavor (*t'u-ch'i**)." He adds that she cannot recover perfectly now, but she will recover thoroughly when she grows up. On two occasions I was told about children with diphtheria or encephalitis who were turned away from the National Taiwan University Hospital because "the doctor" said the case was hopeless. These children came to *Ong-ia-kong*.

(A5) and (A6) (Semi- and non-medical problems.) Social and mental problems (except for psychosis) and non-medical problems are rarely taken to Western-style doctors if there are other practitioners available. Some are no doubt solved through discussions with friends and relatives; others are unresolved till death. Still others, which are best discussed under the classes of the "old-fashioned" taxonomy, are taken to religious and folk practitioners whose methods of description, diagnosis, and treatment are considered more appropriate to such problems.

(B1) (Non-serious, physical ailments.) the Taiwanese "old-fashioned" taxonomy starts with those ailments, usually physical, which are not seen as being serious enough to need the causal explanation "arising from the body." They "just happen," as Ahern notes in her Chapter (2) in this volume, and are usually treated with herbs. This class generally includes colds, menstrual problems, teething, infant diarrhea, and other simple, short-term problems.

(B2) (Disease from the body.) The second class in native taxonomy—"caused from your own body"—may include almost any in the Western list of ailments (1-4). They will all be handled primarily with herbs, *hû-á*, and dietary prescriptions. They may be further explained by reference to hot, cold, and poison, and to body processes. Sometimes *Ong-ia-kong* will also warn the person away from funerals. Other practitioners of sacred medicine who do not dispense herbs would refer an illness "from the body" to a doctor of Chinese or Western medicine.

(B3) (Disease from supernatural problems.) The third native class of ailments handles categories (1) through (5) in Western taxonomy but according to a system of causation not recognized by Western or even Chinese secular medicine. The villagers believe that if the cause of a cold is fright or offense, then you will not get well without treating that supernatural cause. There is no use taking such a problem to a Western-style doctor, since he will not be able to recognize or see its true cause and will therefore be unable to treat it successfully. Many doctors do not come from a rural background. Those who do have been in regular or cram school ever since age 7. Whatever they once knew of religion, folk beliefs, and supernatural danger has been virtually drowned in the secular "rational" theories of Western science and medicine. In fact, young men whose sisters, sisters-in-law, mothers, and grandmothers still went to see gods, bumped into ghosts, made soul baskets, and checked the fates of their children, would confidently assure me, "No one does that anymore." The one market town doctor who appeared to know about these ailments told us in no uncertain terms that, when superstitions were mentioned by the parents, he just informed them they were wrong.

In contrast, when the patient stands before the god, the god first gives his diagnosis of the problem; e.g., a simple cold, a problem arising from the body, or a problem arising from a supernatural cause. The god can see immediately what the true cause of the illness is and is not only able to treat this with appropriate measures but also to prescribe herbs to use on the symptoms.

By far the most common type of supernatural problem which causes illness is *chhiong-hōan*** which means offense to one of 13 malevolent deities called *soah-sîn***. Most prominent among them are the white tiger* and the heaven dog*, though *Ong-ia-kong* also often mentions Highnesses* of different directions or with various colored faces. One can offend them by bumping into them, by being born at a certain time, by building something in the wrong place. A sacrifice to them will usually take away the offense, and then herbs, or even Western medicine are used on the illness already present.[8] The first sentence in diagnosis usually is: "This is offense" or "This is not offense, it is from your own body."

Another ailment is fright, *phàⁿ-kiaⁿ***, which is rare in adults but common in children. It involves the dispersal of the parts of the soul which must be called back together.

A third type of problem involves the *thai-sîn*** which may be loosely translated as fetus god or spirit. This spirit comes into being with pregnancy and is associated with the infant until 4 months after birth. To avoid injuring it, one must not move objects that have not been in daily use. The *thai-sîn* can be located exactly by consulting the calendars or almanacs in every house. However, most people assume that the *thai-sîn* hangs around the mother's bedroom. If she sews there, she may stab him in the eye. If she cuts, she may cut a cleft palate. If she fills in a hole in the earth floor, she may fill in his anus. If she pours boiling water into a long-unused basin, she may scald his skin. All these wounds will be reflected in the unborn or newly-born infant. Therefore, a mother with pain in her abdomen or with a sick newborn is likely to be worried about the fetus-spirit. *Ong-ia-kong* is one of several gods who handle such problems.

(B4) (Fate.) The fate of a child has bearing on its health. One may find out what lies in the child's fate by taking his birthdate and time to a fortune teller. He might say that the child must cross such and such a gate or barrier (*ke-koan**). There are more than 100 possibilities (according to the Taoist priest), but the more common are fire, vehicle, god of hell, and water gate. If the child must cross the fire gate, then he is liable to have injury from fire at some point in his life. If vehicle, then he is likely to be hit by a taxi, train, or bus, etc. If god of hell, then he must not go to his mother's natal home for a certain period of time or he will get sick. If he must cross the water gate, then he is subject to drowning. To prevent such mishaps, the child can ritually cross the gate with the help of a Taoist or other sacred practitioner. If the parents have not gone to a fortune teller, then *Ong-ia-kong* may tell them what is in store for the child and what to do about it in order to solve or avoid problems involving the child's fate.

Sometimes the parents may just be aware that this child is *pháin-chhōa**—hard to raise. This is symptomatically defined as having many small problems—colds, fevers, crying—some of which may arise from contact with pregnant women, with funerals or weddings, with his mother's natal home, with the temple, with distant places—again many possibilities exist. Such a child will come for treatment of diarrhea (or whatever his current ailment) and also for advice and a prescription that will make him easier to raise.

According to the mothers I interviewed, the only one of these problems which is ever taken to a Western-style doctor is fright. I was told by Taipei doctors that the usual treatment is phenobarbital. The other supernatural grievances go exclusively to Chinese sacred medical practitioners, though the illnesses they cause are often treated with Western and Chinese secular medicine.

Adults are also concerned about fate; in fact, getting one's fortune told is a preoccupation of many people, especially girls who work in factories. The knowledge of one's fate and the possibility of manipulating it which *Ong-ia-kong* offers are important assets to his medical practice as they enable people to understand or to avoid traffic accidents, money loss, and sickness. But naturally much of the concern with fate and fortune cannot be regarded as health-related.

(B5) and (B6) (Time and site, social and financial problems). The choices of a good time and a good site for building a factory or storeroom or for digging a well are seen by local people as crucial in preventing disease and the other misfortunes that would result from the offense, fright, or disturbance of geomantic forces, or of harmony ensuing from a bad choice. Patients also present social or mental problems: quarrelling, alcoholism, insomnia, anxiety, disobedient wives or children, a spate of traffic accidents, or flunked examinations. The diagnoses can often be linked to fate, offense, or the actions of ghosts. Lastly, people come in with a host of completely non-medical problems involving business, inheritance, or planning for the future. As there are no secular practitioners to help people sort out these problems, they come to *Ong-ia-kong*.

Prominent in any of *Ong-ia-kong's* treatments is the *hû-á*, a magic character which appears in many variants throughout the spread and history of Chinese religion. In this cult, the efficacious *hû-á* is scribbled with a brush by the *tang-ki* while in trance. A neater version is also written by the assistant with a felt-tip pen on the back of some of the papers given to the patient. The scribbled *hû-á* may be pasted on the wall, worn, or put inside or placed upon a car or motorcycle. It may be burned and added to an herbal brew for drinking or external application. It may be burned with incense and spirit money to propitiate an offended supernatural. There is almost no treatment that doesn't involve at least one *hû-á*. Most of the cases that have anything to do with health also include a list of herbs for brewing and drinking. Herbs, *hû-á*, and dietary proscriptions are most common for "disease caused from body."

Treatments for ailments with supernatural causes generally include one or more of the following procedures:

(1) Instructions on propitiating the malevolent deity in cases of *chhiong-hoan*.

(2) Exorcism of an area—a room, a place outside the house, the child's blankets.

(3) Referral to the market town temple for a regular ceremony performed there by Taoist priests—these include star ritual (*chè-chhi*[n]*), patching of fate (*pó'-un**), and crossing a gate.

(4) Recommending a relationship which resembles godparenthood without, of course, the Christian implications. When a human godparent is chosen, this relationship is called "dry, mother" and "dry child." When a god is chosen, the child becomes a "contract child" *(khè-kiá*[n]*)* or "contract grandchild" *(khè-sun**)* of the god.

(5) Recommending the making of a "soul basket" to cover the soul of the child. This is called *khàm-hûn** "cover soul." The child's name and birth time are written on red paper which is wrapped around some scraps of his hair and fingernails. This package is placed inside a small basket, covered with a cup, and hung from the beam of the family's ancestor hall. The ones I saw were made because of fright or "hard to raise" and were sometimes made in connection with the child's becoming a godchild.

The following case illustrates much that I have written above. A mother has come to ask about her 18 month-old daughter. They live in the market town. The initial question is just about the child's general health. Immediately the *tang-ki* writes a *hû-á* and gives it to the assistant who lights it at the candle, takes it outside burning, and throws it to the northwestern sky.

> *Ong-ia-kong:* The little girl's health is not peaceful (*pêng-an**) because she has seen some unfortunate things (*hiong-sū**, i.e.

funerals), and has offended the devil of the northwest. You must propitiate to the northwestern direction; otherwise it will be of no use to take medicine. This girl is hard to raise.

Mother: Until what age (will she be difficult to raise)?

Ong-ia-kong: Until 5 years old. Afterwards she will be easy to raise. (He gives the mother four hu-á with these instructions.) Burn three incense sticks with 10 sheets of spirit money. With the first hu-a, wipe the girl's forehead three times and the back of her head four times. Then taken the hu-á, spirit money, and incense, go out to the middle of the road, and facing the northwestern direction ask the devil to take back (the problem). Put the second hu-a and these herbs (he names three herbs) into rice-washing water and wash her body. (Rice is washed before cooking; rice-washing water in a ritual context means the water from the second washing.) Burn the third hu-á, put it in boiled water with incense and incense ash, and drink it. (Patients need only sip the water, not consume the ashes.) Burn the fourth hu-á and add it to the (following) herb prescription (he names eight herbs, the quantity of each, and the amount of water to cook them in). And you must put an eight-trigram mirror* over your door. (This makes the family "peaceful," and wards off evil.)

Mother: The girl has liap-a (boils) over her body. Does it matter?

Ong-ia-kong: It does not matter. To have liap-a on head and tail will make the fate develop*.

Mother: Her father is planning to buy a new taxicab. Is that OK?

Ong-ia-kong: Business is good. But after he buys it, he should come here to get a hu-á (presumably to hang in the cab for protection).

Mother: Should he buy it himself or with his uncle?

Ong-ia-kong: Better buy it himself.

3. Ong-ia-kong and Other Types of Health Care

In this section we return to the comments made in the introduction that (1) Ong-ia-kong is concerned with a different area of medicine than is Western medicine, and (2) the kind of treatment offered is very different. In reference to the first, three related conceptual matters must be taken up: (a) The perceived difference between Chinese and Western medicine; (b) the concept of patching; and (c) the concept of harmony (pêng-an*).

(a) In a survey of 300 households, I asked the question, "How would you compare Chinese and Western medicine?" This is a sample of the responses received:

Chinese medicine is slow, Western medicine is fast.
Western medicine hurts the stomach; Chinese medicine is gentle.
Whichever works is better.
Each has its advantages and disadvantages.
Chinese medicine is better for women's troubles and broken bones; Western medicine is better for acute disease.

All these responses I heard many times. But by far the most common was: CHINESE MEDICINE CURES THE CAUSE; WESTERN MEDI-

CINE CURES THE SYMPTOMS.* To "cure the symptoms" means to relieve symptomatic distress. To "cure the cause" means to treat the causative agent and also to remedy the situation that allowed disease to develop or infiltrate. To discuss "curing the cause," one must discuss "patching" and harmony.

(b) The concept of patching is a central one in the native view of health. Emily Ahern (Chapter 2 in this volume) calls patching medicines "tonics," but I have chosen to call them "patching" because one can also patch one's fate or patch one's clothes. I prefer "patch" to the more English "mend" (as in, "His health is on the mend") because it carries the meaning of adding an extra piece of cloth, which is implied by the Chinese pó·*.

When a person becames rundown or ill, then his health needs patching. A woman who has just had a baby needs patching, and some women feel they need patching after every menstrual period. A child who is sickly or too thin needs patching. Anuresis is treated with patching. Old people commonly need patching and almost everyone needs some patching in winter. Patching can be done with foods, especially those that are dry, oily, concentrated, sticky, and meaty. Many Chinese herbs are also used for patching. Chinese medicine, while slow, patches simultaneously, whereas Western medicine may actually harm the general health of the body while it cures the particular disease, or it may leave the patient still weak and vulnerable, then patching is required. Or the patient may fix up some offense against a supernatural and cure the related disease but his fate needs patching. If that is not dealt with, some other misfortune will befall him. Western doctors, because they are either ignorant of or non-believing in Taiwanese dietary and religious practices, cannot patch either the body or the fate.

(c) Pêng-an, peace or harmony, is the state in which one does not need patching. A family is harmonious when everything is going well— people are doing successfully what they ought to be doing at that stage of life—growing up, studying, working, marrying, bearing children, growing old. They are not quarrelling or losing money; they are not getting sick. When illness occurs, particularly if it is repeated, severe, lengthy, or strikes more than one member of the family, then the family has lost its harmony. Sometimes a person feels that his family has lost its harmony and comes to find out if his suspicions are justified and what he can do about it. Sometimes a person comes to prevent the loss of harmony that might result from digging a well in the wrong place or on a bad day. One doesn't speak of patching harmony (to my knowledge anyway), but one can indeed attempt to restore it: putting up an eight-trigram mirror, putting a green tiger head over the door, moving the family altar to face a different direction, following Ong-ia-kong's instructions for propitiation or exorcism—all are ways to restore pêng-an. Western medicine is seen to have no bearing on harmony. Curing one disease will not improve the underlying situation, just as one shot of penicillin for a cold is hardly going to do much to help someone whose health needs patching.

The villagers make use of the concepts of harmony and patching, along with numerous others from Chinese and Western medicine, to decide which medical system to start with when a person falls ill, and when and how to move between systems. The resultant pattern of multiple use relies heavily on self-diagnosis. Some diseases are considered appropriate for Western medicine (appendicitis, syphilis), some for Chinese secular medicine (rheumatism, broken bones), some for Chinese sacred medicine (fright, nightmares). However, most diseases can be seen as having aspects appropriate for treatment in more than one of the different systems. When a disease is seen by only one practitioner (of any type), it is most probably because it disappeared very rapidly rather than because the native taxonomic theory specified the system to which the complaint was appropriate.

The initial symptoms are usually taken to a Western-style doctor. If the Western medical treatment is sufficient, the patient is satisfied. But in the course of a disease or several disease episodes, the patient may feel the Western medicine is insufficient and go to other methods of treatment, perhaps including a visit to *Ong-ia-kong*. The following examples illustrate this point:

(a) One child had frequent colds, fevers, and swollen glands. He was taken for treatment to a Western doctor; but, as the illness kept recurring, both the problem of patching and the problem of harmony became relevant. The mother patched the child's health with ginseng cooked with pigeon. And she heard from a fortune teller that his problems were caused by his father's brother, who had died without issue and wanted this child as his son. The dead man could only get this message across by disturbing the harmony of the family—then they would seek out a practitioner who would make contact with the other world. A contract was drawn up for the child's adoption.* The child's health improved.

(b) In the spring of 1973, the *tang-ki* himself became ill with great pain in the abdomen and inability to urinate. First he saw a Western-style doctor but felt worse after several days of relief. He "went to *Ong-ia-kong*" in the following way: First he told the assistant his trouble, then went into trance. The assistant asked the god about the *tang-ki's* problem, and when the *tang-ki* came out of trance, the assistant gave him the herbal prescription. But since *Ong-ia-kong's* medicine is seen as slow and this disease was seen as fast, the *tang-ki* returned to a different Western-style doctor and, after a total of 5 days' rest and combined Western and herbal medication, got well. The fact that the illness did not clear up after initial Western-style treatment led him to believe that he should see *Ong-ia-kong*. However, the rapidity and acuteness of the disease made him think he needed the rapidity and acuteness of Western drugs even while continuing with the slower, gentler restorative and *pêng-an* producing herbs prescribed by *Ong-ia-kong*.

Ong-ia-kong can refer a patient to another medical system. For the patient who is unsure of how to treat his disease there is an advantage to going first to *Ong-ia-kong* rather than to a Western doctor. A Western doctor does not know anything about sacred medicine and will not refer the patient onward, except within the Western system. But *Ong-ia-kong* does know something about Western medicine and *will* refer. For instance, a pregnant woman came to *Ong-ia-kong* with an ache in her abdomen. Was the fetus-spirit injured or is the pain caused from her own body? she asked. *Ong-ia-kong* answered that the fetus spirit had been hurt and must be propitiated immediately. He gave her an herb prescription and directions for exorcism of the room. He then said, go to Doctor Chen in Pan Chiao to see if the fetus is still alive. Another pregnant woman came from Keelung to ask about her fate. *Ong-ia-kong* said she would encounter troubles and must carry a *hû-á* with her at all times and avoid funerals. She should keep the *hû-á* until the moment of birth. He added, "When you give birth, go to find as large a Western hospital as possible."

There are many higher gods in the religious system, and *Ong-ia-kong* sometimes refers a patient to one of them. For instance, a person who is judged by *Ong-ia-kong* to be headed for a period of bad luck may be referred to the temple in the market town for a ceremony called *chè-chhi^n** (star ritual) in which the names and birthdates of that person and his family members will be read by the Taoist priests to the high Taoist gods for specific protection during this period. *Ong-ia-kong* may also act as intermediary for other gods who are mute. For instance, in one case a person found that the spirit papers under his Earth God statue were mysteriously burned. *Ong-ia-kong* consulted the Earth God and found he wanted the man to move his factory. The Earth God has no *tang-ki,* so except for the yes-no answer system of the divining blocks, this is his only way of communicating with people.

Though *Ong-ia-kong* may refer people to other gods for specific ceremonies or tell them to worship the highest god, *Thi^n-Kong**, for protection against cholera, he does not refer medical cases onward because of their difficulty (as a local doctor would refer them to the university hospital). The religious referral system is specific (certain cases go to a certain god) but is not hierarchical, i.e., harder or more serious cases do not move upwards. The Western medical referral system is less specific, as most local doctors will try their hand at anything, but clearly hierarchical—they will refer the patient to Taipei if the case is too serious.

Occasionally, but rarely, *Ong-ia-kong* forbids Western medicine. He does not say it is not effective. He says it should not be taken at the same time as a particular herb medicine because they do not get along. Many people believe that Western medicine has such a strong effect that it will render herb medicine ineffective if it is taken at the same time; also if the patient has been taking Western medicine for a long time, then his body is considered unable to respond to the delicate nuances of Chinese herbs. In most cases, however, *Ong-ia-kong* does not mention Western medicine and the patient is free to follow his own preference. I have never heard of any prohibitions against taking other Chinese sacred or Chinese secular medicines.

The treatment *Ong-ia-kong* offers is different in various ways from that offered by Western-style doctors. We have already mentioned the differences in diagnosis and materials of treatment—herbs, *hû-á,* soul baskets, and the like—which are not part of Western practice. But differences in medical care cannot be confined to differences in diagnosis, prescription, or fee for service. There is much more that affects the patient: setting, timing, role, and the character of doctor–patient interaction.

It may be of interest first to contrast the styles of the Western and Chinese secular doctors in the market town. Then I will comment on the role of *Ong-ia-kong* and on special features of his care.

The Western doctors that we interviewed in the market town were far wealthier than the villagers. They had considerably more education. They worked hard to reach their positions and some worked almost constantly. For instance, the more popular pediatrician saw patients from 6:00 to 7:30 a.m. before he left in his car (!) for the university hospital. He saw patients again during his lunch period (1:00 to 3:00 p.m.) and throughout the evening (7:00 to 11:00). He also saw patients all day Sunday. He napped at his desk or in the adjoining room when there was no one waiting to see him. The head doctors at the labor and surgery hospitals were also businessmen; they started as doctors and saved money to build a hospital and hire doctors to work for them.

Of the two kinds of doctors in town, the Chinese secular doctor plays a more active role in the town. His shop generally opens on to a street, usually a main street, he is visible from the street, and there are benches to sit on. From sitting in these places, I got the impression that people who are friends or clients often stop by to chat, get their prescriptions filled, see who else buys what for what complaints, and watch the television or the people passing by in the street. The Western doctors are cut off from the street life, socially and architecturally; the Chinese doctors are not. The latter often have several hours of free time which they spend picking over shipments of herbs, watching television, sitting and smoking, chatting, and acting generally in the manner of any small tradesman. A Western doctor is secluded and, given an hour off, seems more likely to retire backward into his private rooms (where we found all those doctors who were not busy when we arrived) than forward into a position overlooking the street (where we found the Chinese doctors who were not busy when we arrived).

In short, a Western-style doctor is often an upper-class intellectual who hopes to become very rich and who keeps himself shut off from most of the ordinary social life of the town. A Chinese doctor is a middle or upper-middle-class small businessman; he hopes to become rich (but probably will not); he is educated, but his education builds on and interweaves with the theories of the "folk" medical tradition common to everyone; he participates in much of the social life around him. The Western-style doctors were mostly outsiders who moved to the market town to work (five out of six interviewed). The Chinese doctors, on the other hand, were mostly local; one came to join his wife's father and three of the five we interviewed were related to each other patrilineally.

From the point of view of the villagers, the Western-style doctor is merely a doctor, and as a businessman he is out of their class. The Chinese doctor is both a doctor and a small tradesman, and he may be a friend or distant relative as well. But the god belongs to the village; his cult is a focus for village life.

In his non-medical role, *Ong-ia-kong* has two personalities: that of the deity and that of the *tang-ki*. The deity is outside and above the local system; somewhat as an official under the imperial system had to be a foreigner in the province where he served so that he would not be subject to local influence. *Ong-ia-kong* cannot be bribed, he has no personal stake in decisions, he is a truly impartial judge and mediator. The *tang-ki*, however, is undeniably local. He is an illiterate laborer, father of four children, member of one of the four major surnames in the village. When he is *Ong-ia-kong*, he is far above his neighbors. But when he returns to himself, he is merely one of them—no better or wiser or richer—though they are grateful for his exertions. Similarly, the wisdom of *Ong-ia-kong* that emanates from his dual personality consists primarily of local community values given sanctity and impartiality by the god. *Ong-ia-kong* says what everybody, in some sense, knows, but he says it in cases where others are afraid to offer their opinions with authority and without suspicion of bias. In case after case the advice about personal problems and business seemed to me sensitive and reasonable, and firmly rooted in the traditional culture yet in touch with the changing values, both moral and economic, of modern Taiwan.

Within the religious system, this particular *Ong-ia-kong* holds no high position—in fact, very few non-village people have heard of him. On the other hand, he is a proud, powerful, and personal god. On the birthdays of other gods, it is *Ong-ia-kong* who holds the front seat, displacing the god whose birthday it is. The village participates in the worship of the more important gods of the Chinese pantheon, but this one is singularly their own though they share him with others. He takes their children and grandchildren as his contract godchildren. He gives the village an annual birthday celebration with feasting, firewalk, opera, and paid Taoists. During the dark nights, his altar is the only community gathering point. How can any doctor, however mighty his injections, compare with this physician, advisor, mediator, and deity?

It seems clear that, within the system of Western medicine available in Taiwan, the doctor–patient interaction does not provide much reassurance. The patient is unable, through ignorance and minimal personal contact, either to hand himself over confidently to the doctor's care, or to take charge of the disease himself, with the doctor's help. The Western doctor does not, and feels he cannot, allow the patient to participate in his own diagnosis, treatment, and cure: the doctor ignores the patient's statement of self-diagnosis and does not explain his own diagnosis.

The Western doctor in diagnosis uses a body of medical theory which is largely inaccessible to the patient. He rarely attempts to explain even the simplest parts of it: transmission of disease, purpose of test, side effects of medicine. He often does not even name the disease or the drugs or tell why he is doing what he does. The doctor plays no other role in the patient's life and pays no attention to the other aspects of the patient's life. Most doctors said they did not ask whether a woman was pregnant or ask about the home situation. Many problems having bearing on a patient's illness or state of mind are not considered relevant to Western medicine and are not brought up by either doctor or patient. Oral treatment is generally given on a daily basis so that the patient must return to get more medicine, instead of being instructed and then allowed to carry out his own treatment at home. The patient is questioned, manipulated, and injected as an object. In the end, the doctor's interaction with the patient often does not make the patient *feel* any better. He goes home not knowing what is wrong with him, what the doctor did or why, what the medicine he is taking is called and what it is likely to do to him. There is nothing he himself can do for his illness except finish taking the medicine and return to the doctor, or seek out a different practitioner. I don't know if this professional remoteness is modelled on traditional Chinese practice or is a product of Western training. However, it characterizes every Western doctor I met in Taiwan.[9]

The situation at the *Ong-ia-kong* cult is quite different. The patient appears before the god in the company of friends. He gives as much or as little information as he chooses. He is not handled or manipulated or injected. He can ask questions that occur to him and suggest his own explanations. Even the most petty of his grievances are dealt with, if not by the god, then by the assistant or the sympathetic onlookers who have experience in these matters. The theory which *Ong-ia-kong* relies on in diagnosis and treatment fits within a coherent world view which explains most of the major and minor events of life. The patient participates in this world view, and anything he does not understand he can ask of older friends and relatives.

Furthermore, the treatment is cooperative. If there is an herb prescription, the patient is given a detailed list of the herbs, the proper amounts, and the way in which they should be brewed and taken. After each instruction he is asked, "Do you understand?" Few people know all the herbs, but most people know some, especially older people. Anyone with an herb prescription relies on friends, relatives, neighbors, and the other people at *Ong-ia-kong's* house to help him collect all the ingredients of his prescription. One old man comes every night just to worship *Ong-ia-kong* and help other people find herbs.

The treatment is active. If, for instance, you are to propitiate a malevolent deity who is troubling a child, then even the child must sit up in bed while the ceremony is being performed for him. The patient and his family must follow a rather detailed set of instructions and prohibitions by themselves or with the help of neighbors. When they leave *Ong-ia-kong,* they believe they know what went wrong and what to do about it, they have people to help them.

There is also, within *Ong-ia-kong's* cult, the possibility for a person to affirm his ties to his friends and relatives in the countryside, and to Taiwan's religion——which is at present the only legal expression of Taiwanese nationalism. Almost every Taiwanese has friends and relatives who are part of such a cult. Many of the outsiders I saw, like the pregnant woman from Keelung or the rich businessmen from Taipei who donated the incense pot, come to their natal home or to the home of a good friend when they come to *Ong-ia-kong.*[10]

In the introduction, I said that the Plague God and the associated sacred medical system exist behind, beyond, and under the modern one. Let me summarize the ways I have tried to show this. *Ong-ia-kong* handles cases Western medicine cannot, either because they are incurable or because they are not part of the complaints that Western medicine recognizes. *Ong-ia-kong* handles underlying conditions—weakness of health or fate and loss of harmony—that Western medicine does not. Perhaps when practiced ideally, Western medicine would treat these problems too; but in Taiwan, and among most populations, it rarely goes beyond the surface complaint. *Ong-ia-kong* provides a theory which the patients understand so that they can participate in their own diagnosis and cure. Here again, perhaps an ideal system of Western medicine would provide this, but few actually do. *Ong-ia-kong* provides an active and positive stance against disease and misfortune. His treatment calls upon community beliefs, values, resources, and members. Sickness is often caused by and causes disturbances in the patient's social, economic, and religious life. But only if he goes to *Ong-ia-kong* will this interaction of health and daily affairs be recognized. Perhaps *Ong-ia-kong* will one day cease to be a physician and a part of Taiwan's medical picture. But unless Western medicine on Taiwan changes radically, his departure will represent a great loss. In his current practice, he does not interfere with Western medicine; he "patches" it.[11]

NOTES

1. My fieldwork was supported by the National Institute of Mental Health, Public Health Research Fellowship Number 1-FO-1-MH53580-01.

2. The asterisk indicates terms found in the Glossary. Romanization of Taiwanese terms follows the so-called Standard (church) romanization system, as in the *Dictionary of Amoy Vernacular* by Rev. Charles Douglas (Taiwan reprint). Taiwanese terms are underlined, and given tone markings on first appearance. Mandarin terms (except place names) are not given tone markings; they appear in the Wade-Giles romanization unless another spelling has become standard (e.g., place names). In some cases, the characters appropriate to the Taiwanese term do not really make sense in Mandarin, either because the referent itself (e.g., the *tâng-ki**) is not part of Mandarin-speaking culture or because it is called by a different name: e.g., a *khè-kía^n** is called an I-tzu* in Mandarin.

3. Although the subject of trance is an interesting one, I did not pursue it. No one I spoke to, including people who did not "believe," ever expressed doubt that this *tang-ki* was in trance. Furthermore, advice which came from his lips was never attributed to him but always attributed to *Ong-ia-kong*. People go to hear and see *Ong-ia-kong*. The *tang-ki* functions somewhat as a telephone and is not considered personally responsible. Because I have no grounds for doing otherwise, I have followed the native idiom and written of what *Ong-ia-kong* said. Where I write of the *tang-ki*, it is of him as a man, not as a god-substitute. Appropriately, the *tang-ki's* status in the community does not seem much affected by *Ong-ia-kong's*. It is relevant to mention that Taiwanese consider it quite easy to go into trance. Becoming entranced is even part of a children's game (Diamond 1969:35).

4. The *hu-a* drawn by the *tang-ki* is a scrawl which represents a multi-unit Chinese character. This *tang-ki*, according to the registers, actually received a primary school education, and although he may still recognize a few common characters, writing and reading such complex characters is clearly beyond his ability. Thus the *hu-a* as written by him is a magical symbol.

5. The economic and business aspects of some cults of this sort have been thoroughly explored by Elliott (1955). In regard to the *Ong-ia-kong* cult, I ascertained that (1) the patient's payment was optional, (2) usual payment was approximately the same as for a doctor's examination, injection, and prescription (40–50 NT or about one U. S. dollar), (3) the three men most involved in the cult were not becoming noticeably wealthy, and (4) nobody commented on their use of the money except as it was spent on the

cult, e.g., "Wait and see what a big birthday celebration we have for the god this year." Many of the gifts to the god are either not negotiable (the incense pot) or are spiritual (the essence of a cake, the rest of which the donor takes back home to eat). These may be expensive for the donor, but do not enrich the men involved in the cult. Obviously, I was worried about charlatanism, but I detected no signs of it.

6. *Tang-kis* are common throughout Taiwan, Singapore, and Hong-kong; and they once practiced on the Chinese mainland (Osgood 1963:304–316). Almost every anthropologist who has worked in Taiwan has written about them; even those who worked in large cities have found them practicing (Hill Rohsenow, personal communication). Some social surveys, such as Grichting's (1971:389, 397–399) claim to show that almost nobody goes to a *tang-ki* now. However, there are numerous problems involved in asking and answering such a question with a survey. (a) The question does not make sense, since in the local dialect, one goes not to a *tang-ki* but to a god and there are numerous ways of doing that. (b) Faced with an educated interviewer who represents the government, the church, or some other institution with a known bias against folk religion, many people would not confess to going; still they may go. (c) Many people, especially, I suspect, young men, do not go to the *tang-ki;* but their grandmothers, mothers, and wives go for them, to get them herbs, patch their fates, cover their souls, and work other rituals upon subjects who would publicly claim not to believe in such things.

Two of the Western-style doctors we interviewed talked about *tang-kis:* A pediatrician said that 60 percent of the sick children are taken to a *tang-ki* before being taken to a doctor. Another older doctor, whose father worked in this town before him, estimated that when people in this area get sick, 10 percent go to a Western drugstore, 10 percent to a Chinese drugstore, 10 percent to a *tang-ki,* and 70 percent to a Western-style doctor. He added that he thought 1/40th to 1/50th of his patients were referred to him by a *tang-ki.* I doubt that the doctors, or anyone else, really know the incidence of use of *tang-kis* or know how to find out.

7. Although it would be interesting to do so, I have not made a thorough investigation of the herbs, nor am I competent to do so. I tried to obtain standard Chinese names for those herbs prescribed by *Ong-ia-kong.*

8. I believe *thó·-soah** to be a subclass of offense, i.e., offense of those *soah* specifically concerned with wind, water, and the geomantic features of landscape. I was told by one ritual practitioner that it is treated with *khi-thó·**; by another that *khi-soah** is the proper ritual.

9. My observations on doctors were made when seeing them as a patient, when accompanying a patient, and during interviewing. I often asked mothers about visits to physicians. Furthermore, I remembered the records of doctor–patient interaction made by Emily Ahern and Chou Pi-se.

10. Of course such reasons may keep a person from using *Ong-ia-kong's* services. He may be unable or unwilling to muster the social network necessary for gathering and brewing the herbs. He may not wish to associate with the farm people who go to *Ong-ia-kong,* to air his problems in their presence, or to have to listen to their advice and rely on their help. He need not understand modern medical theory, but simply wish to claim for himself a certain level of education, modernity, and progress where "no one does that anymore." Still, his peer in education and wealth may see *Ong-ia-kong* as an expression of Taiwanese essence and community, and therefore value his contact with the god and with the cult members. It is not that there is any specific political content whatsoever in such a cult—but in a country where many institutions are run primarily by non-Taiwanese, only folk religion, and in particular this kind of local cult, is exclusively Taiwanese.

11. I wish to acknowledge the help I received from E. M. Ahern, M. Clark (Clark 1970), E. V. R. Gould, C. S. Harrell, D. K. Jordan (Jordan 1972), Kuo Chau, R. L. Martin, L. Tiger, M. Topley, and M. Wolf (Wolf 1972). I am deeply indebted to a fellow anthropologist, Mr. Huang Tao-lin, who made detailed maps of the medical and religious facilities in the market town, conducted and translated the interviews of Western and Chinese doctors, and made verbatim recordings of evenings at *Ong-ia-kong.* Most of the data in this paper are as much his as mine, though any mistaken conclusions drawn from them are mine alone. Some of this material is included in my thesis (Rutgers University, 1976).

GLOSSARY OF SELECTED TERMS

(Taiwanese terms are underlined.)

Plague God 王爺公 *Wang-yeh-kung* *Ong-iâ-koñg*
San Hsia 三峽
Pai Chi 白鶏
a goddess 媽祖 *Matsu Má-chó˙*
god of war 關公 *Kuan-kung* *Koan-kong*
a district 里 li
three happinesses 財子壽 *ts'ai, tzu, shou*
fortune sticks 籤 *chhiam* (also 簽 and 韱)
divination blocks 筊 *poe* (also 杯 and 筶)
surname of Heng 邢府 *Hsing Fu Hêng-hú*
shaman/spirit medium 童乩 *tâng-ki*
divination chair 轎仔 *kio-á*
assistant to spirit medium 監桌頭 *khīa-toh-thâu*
believing man or woman 信士信女
magic character 符仔 *hû-á*
yin of yin/yang 陰 *yin im*
Glycyrrhiza glabra (liquorice) 甘草 *kan-ts'ao* *kam-chháu*
earth flavor 土氣 *t'u-ch'i*
offense 冲犯 *chhiong-hoan*
malevolent deities 煞神 *soah-sîn*
white tiger 白虎 *pai-hu*
heaven dog 天狗 *t'ien-kou*
Highnesses 太歲 *t'ai-sui thài-soè*
fright 怕驚 *phàⁿ-kiaⁿ*
fetus spirit 胎神 *t'ai-shen thai-sîn*
cross a gate 過關 *kuo-kuan kè-koan*
hard to raise 歹導, *phaíⁿ-chhōa*
(equivalent Mandarin terms) 難帶 *nan-tai* 不好養 *pu hao yang*
star ritual 祭星 *ché-chhiⁿ*
patch fate 補運 *pu-yün pó˙-un*
contract child 契囝 *khè-kíaⁿ*
contract grandchild 契孫 *khè-sun*
(equivalent term) 義子 *I-tzu*
cover soul (basket) 蓋魂 *kai-hun khàm-hûn*
peaceful, harmonious 平安 *p'ing-an pêng-an*
unfortunate things 凶事 *hsiung-shih hiong-sū*
eight trigram mirror 七星八卦鏡
to have *liap-a* on head and tail will make the fate develop.
生頭發尾才會發運

harmony 平安 *p'ing-an* *pêng-an*
Chinese medicine cures the cause, Western medicine cures the symptoms. 中藥治本西藥治標
to patch, patching restorative, tonic 補 *pu pó·*
adoption between brothers or patrilineally related male cousins
過房囝 *kè-pâng-kía*[n]
star ritual 祭星 *chè-chhi*[n]
Heaven God 天公 *T'ien-kung* *Thi*[n]*-kong*
contract godchild 契囝 *khè-kía*[n]
(equivalent term) 義子 *I-tzu*
offense to earth 土煞 *t'u-sha thó-soah*
(De Groot writes: 地煞 *ti-sha té-soah*)
ritual to fix offense to earth 起土 *ch'i-t-u khí-thó·*
起煞 *ch'i-sha khí-soah*

REFERENCES

CLARK, M.
1970 Health in the Mexican-American Culture. Berkeley: University of California Press.

CROIZIER, R. C.
1968 Traditional Medicine in Modern China. Cambridge: Harvard University Press.

DIAMOND, N.
1969 K'un Shen. New York: Holt, Rinehart and Winston.

ELLIOTT, A. J. A.
1955 Chinese Spirit Medium Cults in Singapore. Monographs on Social Anthropology No. 14 New Series. London School of Economics and Political Science.

GRICHTING, W. L.
1971 The Value System in Taiwan 1970. Neue Zeitschrift für Missionswissenschaft CH-6375. Beckenried, Switzerland.

JORDAN, D. K.
1972 Gods, Ghosts and Ancestors. Berkeley: University of California Press.

OSGOOD, C.
1963 Village Life in Old China. New York: Ronald Press.

TAIWAN DEMOGRAPHIC FACT BOOK
1970 Department of Civil Affairs, Taiwan Provincial Government, Nantou, Taiwan.

WANG, S. C.
1972 *Min-chien hsin yang-tsai pu-t'ung tsu-chi yi-min te-hsiang ts'un-chih li-shih.* Taiwan Wen Hsien 23 (3).

WOLF, M.
1972 Women and the Family in Rural Taiwan. Stanford: Stanford University Press.

CHAPTER 4

FOLK DIETETICS IN TWO CHINESE COMMUNITIES, AND ITS IMPLICATIONS FOR THE STUDY OF CHINESE MEDICINE

E. N. ANDERSON and MARJA L. ANDERSON

Diet and Health: Dietetics and Dyadic Classification

The close relationship of diet and health, and the vital importance of nutrition in medicine, are becoming better recognized in modern medicine (Berg 1973; R. Williams 1971; S. Williams 1973). Even so, as these cited works point out, nutrition is still not taken very seriously by many or most modern doctors. In China, by contrast, the importance of diet has never been ignored. It is reported that in imperial days the government ranked nutrition as its highest among medical authorities (Wong and Wu, 1932:25). Much attention was always paid to diet; books were written on it, and malnutrition syndromes such as beriberi were recognized (Said 1965). If there is one thing universal in Chinese medicine, classical or folk, professional or self-managed, that one thing is diet therapy. Modification of food patterns is part of medication, not to be separated from use of drugs. Not only doctors, but also spirit mediums and other faithhealers, usually prescribe teas, special foods, special "wines," and/or modification of diet, whatever other methods they may be using to treat patients' problems. Yet nutrition and diet therapy, like spirit medium curing (see chapters by Ahern (2) and Gould-Martin (3) above) have been neglected by most outside observers of Chinese medicine, who seem more interested in acupuncture, disease classification, and the like. Possibly the low prestige nutrition often has in Western medicine (Berg 1973) is a factor.

In this paper we begin an analysis of folk dietetics in two communities of south Chinese background. We use "folk" here to refer to the behavior of the ordinary community member, the man-in-the-street, as opposed to the medical experts (of whatever school or type) who are carriers of a classical or great tradition, or some similar body of highly specialized lore. Our justification in focusing on the folk is twofold: first, we lack the competence to discuss the classical traditions (having had neither field nor library opportunities to study them) and, second, since almost all of the literature on traditional Chinese medicine refers to the classical tradition, we feel that further exploration of the ordinary person's behavior and beliefs is worthwhile as a counterpoise. The folk system is not merely a depauperate version of the classical ones; it has its own logic. For example, the extreme fascination with the number 5, which

69

leads to an apparently arbitrary classification of foods and their relationships in the Yellow Emperor's classic (Veith 1966; Croizier 1968—but
see Palos 1971:184, for a rationale of the basis of the system in modern
scientific terms), is lacking in the folk tradition. Instead, dyadic classification is especially important, e.g. the division into "hot" and "cold" foods.

The communities to be described here are: Castle Peak Bay, a Can-
tonese community in the rural New Territories of Hongkong, where we
carried out field research (primarily on the fishermen) in 1965-66; and
"Kampong Mee," a similar community—rural, fishing-centered—in
Penang state, Malaysia. The Chinese of Kampong Mee are primarily
Hokkien from villages near Amoy, Fukien Province, China, and their
descendants; other Chinese of Kampong Mee come from Cantonese,
Hakka, and other backgrounds, but have more or less acculturated to the
Hokkien lifeway. In both communities, most people were poor enough
to find food a major expense, but well enough off to eat a varied and
potentially adequate diet, especially since most of them fished or were
connected with the fishing economy, and thus could obtain sea foods
free or at low prices. In the main, the towns were comparable: both
Chinese, both fishing-oriented, both similar socioeconomically, both
linked by similar bonds to bigger cities (Georgetown, Penang, and Kowloon, Hongkong) at similar distances from them. Besides the ecological
differences between them (Hongkong is barely within the tropics while
Penang is equatorial, and foods raised are correspondingly different),
the only striking differences between them are the differences between
Cantonese and Malaysian Hokkien culture, and between Hongkong's and
Malaysia's courses toward modernization. Thus we have an interesting
comparison between these two communities, both changing slowly from
a traditional to a modern industrialized world.

This opportunity for controlled comparison affords us the chance to
speculate on process and change in foodways. Why did the Chinese diet
develop as it did? Why did the beliefs about diet and health come to be
as they are? Above all, what causes the changes that are taking place
now?

Our interest is not solely in the dynamics of the south Chinese dietetic
system. We are also interested in what the dynamics tell us about culture
change and development in general, and above all we are interested in
understanding changes in nutrition and associated behavior. One striking
phenomenon is that as modern scientific nutrition is promulgated, the
diet in these two communities deteriorates, because white sugar, white
flour, soft drinks and the like travel along with nutritional science and
are far more quickly adopted by the ordinary people. Why is this so?
To understand it, we must place it in perspective.

Ethnodietetics and Beliefs About Food

Let us begin with the traditional belief system—ethnodietetics (the
folk science of dietetics) and related beliefs about food. (See Anderson
and Anderson 1973a & 1973b for further discussion of food and diet in

these communities. The first cited work reprints our earlier articles on the subject, with considerable new material.)

The general rule is that food is clearly necessary to maintain health, and specifically that a balanced diet (balanced in terms of traditional Chinese medicine) creates, restores or preserves a balanced physical being. In particular, one's *ch'i* or vital energy must be kept in good health, by harmonious balance of all inputs to the body, so that a sort of dynamic equilibrium is maintained—the body can meet all the constant variations and fluctuations of the environment. Good health involves real strength, energy and power, not merely the absence of disease. Similarly, good food tastes good. Healthy foods should in general be good-tasting, and bad tasting foods are often considered poor in quality, although there are of course some foods that are healthful but unpalatable, while any food—no matter how tasty—can be bad for health if taken to excess. Moderation, diversity, and taste quality, in about that order, are sought in food consumption. This is so partly because such things serve to maintain the natural order, but partly for the very sound reason that a gourmet diet is one of the most easily and generally available ways (given Chinese culinary skill) to achieve happiness, and the connection between psychological contentment and physical health is well enough recognized that the same word, *shu-fu* "comfort" or "contentment," is used for both (or, in the folk concept, for these two aspects of the unity that is our life).

Some foods, notably protein foods and especially meat broths, make or strengthen *ch'i*. Other foods, especially those too "cold" (see below) for a given individual, weaken it. During convalescence or after childbirth, individuals must be especially careful to eat strengthening foods and avoid weakening ones. Certain foods are especially rich in *ch'i* and build it in an individual who eats them; among the fishermen at Castle Peak Bay, the maws of large fish, especially sea bass and similar fish, were thought to have this property. These fish were thought to grow large and powerful because they had very strong *ch'i*. The giant croaker or jewfish sometimes had commensal crustacea living in its gills; when this fish died, these were thought to take up all its *ch'i* and thus become the most concentrated source of all. Another fish with special properties was the snakehead or walking catfish (*Ophicephalus*), able to breathe air and very tenacious of life, so that it lived for hours out of water. For this it was called the "living fish" and considered to have a great deal of power. It was eaten as soup. It was often considered poisonous, however, in terms of the Cantonese medical system, and thus care was taken in consuming it. Like other catfish, it was very hot and wet in terms of the hot-cold system described below.

This dichotomizing of foods into "hot" and "cold," or "heating" and "cooling," is widespread in Old World civilizations (Hart 1968; Wilson 1970 and personal communication), and has spread to the New World, where it is now exceedingly important in many areas, e.g. Mexico (Foster 1953) and Guatemala (Logan 1973; note references therein). In Europe it is traced back to ancient Greek medicine, and still survives (often transformed or absorbed into the "rich"–"bland" dichotomy, but also in such phrases as "cool as a cucumber"). The ancient Greeks may well have acquired it from Asia, where it is very widespread. It has been known in China since the earliest time that such things were recorded. In the two communities described here it was by far the most well-known and elaborate system of dietetics. The basic tenet of the system is that certain foods have body-heating qualities quite apart from their actual temperature, while others have qualities that cool the body. The heating and cooling can be literal, as in fevers, or it can refer to spiritual or metaphoric heat. Sometimes (in China and elsewhere) a "wet"–"dry" dichotomy, similarly spiritual or symbolic, is found, cross-cutting or supplementing the "hot"–"cold" one. Also associated, as a cross-cutting dimension, is the "poisonous"–"non-poisonous" contrast, covered in other papers in this volume. It is rarely important in China, but has its own interest. In general, heating foods give strength and blood, but can cause fevers and fever-associated diseases. Some heating foods give strength with minimal risk of disease; others are more prone to cause disease, while giving less strength. Cooling foods reduce temperature, help to cure "hot" diseases, and bring rest and relief; they may also produce weakness and chill, even to the point of death. Again, some are more prone to relieve without damaging, while others weaken without a corresponding strength in relieving. Diseases characterized by depressed temperature, weakness, lassitude, and wasting (such as some phases of tuberculosis) are "cold" diseases, often identified as due to eating too much cold food and too little hot food. The ideal is to keep a balance; good health is proof that a balance has been maintained. General balancing rules cannot be set, since each person is thought to differ in his ability to tolerate heat and cold in foods. Many foods are balanced in themselves, and thus neutral. In China, the hot–cold dichotomy has been assimilated very naturally into the classic *yang-yin* dichotomy, with hot, of course, being *yang,* while cold is *yin.* The heating and cooling act on one's *ch'i*—vital energy—which in its own right may be strengthened or weakened by various factors, including dietary balance or imbalance.

In spite of the universality of this system, most people fail to agree with each other on what foods are hot and cold, and what foods are the hottest and coldest, or are the most dangerous. This is true not only in China, but apparently everywhere that the system is found such as in Mexico (M. Kearney, personal communication), Malaysia (Wilson 1970 and personal communication). Most people are vague about lists. Herewith we give partial lists for Castle Peak Bay, Hongkong, and for Kampong Mee, Malaysia. We list items in approximate order of agreement among the informants.

Hot foods

(1) Strong alcoholic beverages; universally considered heating. Hang-

overs and upset stomachs from too much feasting were identified as hot diseases caused by overindulgence.

(2) Spicy and fatty feast foods; these are especially characteristic of feasts—*yang* occasions.

(3) Foods prepared by long cooking at high heat; these were thought to have absorbed much heat from the cooking process. Western foods often fell into this category: baked foods, Western-styled fried foods (deep-fat fried for a long time), and so on. Chinese food, being usually cooked for much shorter periods or in a less hot situation, was much better balanced. Westerners, with their rich and long-cooked diet, were usually thought to suffer from chronic overheating; the Westerners' proneness to dysentery, digestive upsets, and flu in Hongkong was traced to this, since all those are hot diseases.

(4) Spices, spicy foods—notably chili pepper. (We suspect that the English use of the word "hot" to describe the sensation produced by pepper is traceable to a similar belief in earlier European medicine. Neither Chinese nor Malay describe pepperiness with a word for "hot," they have separate words for it.)

(5) Fatty foods generally, notably dog meat. For this reason, dog meat is eaten in winter, rarely in summer. Its fattiness does indeed provide many calories to burn metabolically.

(6) Protein foods—meat, fish. Considered strengthening, and not hot enough to be dangerous. Thus when someone was "cold," or at risk of becoming sick from overcooling, these were administered. Particularly important was to give chicken and/or fish stomachs or the like, in soup, to parturient women to restore strength and "heat" loss in childbirth.

(7) Various other foods, such as beans, onions, etc., sometimes considered heating, usually not worried about.

Hot and wet foods—sluggish marine animals—specifically, crabs, mollusks and catfish. Venereal diseases are *the* famous hot-and-wet diseases. This leads, among other things, to a lot of good-natured teasing of anyone who turns down the shellfish at a feast, particularly if he is male and a known womanizer. The implications is that he avoids them because they would aggravate his condition.

Hot and dry, cold and wet, and cold and dry are empty cells in this system, and no one sorts foods thus.

Cold foods (not differentiated as wet or dry)

(1) Herbal teas. Most of the herbs obtained from herbalists are regarded by the ordinary people of Castle Peak Bay as valuable primarily for their cooling qualities. They are said to be very cold, and to be used in small quantities for hot diseases. (By contrast, protein-rich medicines, often acquired from roving vendors, are strengthening and mildly heating: monkey brains, boiled "cranes" (egrets) and other powerful birds, such as birds of prey, and the like.)

(2) Bland, low-caloried vegetables. Most famous and widely accepted as very cold are carrots and watercress. It can safely be said that more Castle Peak Bay self-medication is in this form than in any other. Most of the ordinary diseases of the Bay folk are considered hot—colds (which apparently got their English name from exactly the opposite belief among the old English!), flu, digestive upsets, and the like. Watercress and carrots, appropriately prepared (see next paragraph), are continually used for these, and one of us (M.L.A.) suffered through enormous doses of carrot soup during colds. Turnips, etc., also fall in this category.

(3) Infusion in cold water is considered the coldest preparation process; boiling in lots of water is second. Thus foods used to cool the individual are prepared in these ways.

(4) Beer. Although an alcoholic beverage, this is often considered cold, being weak, always served chilled, and watery. At Castle Peak, it was often thought to be the salvation of Westerners, who would die of the heat from their hot diet (see above) if they did not drink so much cold beer. This, in fact, was given as one reason beer was assumed to be cold.

(5) Rice congee—often regarded as neutral (especially in Kampong Mee), but involving boiling in a lot of water, so sometimes considered cold (Castle Peak).

Neutral foods

Rice, the perfectly balanced food, was the main neutral food. Many people, especially those not very concerned with heat-cold problems, lumped the more lean meats and more substantial vegetables (potatoes, cabbages, beans, and the like) as neutral.

Food associations

Looking over the above list, one quickly sees that foods regarded as especially good, or festal, are at the top of the "hot" list. This is not unconnected with the indigestion that results from overindulging, but it also provides useful insights into the whole system as it is seen. Feasts are yang events—pleasant, noisy, bright, and usually marking major festivals or events of rejoicing. Thus the foods criterially associated with them are also yang. Such foods are also associated with the extroverted, male, the outside-the-house world of restaurants, dinners out, the noisier and more playful sorts of enjoyment, and excess (albeit pleasant excess). It is no surprise to find that men (maleness is yang, of course) are in general more prone to hot diseases, women to cold ones. Cold foods are bland, not very calorie-rich or filling, not marked in taste, not marked in color, and not associated with feasts or away-from-home occasions. The herbs come from the dark interior of the herbalists' shops, with their subdued, sombre decor. The vegetables most often considered cold are not only bland; they tend to grow in cold water (watercress) or underground, in the yin region (carrots, turnips).

Nutritional considerations and food beliefs

This cosmology could be followed up in much greater detail (see the discussion of *yang* and *yin* in Saso 1972) but we must turn to nutritional considerations here. First, though, a contrast with the Penang Hokkien system as found in Kampong Mee. In this latter town, similar beliefs are held, except for the following: Vegetables are not of much concern or common use as producers of cold; fatty foods and long-cooked foods are not avoided or considered so dangerously hot; and, above all, ordinary steamed rice is hot, while *congee* is neutral (a hotward shift from the Hongkong belief that ordinary rice is neutral and *congee* cold). *Congee* may even be considered slightly hot. Mee, the wheat noodles that are almost as important as rice among Hokkien (and, in their Malaysian spelling, give the village its name in our pseudonymy), are usually considered neutral. (Fried *mee* are hot from the frying process, though). It would seem that the Hokkien prefer to be more hot, more *yang,* than the Cantonese, since the basis of the Malaysian Hokkien diet is considered somewhat hot (boiled or steamed rice, fat, deep-fried foods, and so forth). Children and recent mothers, however, are made to keep their balance better, and thus eat more *congee* and *mee.* Sickly people of all walks of life are apt to do this also; breakfast, eaten at what is often considered a vulnerable time of day, is also *congee* or *mee* or the like, though it may include relatively hot foods such as cakes and bread. This latter touch is possibly a recent innovation related to a breakdown of the hot–cold system beliefs.

Nutritionally, the effects of the system were good. Everyone was forced to vary their diet, eating meats, vegetables, and starches—in so far as they believed in the system. In Hongkong especially, easy-to-digest, protein-rich foods went to the sick and the weak, while vitamin-rich vegetables (such as carrots) were the food of those with the commoner diseases. Excess of any one thing, especially repeated excesses of alcohol and rich food, was avoided. At the same time, almost no foods were tabooed by the system, and we observed none of the problems found in Malay villages (Wilson 1970 and personal communication) where many nutritious foods are denied to the weak (especially parturient women) and sick because they are too hot or too cold, or otherwise dangerous. Care was taken in such cases by the Chinese, but the diets planned were nutritionally fairly good; women who had just borne children, for instance, were fed on chicken, rice, cabbages, bean curd and the like, avoiding rich foods and above all very cold foods, but still getting a reasonable diet. This was less true in Kampong Mee, because the Malay-influenced diet of the adults ran heavily to chili peppers and curries and other rich spicy foods, difficult for the children to take; the children got far too little meat and vegetables, and far too many carbohydrates (they lived mostly on *congee, mee* and sugar). But the hotness of the adult food in Western terms put off the children in any case, to say nothing of its hotness in Hokkien terms. Still, the difference is significant; of this more anon.

Other nutritional beliefs of significance were few. Far and away the most important was the belief, so widespread in east Asia, that rice in itself is a perfect food—or, as one Western-trained doctor in Hongkong put it to us, "Chinese babies don't need vitamins; they get *rice.*" In Kampong Mee, the *mee* shared much of this cachet. About half as many calories in their diet came from *mee* as from rice; the two together providing at least half of calories required (Anderson and Anderson, 1973b). Thus when people were really poor, they first tried to ensure themselves a supply of rice or equivalent starch. Of course, there is some justification in this, rice was a cheap way to get calories. In Hongkong, the first thing done with any extra money is to obtain some *sung* (food eaten with rice)—cabbage, bean curd, onions and tomatoes being about the first to be bought, in that order, as the poverty level is gradually passed. In Kampong Mee, commitment to starches is greater and to other foods less. Carbohydrates—rice, *mee* and sugar—are the staples, and an increase in food expenditure tended to be an increase in the amounts of these eaten and in dietary fat, especially lard; there was much less tendency to diversify into vegetables. In neither case was the need for added nutrients (apart from those in rice) well recognized; it was food preferences (conditioned, to be sure, by thousands of years of peasant experience) that made the Cantonese poverty diet more adequate. Again, this point will be developed later.

In short, the dietary beliefs center around maintaining harmony, conceptualized as part of the need to maintain general harmony of *yang* and *yin* in the system, and balance. Rice is perfectly balanced (depending on cooking style); other foods depart from balance and must be themselves balanced out. Some people are more vulnerable to disturbance of balance, and no two people have quite the same requirements.

Some other food beliefs are relevant to our concerns—not because they form part of the Chinese systems, but because they affect nutrition by medical standards. Such beliefs include attitudes toward food in which food is removed from nutrition and made into a social marker or a religious marker. Social correlates and determinants of Cantonese and Malaysian Hokkien diets have been discussed by us elsewhere (Anderson 1970; Anderson and Anderson 1973a and 1973b). A very interesting beginning at analysis of food as a religious marker has been made by Emily Ahern (1973). A brief *ad hoc* classification of such uses of food is given here:

Food As Religious and Social Markers

(1) *Marking social context*

Rice marks a real meal as opposed to a snack (Anderson and Anderson 1973a). A profusion of meat-rich dishes marks a feast (Frake 1964). At Castle Peak Bay, there is a hierarchy of feasts, ranging from ones with only three or four meat dishes up to highly elaborate ones marked by shark fins, a bowl of shark-fin soup being the commonest and most explicit way of marking a really special occasion, such as a wedding (or in less well-off families its cheaper replacement, chicken-and-corn soup). A fairly elaborate meal is also obligatory at any major business transaction; deals are closed over lunch or dinner. Less important business is transacted over breakfast or snacks. There are quite elaborate rules for this, both at Castle Peak and at the Kampong Mee coffee shops (see sources cited above). This use of food as social marker distorts the diet in a predictable way: it means that much of the family's food money is spent by the adult male head (and to some extent other adults in the family) on meat dishes and other restaurant goodies, while the ordinary daily diet is sometimes cut to make up for this. On the other hand, there are many feasts in which all members of the family take part, and this leads to higher consumption of meat, and to some extent other protective foods—thus the nutritional effects are, on balance, usually good.

(2) Marking reference group affiliation

This may be subdivided into two things: Marking one's ethnic affiliation publicly by consuming foods associated with a high-status group which one respects and wishes to emulate. Both are more important in Kampong Mee, or at least more self-consciously cultivated. Cantonese in Hongkong eat Cantonese food, and do mark affiliation thus, but there are not enough members of other ethnic groups to make this an issue at Castle Peak Bay (an area of virtually 100 percent Cantonese population). Status emulation is found, but it consists of eating more feast-type foods as opportunity affords, because the rich do; it does not introduce anything new into the diet. In Kampong Mee, the Chinese must coexist with Malays and other people of different culture. They cling, often very militantly, to certain traditional Hokkien features of diet: pork, *mee,* and the like. Particularly important is pork, favorite meat of the Hokkien, since it sets them off very sharply from the Malays, who are Muslim and thus refuse contact with pork. (Malays did not even eat in Chinese cafes at Kampong Mee, since all the pans and dishes therein were well seasoned and coated with lard.) Similarly, the Hokkien consciously showed their Hokkien affiliations, when in areas of mixed Cantonese-Hokkien-Teochiu-Hakka settlement, by resorting to Hokkien dishes contrasting with those of the other Chinese groups. Conversely, the latter used their own dishes as markers. All relished each other's cooking occasionally, however. Noteworthy is the very strict identification of blood coagulated with alum with the Southern Min language group: Hokkien, Teochiu and Hainanese. Among these it is a very popular dish, found in every cafe and in better-off homes; other Chinese groups do not eat it unless dining out in such cafes. It clearly is exceedingly important in nutrition, especially by providing iron in the otherwise iron-poor Hokkien diet.

Status identification among the Hokkien of Malaysia includes the consumption of various Chinese foods thought characteristic of the rich, but is primarily a matter of eating Western foods, especially sweets. Candy, cookies, soft drinks and bread all have exceedingly high prestige value because of their identification with the British, former colonial masters of Malaysia and still the high-status group in Hokkien eyes.

In addition, self-conscious consumption of Malay food is done on some Malay festal days, to mark affiliation with Malays and with Malaysia. This is distinguished from the Sinified Malay food (called *Nonya* cooking) developed over centuries by the Malayan Chinese community; such food is ordinary everyday fare, considered part of the ordinary Chinese diet.

(3) *Marking religious contexts*

Certain foods are requisite for certain religious transactions. Others are taboo for religious or quasi-religious reasons (Anderson 1969). Some foods sacrificed to spirits in religious rites are not eaten, but most, especially the expensive ones, are eaten by the worshippers after the spirits have eaten the spirit of the food. Full discussion of this in Castle Peak has been given elsewhere (Anderson 1969; 1970); a really excellent analysis of religious marking by food, but from a social rather than a nutritional viewpoint, is given by Emily Ahern (1973). For our purposes here it is important only to note the nutritional consequences, which are a considerable increase in protein consumption over the ordinary diet; the spirits, especially those more powerful or more directly relevant to the worshipper, demand the best and most *yang*-related of foods, and these are most importantly pork (criterially in the form of "golden pork," a whole pig roasted in a sugar glaze that makes the outside of the roast golden red) and secondarily poultry: chickens and ducks. The only meat that the poorest Chinese get, traditionally (and often today) is at ceremonies. Ritually-forced expenditure on, and consumption of, high-quality protein may have been the difference between life and death for millions of people over the millennia.

Food in Chinese and Western Medicine

Food therapy is closely tied in to the whole complex of folk medicine available to the Chinese of these communities. In both communities Chinese folk medicine and Western medicine flourish side by side, though special trips to larger towns are necessary to obtain anything beyond the most elementary of Western medical attention.

We use "Chinese medicine" to refer to medical traditions found in China over the centuries; "Western medicine" to refer to medical practices and beliefs, whether right or wrong, typical of the European world; and "modern medicine" or "scientific medicine" to refer to the corpus of scientifically tested, proven, and currently adopted practices of whatever origin. Thus the hot-cold system is part of Chinese medicine but not usually incorporated in modern medicine; the belief that doctors should not concern themselves with patients' lives or diets or psychological states is part of Western medicine (as practiced in the communities described here, and in much of the West) but not of scientific medicine; both modern acupuncture (of Chinese origin) and bacteriology (of European origin) are part of modern scientific medicine.

The Western medicine available to the folk of our communities was often very different from scientific medicine. Too poor to go to the more competent Western-style doctors, the villagers had recourse to over-crowded clinics where they would wait for 8 hours to see a medical technician for 2 minutes; they would go to medical personnel who gave chloramphenicol for pinworms—we saw this occur—they would resort to out-and-out quacks who gave injections of normal saline claiming these were penicillin shots and would cure everything. To the villagers, any medicine practiced in a modern-looking office with fancy equipment and many pills and shots was "Western." (See chapters by Ahern (2) and Gould-Martin (3) in this volume.)

The vast majority of health-related activity was self-therapy by keeping in nutritional balance and otherwise staying healthy, or treating one's own (or one's family's) minor diseases and other insults. Only serious or chronic illness took people to medical practitioners, traditionally, though this was rapidly changing as inoculations, maternity clinics and the like brought organized preventive medicine to areas the villagers could reach. Recourse to traditional Chinese medicine was also limited by spatial and financial considerations; only at Castle Peak were there herbalists, and neither Castle Peak nor Kampong Mee had acupuncturists or other traditional practitioners. Kampong Mee, in fact, had no professional medical practitioners at all, not even spirit-mediums. At Castle Peak, our informants were usually not sufficiently well off to patronize the herbalists except in cases of severe illness that appeared otherwise incurable. More popular were the roving peddlers of nostrums: sellers of black medicinal plasters for sores; sellers of animal or plant drugs. At Castle Peak these included sellers of monkey bones, and of herons, live monkeys, live civet-cats, kites and other hawks and similar creatures, boiled to make a soup that cured soul loss and related conditions (see below). At Kampong Mee, peddlers were rarer, but villagers who went to the city returned with various herbal drugs, usually obtained from peddlers rather than herbalists, and also bought great quantities of patent and/or herbal medicines such as Tiger Balm. Finally, in both communities, recourse was very commonly to spirit mediums. These practitioners were primarily religious, rather than curing, personnel, but most of the questions addressed to them concerned health. They were consulted most often when the condition involved was chronic and had resisted other treatment, or when the condition was diagnosed as "soul loss" or haunting by ghosts. "Soul loss" was the diagnosis in cases of anaphylactic shock, amnesia, (even very transient fright-induced amnesia such as "blanking" on tests, among schoolchildren), and sudden conditions of hysteria or other mental derangements. Soul loss was thought to be caused by fright. The soul, or one of the souls, or an aspect of a soul (there was no agreement on the nature of the human soul or souls) was scared out of the patient. People who were diagnosed as being haunted or bewitched were, in our experience, people who showed mental aberrations (especially paranoia—the belief that they had ghosts haunting them or evil spirit-mediums bewitching them apparently being a paranoid fantasy). Some had been in and out of mental hospitals. Hysterical paralysis was another condition in which spirit-mediums were resorted to, though it was not regularly considered to be a result of the above magical causes. Spirit-mediums were far more often resorted to than were traditional Chinese medical practitioners. In general, medical care-seeking behavior in these two communities was similar to that described for Malaysia, Taiwan, and Hongkong in the other papers in this volume.

The connection of all of these structures of medical care with food and nutrition is via the fact that direct treatment usually (if not always) involved the use of remedies taken by mouth. Spirit-mediums wrote charms, often cutting themselves and using their blood; these charms were burned and the ashes drunk with medicinal tea. Often the mediums would prescribe a course of medicinal teas and diet reforms. The menageries of bizarre animals sold by the peddlers were used to make soup. There is only the thinnest of lines separating, say, kite soup or "white crane" (egret) soup from food. Soup of snakehead catfish, noted earlier in this section, was a food that was used as a medicine, soup of white cranes was a medicine appearing like a food. The boundaries of *ye shih* ("things to eat"—the broadest term for foodstuffs) and *yi* "medicines" were ill-defined and subject to debate, and on the border were soups that could be labeled either way. In other words, food graded into medicine and medicine graded into food, thus showing very clearly the extent to which food and health were connected in folk thought. Conversely, many herbal remedies are possibly best analyzed as foods; many of them may derive their medicinal reputation from their protein content (e.g. the soups of birds and animals) or their vitamin and mineral content (many of the vegetables, e.g. carrots, and the herbs).

It will be noted that most medicines were made into teas either by boiling the water or by cold-water infusion, the latter, of course, being a "colder" method. For many medicines, especially poisonous ones or ones in which a more "heating" medium was useful (e.g. to counteract their excessive cold), tinctures were used. These were called *chiu* ("alcoholic drink," usually mistranslated "wine") or sometimes, at least in English, oils or balms. Sometimes oil was used as the medium. In any case, medicines and remedies were usually taken in a liquid preparation of some kind, when they were specifically intended to cure or strengthen a patient. By contrast, foods for maintaining a healthy person in good health were, of course, usually solid; though even the healthy would very often consume soups, and typically comment on their healthful qualities. Tinctures of poisonous snakes, or at least of supposedly poisonous snakes, were especially sought after by the people of Castle Peak; "five snake *chiu*" was regarded as a powerful cure-all. (It was forced on one of us (M.L.A.) who caught leptospirosis; it seemed to aggravate the condition. The leptospirosis was cured (?) by a method that will give some incidental insight into Western-style medicine in isolated rural Hongkong in 1965; the doctor mixed all the kinds of antibiotics he had on stock—about a dozen—into one super-shot, and administered it. M.L.A. survived.) Again, the tinctures are not foods; yet ginseng "wine" and many other medicinal "wines" are often drunk simply for pleasure, with a side comment on their health value, just as many liqueurs are in Europe. There is, in drinks as in foods, no real dividing line between *ye he* and *yi*.

Diet and Nutritional Science

We turn now to some considerations of the diets of Castle Peak Bay and Kampong Mee, as viewed from the standpoint of nutritional science: modern as opposed to traditional.

The south Chinese diets are variations on a basic theme: The wet-rice agriculture food systems of monsoon Asia. This food system is able to feed more people on less land than any other agricultural system known, except for extremely high-cost laboratory or hydroponic systems. Moreover, it has been adapted over the millenia to southeast Asian conditions: lots of labor, little good land, little capital for such inputs as fertilizer, and little political stability or equity (resulting in problems of coordinating or planning activity above the village level). The goal of the system can be viewed as maximizing the use of labor while mini-mizing consumption of anything else. Thus the system tends to develop in a way that Geertz has called involuted (Geertz 1963)—more and more people are fed from less and less land, but only by increasing the amount of labor per unit of land, so that more and more people are needed, and a vicious cycle results. No one becomes much richer; in fact, the price of labor goes steadily down, as less and less land and capital is required to provide subsistence and the labor force grows larger and larger in a bureaucratized economy where any economic growth benefits only a conservative (or alien) elite. We have analyzed this system elsewhere, from both production and consumption view-points (Anderson and Anderson 1973a). It follows from the model that the diet must be selected such that the staple foods are those most economically produced on the least land, while still affording adequate nutrition—the minimax game here being to maximize "balanced diet" for minimal cost of inputs other than labor. Each region within monsoon Asia has a slightly different variant of this, adapted to local conditions. The most successful variants are those found in Java (Geertz 1963) and south China. Among the latter are the traditional diets of Castle Peak Bay and of the Hokkien who settled Kampong Mee. The Castle Peakers are still eating about as they did a hundred years ago, though changes have occurred; the citizens of Kampong Mee have changed greatly. This is a point of interest, as will be seen.

The traditional Cantonese diet had its own process: adopting tropical crops and, since 1500, New World food crops, acceptance of which has steadily increased since their initial arrival. These New World crops provided a number of options hitherto unavailable, at a time when population was increasing, and allowed the increase to become rapid and sustained from late Ming times on. As of the end of Ch'ing, the diet was based on wet-grown rice (the most productive of all crops that have significant vitamin and protein content, in terms of calories per acre), corn and potatoes (most productive of dry-grown crops, these being the upland staples), soybeans (most productive of usable protein per acre of any crop; also, the protein is well balanced, fairly rich in amino acids such as lysine and methionine that are scarce in other plant proteins), fish (often pond-grown), cabbages (most vitamin-rich of cold-weather crops, especially in vitamins C and A, otherwise scarce in most foods), and other vegetables (added protection, and safety valve if the main ones failed). Feasts added chickens, ducks and pigs; these, with fish, being the most efficient at converting feed into meat, and able to live on feeds that would otherwise be a problem for the system: excrement, weeds, insect pests, etc. Thus even the pests were used as food, while all nutrients were recycled as often as possible.

The traditional Hokkien diet differed from this in a few ways. Wheat was a secondary staple of considerable importance, because the Hokkien lived farther north, where wheat grew better; vegetables (corn and potatoes as well as protective vegetables) were less in evidence. Blood was a major food. The Cantonese do not use blood to any extent, probably because they did not traditionally slaughter animals often enough to make the blood worth capturing and preserving, while the Hokkien and their linguistic relatives, almost alone among Far Easterners, relish it and use it as a staple food. Here we have a puzzle: Why don't the Hokkien adopt more vegetables, and obtain more vitamins, especially C (often in short supply in their diet)? Why don't the Cantonese use blood more, thus obtaining more protein and iron? The Teochiu—Hokkien-speakers in the Cantonese homeland of Kwangtung Province—have more or less obtained the best of both worlds, judging from our rather limited knowledge of their diet (basically Hokkien-type but with Cantonese borrowings). Why don't their ways spread? Obviously the food system can approach perfection, but does not quite reach it. (For further notes on diets and their relation to agriculture, see Anderson and Anderson (1937a and 1937b).)

In Malaysia, the Hokkien adapted to tropical conditions by using local fruits and vegetables, and by using the Malay condiments which are exceedingly rich in vitamins and minerals. It remains to relate this brief overview to the medical beliefs of the folk, and to our other concerns. Seen against the background of high-nutrition diet, the medical beliefs (hot-cold system, etc.) serve to increase diversity, thus increasing the possibility of getting more balance in nutrients, in modern scientific terms as well as in traditional Chinese terms. Also, protein is channeled to those in need, such as parturient women, because of the use of chicken soup, fish, etc., for restoring heat; while an overly rich diet is balanced by the bland, low-calorie cooling foods. Also, many cooling foods are rich in vitamin A and C and some minerals, and no doubt help in cases where a "hot" disease is complicated by deficiency thereof. (This is our guess, at any rate; we have no clinical data on this. We hope to collect relevant data when we return to the Orient for fieldwork.) Status foods and religiously required foods can be seen as working in the same direction; most specifically, they force consumption of more high-grade protein than would otherwise be eaten. (This statement *does* have hard evidence from our fieldwork.) Lastly, the beliefs about the perfection of rice have kept the people from switching to cheaper but less nutritious starch staples when such are available, e.g. tapioca (manioc, cassava) in Malaysia. Unfortunately, high regard for white rice (not originally dysfunctional in an area where rice is apt to be dirty and before polishing machinery was invented) and the millers' discovery that overmilled rice stores longer has led to the decline in rice quality, due to milling off all the seed coats, a process that seems so universal and so difficult to reverse in modern Asia. The same process has happened to the wheat of the Hokkien diet. The Green Revolution has not helped so far; it has produced higher-yield but also higher-starch grains, thus diluting still further the nutrients in the grain. Fortunately, both at Castle Peak Bay and Kampong Mee, the nutrients lost by milling are not those in short supply in the diet.

This introduces us to the modern changes in the diet and in medical beliefs about it. At Castle Peak, as of our work in 1965-66, the only changes of importance were the overmilling of rice and the widespread consumption of soft drinks and beer. At Kampong Mee the situation was very different. As well as overmilling of wheat and rice, much else had happened. We have space here only to summarize the changes (see Anderson and Anderson 1973b for a fuller story). The main one is an enormous increase in the consumption of white sugar. In traditional south Chinese diets, e.g. the diets of most people at Castle Peak Bay, sweets did not rank high; fruit was about the only source of sugar, and it was often eaten unripe and/or salted, very sweet fruits being disliked. Desserts did not exist, nor were sweet drinks common. In Kampong Mee, about a quarter of the calories in the average diet came from white sugar, fewer for adults but more (up to one-third) for children. Soft drinks, candy, sweet cakes and cookies of various kinds, and sugared coffee and proprietary drinks (Horlicks, Milo, etc.), were the main sources. Children lived on rice *congee, mee,* bits of very fat pork, sweet cakes, candy, extremely heavily sugared condensed milk or proprietary drinks, and soft drinks. Children's breakfasts, for example, often consisted of unenriched white bread heaped with white sugar, or of heavily sweetened rice-flour cakes. Other changes from the traditional Hokkien base (as near as we could reconstruct it) were: higher consumption of wheat flour (in *mee,* bread, cookies, etc.); high consumption of meat, especially pork fat, lard being the preferred cooking oil and fresh bacon the preferred meat; and higher consumption of chili and curry spices (turmeric, cumin, anise seed, cloves, cinnamon, etc.) incident upon adopting many Malay-derived dishes. Fruit was being replaced in the diet by purchased sweets, which had more sugar by far, and none of the vitamins and minerals present in native fruit. Malayan fruits are on the average far more nutritious than American fruits—part of the mini-max strategy of the south Asian rice dietary. Much of the vitamins A and C in traditional tropical Asian diets are derived from them, apparently (Wilson 1970).

On balance, the changes in the diet were disastrous, especially the increasingly rapid change from fruit and vegetables to white sugar. This and many other changes were due to status emulation of the British. The Hokkien had all too correct an idea of the British diet: bread, fat meat and sweets (Yudkin 1972), and ate accordingly, to an increasing degree. Their own culture was a subject of loyalty, but they were deeply ambivalent toward it, had deep insecurity about it; were antagonistic toward the Malays, and thus acculturating little in their direction, they could only change in the direction of the rich, prestigious former rulers of the country. Thus a use of food for symbolic purposes led to deterioration of diet, due to sacrifice of a better but "peasant" diet for a worse but more prestigious one. The effects were visible most clearly in their teeth—all persons observed had much tooth decay and the teeth of babies and children often rotted as fast as they grew in. This was evidently associated with a soft diet rich in sweets. The general health of the villager was poor, evidently due in part to poor diet. Obesity was common, due to high carbohydrate and fat consumption and lack of exercise among those whose work did not require high calorie expenditure. Unfortunately, we were unable to measure nutritional deficiencies.

As to the traditional medical nutritional belief system, it too was fading, without being replaced by modern nutritional science (which was *completely* unknown to the people of Kampong Mee, except for a belief, derived from advertising, that milk and the proprietary drinks were good for children). Not much attention was paid to the hot-cold system, though it was still invoked in sickness. Herbal cures were less numerous and less important than at Castle Peak Bay, and there was a strong tendency for patent medicines to replace the old remedies and the herbalist. (There were no herbalists in the community, and those in town were few and expensive. By contrast, the Castle Peak Bay area had several large, well-stocked shops, but its population was larger, also.) Spirit-mediums at Castle Peak almost always prescribed herbal and dietary aids for their clients, but this was not true at Kampong Mee (though spirit-medium curing was as important as at Castle Peak, being one part of traditional culture that emphatically had *not* faded (see Elliott 1955) for spirit-medium curing in Singapore). In general, the fact was that both the traditional diet and the traditional diet-therapy beliefs had broken down, the one being linked with the other. Much of the old system persisted, including a general belief that balance in diet was absolutely basic to health and that foods and herbs could cure, but no one professed great knowledge about this, or indulged in self-treatment, which was so frequent and detailed at Castle Peak Bay. The basic principles of the old system were still accepted; the knowledge and initiative necessary to use it were running out. The reason given for this was that the community, being small, poor, isolated, and far from China, had forgotten much. The anthropological question is why this particular thing was forgotten, when much else was not; the reason, in our opinion, is that this community was so shattered by its economic and political problems that the people had given up hope in themselves, and hope in the future; thus they had no more confidence in their ability to manage their lives or bodies. They left the care thereof to the mercy of the gods (via religious curing rites) or of city doctors or patent-medicine makers, while they copied the diet of the prestigious West. We have a mass of evidence on the point, based on analysis of many systems and on the testimony of informants (Anderson and Anderson 1973b).

Conclusions

We come now to conclusions. What can we say about the material summarized herein?

First, it is desirable to analyze traditional beliefs—here, medical and food beliefs—as systems, and as part of behavior systems. There has been too much tendency in the literature to list beliefs like items of laundry. There has been even more tendency, even in the best and most recent works, to ignore the relationship of beliefs and behavior, and to describe either one or the other without showing interrelationships. In Chinese medicine, this has taken the form of describing the teachings of the medical system without showing how they related to the realities of Chinese life and its medical problems. We have tried to make a bare beginning here and elsewhere (Anderson and Anderson 1973a) at showing the relationship of the hot-cold dietary belief system to the facts of diet, showing how the beliefs increase dietary diversity, bring about a real balance in the diet (e.g. religion, with its prescribed protein feasts) and thus reinforce highly adaptive behavior. Viewed this way, dietary beliefs are part of an adaptive strategy, based on the economic or, more accurately, ecological realities of south China.

This raises the question of how we can identify beliefs, and how we can say that beliefs are shared (or not shared), in a community. We have access to what people say, and we can observe their behavior. If they tell us they will behave a certain way, and then do so, we have a fair fit; can we work back to the belief system? If they say one thing and do another, how can we reconcile it? Our strategy is first to collect data on many systems of behavior, and then find common threads running through these, implying a single underlying cognitive pattern; then to seek situations in which only this pattern (and no other) could produce a certain behavior. This is tricky and may not really get into people's minds. At worst, though, it does produce a description of the system. We also engaged in detailed frame interviewing, to get as far as we can into "what people say" (Frake 1964).

Granted that the cognitive system exists and is relevant, we can see how changes in ecology or economy are filtered through it and then expressed in behavior. In Kampong Mee, we have seen that the foods eaten and the extent of self-doctoring by dietary devices have both changed. Specifically, the Chinese found themselves a poverty-stricken and insecure minority in a country ruled first by the British, then by their traditional opponents the Malays. (In fact, Chinese have a share in Malaysian politics, but the Chinese of Kampong Mee see the government as Malay, and refer to it as such.) They thus faced loss of self-confidence and security. To this they reacted by, among other things, losing faith in their self-medication practices and in the virtue of their traditional diet. They then moved (and are still moving) toward using medical resources external to the community and toward emulating the foodways of their neighbors and superiors in the political hierarchy as they saw it. In short, considerations of status and security, in an environment of political and economic worries, led to great modification of the diet, usually in a way that would be considered exceedingly unfortunate indeed by both traditional Chinese and modern dietitians.

We must now place these foodways in the context of the traditional folk medical system of China. When a person was sick, treatment began with self-therapy by diet, and went on to other treatment based on the hot-cold system, and/or other home remedies. Then recourse was had to medicines or other curing items from vendors (often roving peddlers) if the sickness got worse; then, if it became really acute, to a doctor—Chinese-style, Western-style, or mixed, or sometimes two or three different sorts to cover all the odds—last, if the condition became chronic to a spirit-medium, who became possessed by a spirit able to explain and tell cures for the ailment. (A spirit-medium curing rite is exceedingly dramatic and vivid; it makes the patient feel the center of attention, and brings all the supernatural forces down to deal with his or her problem.) Most questions asked of "legitimate" spirit-mediums in areas we know dealt with health (Elliott 1955 and our field notes). (The spirit-mediums considered less reputable gave out gambling tips, invulnerability, and the like, and practiced magic to harm victims, but they too did a great deal of curing.) The whole curing nexus of religion deserves the most serious and thorough study from a medical point of view. In regard to food, as noted previously, the spirit-medium returns the course of medical care-seeking back to the start, by telling his clients to eat certain foods and drink certain teas. At least most spirit-mediums do this, and all, or almost all, give out charms that are to be burned and the ash drunk in a tea. This may be nutritionally trivial, but it stresses the point that at the last analysis it is what goes down the patient's throat that really cures.

Traditional Chinese medicine, as everyone knows, focused on the patient. This can be seen as a rational strategy in the Chinese context. Western medicine is apt to focus on the disease, or whatever insult is being treated, and ignore the patient's psychology, life-style, and diet. This is changing, but not fast enough, we feel. Chinese medicine is best where Western is worst—at taking account of the patient's total way of life, from interpersonal relationships to diet (both are always talked about in curing contexts, and by spirit-mediums in long curing rites). Western medicine is best where Chinese is worst—at fighting the invaders of the human body, the bacteria, parasites and so on. All medical books that deal with the comparison of the systems stress this, pointing out that Chinese medicine seeks to strengthen the patient (so he can fight off disease or whatever insult he has sustained), while Western medicine seeks to deal with the insult.

Wider Implications of Study

There are wider implications from this study of folk dietetics. Such a bottom-up view, in terms of social status, can be a partial corrective to the focus on elite or at least professional medicine that is found in all general works on Chinese medicine known to us (Beau 1972; Chamfrault 1963-64; Croizier 1968; Huard and Wong 1968; Hume 1940; Mann 1963; Morse 1934; Palos 1971; Veith 1966; Wallnofer and Rottaucher 1965, in spite of the title of their book; Wong and Wu 1932). Books dealing with herbs have similarly concerned themselves primarily with the herbals, not with actual practice or folk remedies in current use (Gan 1958; Hu 1969; Ibragimov and Ibragimova 1964; Read 1931-32, 1936, etc; Roi 1955; Stuart 1911—these works, especially the last four, giving a good cross-section of the *Pen Ts'ao K'ang Mu*). We still lack an analysis of an herbalist's shop, or of a set of household medicinal herb gardens. Many actual field observations are buried in the brief botanical-label notices collected by Altschul (1973) and in other compendia of economic botany such as Uphof (1968), but these are fragmentary notices, with little value out of context. Works on modern Chinese medicine (Said 1965; Horn 1969) do not deal with food in much detail; works on traditional Chinese folk medicine are few and far between. Said refers to Hu Ssu-hui's great Ming tome on dietetics and nutrition, but says little about it (Said 1965:192-234). Besides the papers for this volume and other papers cited in it, there is the work by Hsu in Yunnan (Hsu 1943, n.d., 1952, 1961) and little else; most of the earlier work, including Hsu's, is somewhat handicapped by intolerance for and consequent lack of interest in the folk medical system. There are some interesting items about food in Li (1964). The colossal task of separating the valuable traditional remedies from the chaff has fallen to the modern Chinese, especially the medical establishment (if such it can be called!) of the PRC. In this connection, it must be remembered that the traditional system had accumulated a lot of chaff—Lu Hsun's classic story "Grandma Takes Charge" is all too accurate a picture of family medical practice. (We have seen women very much like the Grandma of the story, doing things not significantly different from what Grandma did.) Assessment of the PRC effort has only begun; in addition to this volume, Croizier (1968) and Quinn (1973) are important sources. Other chapters in this volume cover the People's Republic; we need only add the point that very valuable sources are *China Pictorial* and *China Reconstructs,* not just for their information on medical practice, but because they are specifically intended to provide to the world the current "best of China." Thus they give a very clear picture of what are currently regarded in China as the models to follow, the correct ways of doing things, and the correct ways to talk about them.

In any case, study of the actual practice of traditional medicine, in the villages where most of China's population has lived throughout history, is particularly useful in showing why the system developed as it did. If we see the needs of the peasants and craftsmen, the ordinary people of old China, and see how the system was able to respond to those needs, we can provide a broad and general yet possibly useful view of the dynamics of change in China's medical tradition.

Particularly significant is the pattern of strengths and weaknesses—the pattern of areas more developed and more competent in their curing, and of areas relatively neglected or unsuccessful. Looking over China's record in this field, we can see that diet and herbal therapy were relatively highly developed, and, as we have noted, had both high prestige and high popular interest. Pulse diagnosis and acupuncture represent other areas in which Chinese medicine excelled. Closely related are the exercises of the *T'ai Chi* variety, massage, and other physical therapies. The focus was, as every source stresses, on maintaining health or on strengthening the patient, not on attacking the disease itself, as is said to be the case with Western medicine. The disease is generally supposed to be the result of some part of the body being out of harmony or weak; either the disease is the direct result of this, or it can take hold because the body is weak. This belief is not unreasonable in regard to many infectious diseases, such as tuberculosis, in which a well-nourished individual living in good housing and with other physical amenities is much less susceptible than one in the opposite situation. In fact, since every disease is a matter of insult, environment and patient, rather than just the insult (Burnet and White 1972), there is much to be said for the strategy of treating the patient and the environment rather than the insult, in a situation like that of traditional China where bacteriology and other relevant sciences could hardly be expected. This point leads us to considerations that will be discussed anon.

The other great focus of traditional medicine was on psychological, psychiatric and psychosocial curing. Most of this was done by the spirit-mediums, though the traditional doctors knew its importance, and of course, the family of the patient would be expected to give supportive care. But as noted above, our experience is that spirit-mediums were the "medical practitioners" who were sought out when functional disorders, from soul loss to hysterical paralysis, were involved. No doubt they were more often sought out for organic disorders before the coming of modern medicine, but even in the old days they clearly had a clear role in the treatment of psychological and psychosomatic problems. Anthropology has recently focused in some detail on the shaman and the spirit-medium as psychiatrist (Eliade 1964; Kiev 1964; Kiev 1972: M. Kearney personal communication). Whether the spirit-medium did any good, of course, is an empirical question (we think a good spirit-medium can be quite effective in such cases, based on our observations and findings, but we have no hard evidence). The important fact is that there were a great many other kinds of supportive care for people with functional disorders—in short, the people tried hard, whatever their success rate. Today, in the PRC, acupuncture is combined with social and ideological methods in treating mental problems (R. Sidel 1973); the use of a supportive social environment is clearly a carry-over from the past.

By contrast, China's medicine traditionally relegated surgery to a lowly and minor status; failed to develop scientific bacteriology, parasitology and the like; failed to devise the medical machines and the more sophisticated mechanical aids and tools found in the West (and, today, in China as well, of course) and, after a promising start (e.g. in the *Shang-Han Lun*), did disappointingly little more with epidemiology and studies of specific diseases. It is interesting to note that the traditional prestige hierarchy alleged for China (Wong and Wu 1932) put nutrition at the top and surgery at the bottom, exactly the reverse of that alleged for the West (Berg 1973)! Clearly we are dealing here with a distinctive pattern inviting explanation, not with simply a system that made a good start but failed to keep up with the West and instead deteriorated into mumbo-jumbo, as Westerners' descriptions of Chinese medicine often seem to be saying (Morse 1934; Hume 1940).

The pattern can be understood if one puts oneself in place of a Chinese doctor in traditional times. Without modern technology, mass production, and quality control, how could bacteriology or advanced surgery develop? Without prior advances in theoretical biology and related sciences, how could diseases be well understood? It is well to recall Kenneth Boulding's perhaps exaggerated but effective line: "Indeed, it is said that the medical profession started doing more good than harm only about 1910 and that this is mainly the result of influences from the pure sciences, quite outside the medical profession." (Boulding 1973; xviii-xix.) Without journals, telephones, linotypes, and so forth, the information crisis and the problem of getting new knowledge diffused rapidly was even more difficult in an empire as huge as China than it is in the world today. Indeed, with the store of information limited and only haphazardly expanding, a doctor knew that he must keep his own lore secret, for this could well pay off better than trying to keep up with the latest information. Without techniques for maintaining a sterile field, how could surgeons keep producing good survival statistics? On the other hand, building up the patient, especially with food, herbs and exercise, was a universally available and cheap strategy. Food was available in great variety and at reasonably low cost (compared to other things), due to the fantastic sophistication of China's agriculture (Anderson and Anderson 1973a). Herbs were free for the gathering, and exercise free to all. Manpower too was cheap, so that a doctor would spend hours with his patient, or make many visits, while spirit-mediums also gave freely of their time. As in so much of the world, medical time was expensive as time went but it certainly was not disproportionately more so than other skilled craft work, as it is in our society. The relatively low status of doctors guaranteed (and was closely related to) that situation.

In short, the system produced a cost-effective strategy. As a result of millions of small choices, over many centuries, and as a result of the limits on choice set by sheer necessity, the system specialized in doing what it could do with the materials and operations cheaply at hand; doctor's time, spirit-medium's time and trance, patient's effort and lifestyle. In a world where labor was cheap, relative to capital or factor inputs, and where biological goods (such as food and herbs) were cheap and easily modified while mechanical goods and technology were less so, the most reasonable choice was always for the practitioner to work with the patient to modify the latter's lifestyle in the name of health, or for the patient to do it himself. The Western world faced the opposite choice over the last couple of centuries: As more and more technology became available at lower and lower real cost, while medical practitioners' time became almost prohibitively expensive, the only possible course was for a doctor to preside over a vast world of machines and mechanics or machine operators. Chinese medicine makes sense in a society where labor is cheap and other inputs expensive, where elaboration of the system is easy but coordination of huge efforts over long distances is difficult and expensive. We have seen that this is true of the food production system. It is also true of the medical system. Where labor is cheap and abundant, but other capital sparse, it is more rational to have many curers than to have huge hospitals and laboratories. Where coordination is difficult over long distances, while population density makes contagion almost inevitable unless really heroic mass measures are taken (as they have been by Chinese governments of late), combating of infectious disease is difficult, public health more so, and elimination of the diseases themselves next to impossible. Under the circumstances, it is incredible that the Chinese have done as much as they have done, both recently and in dynastic times. With abundant labor and little capital for hospitals and laboratories, it is more reasonable to focus on diet, psychological and psychosocial problems and the like, than on developing expensive and complex equipment and drugs. The former take more of a doctor's time, but less resources. In the West, increasingly expensive labor, especially in the medical field, has made opposite strategies increasingly attractive—treat with drugs, equipment, public health measures, etc., strategies that require great amounts of resources, great coordination of communication and planning, but very little of a doctor's time and mental effort per patient. The contrast is spectacular to the Chinese themselves! They know very well indeed which system involves waiting 8 hours in a multi-million-dollar hospital to see a doctor for 5 minutes and to get an injection, and which system involves hours and hours of curers' time and effort (be it herbal, acupuncture, or religious and ceremonial) in a tiny room with the barest of goods. This does not exhaust the extent of correlation between medical development and ecological development. Consider how reasonable it is to work through dietary modification in a diet already made maximally nutritious and rational by millennia of sheer desperate need; by contrast, consider the difficulty of working through dietary modification in modern America, where diet is far less rationalized and the prescribed changes are beyond the patient's ability to stand. By contrast, consider how naturally heart pacers, sterile fields and other wonders of modern surgery follow from an economy in which expensive labor has led to increasing reliance on machines and precise techniques, and how impossible they would be in the world of the Ch'ing Dynasty, when the cheapness of labor was leading to the abandonment even of such machines as the Chinese had before. Eastern and Western medicine started from very similar roots. Ancient Greek medicine was much like early Chinese medicine, hot-cold dichotomy and all; they have tended to diverge since, each adapting to the realities of medical problems and patients' needs in the two areas.

In so far as we are correct in our analysis above, we have developed some new theories of why diet and medicine change as they do. Specifically, we have tried to become a little more precise about the "social factors" and "economic factors" that are always mentioned but never explicated in discussions of nutritional and medical change. We trust this will be useful in planning change, and in helping the world to eat better and suffer less sickness.

The Chinese abandonment of "science" in the Western sense, and of much technology, has been viewed as the effect of "ideology." The Chinese pattern of focusing on strengthening the patient, rather than on combating the insult, has also been explained by recourse to that question-begging and ill-defined word. In recent years, however, the actual factors operating on the Chinese economic system have begun to emerge, and solid economic explanations have been advanced for what was once considered ideological. In particular, Mark Elvin, drawing on Japanese economic historical scholarship, has coined the term "high-level equilibrium trap" to refer to the Chinese case (Elvin 1972; 1973). He argues that the falling price of labor relative to capital and technology led to a process of substituting the former for the latter. To oversimplify a bit, it was cheaper to hire workers than to use machines. Thus many Chinese technological innovations, in textiles and agriculture and elsewhere, actually went out of use, because they were more expensive than a group of workers doing the same thing. This is precisely what seems to have happened in medicine. Elvin's case can be seen as one corollary of the induced development hypothesis of economic change (Hayami and Ruttan 1971). According to this hypothesis, people will try to invoke a cost effective strategy, reducing the cost of expensive inputs by using them more efficiently or substituting cheap inputs for them. Thus the use of the cheap factor inputs increases, while the amount of expensive inputs used falls. Hayami and Ruttan compare American agriculture with Taiwanese and Japanese; in the former, land and machines were cheap and labor expensive, so a mechanized, land-extensive agriculture developed, with output *per worker* rising constantly. In the latter, land and machines were expensive and labor cheap, so a labor-intensive, land-intensive system arose, with output *per acre* rising constantly. This comparison is also true of the medical systems, *mutatis mutandis*. In America, the doctor presides over a huger and huger physical plant, and cures most effectively those problems that can be cured by applications of enormous technological resources by skilled technicians. In China, the doctor had minimal equipment, minimal contact with other practitioners, maximal time at his disposal; and he used that time to advise the patient in the art of living well. In regard to food specifically, the poor variety and poor quality of Western food compared to Chinese food is clearly a factor—especially when one talks of the ordinary diet of Britain or America a century or two ago, when modern medical ideas were forming. It is easier to modify a basically good diet plan than to tell people to throw out their diet and get a new one; when one works with people who perversely refuse to eat well in modern times, it is more reasonable to prescribe vitamin pills (Berg 1973; Yudkin 1972). Obviously this last point is overdrawn for many of us and for many purposes (we are deliberately exaggerating the differences), and there is much in the Chinese system that cannot be explained by the high level equilibrium trap and the induced development hypothesis—*so far*. But in the main these models predict the system's broad pattern extremely well. Details can be investigated in the light of these overall generalizations.

The same outlook can be used to explain the differences between classical and folk traditions in Chinese medicine. The folk traditions elaborated the hot-cold dichotomy and diet therapy in general; it was much concerned with herbs and the like as well; and it was very heavily involved with spirit-curing and other curing of psychological, social, and interpersonal disorders. In this latter, it was probably more elaborate than the classical or elite tradition. The latter, by contrast, was far more detailed about the fivefold classification of the universe, about specific man-cosmos parallels and the whole cosmological theory of medicine, about acupuncture and other somewhat "technological" medicines, and about overall explicit medical philosophy. This we consider to be another case of taking advantage of opportunities and invoking a cost-effective strategy. The folk system worked best, or at least tried hardest, on chronic ailments and on socially crippling ailments. These had more effect on a small personalistic society than did conditions that either killed quickly or passed off quickly. A victim of the latter conditions was either lost or healthy in short order, but a victim of the former would be a drag on the community indefinitely. Also, the folk system excelled in the very least expensive and technologically demanding of practices. The elite system differed from it in that the elites could get information more readily, and distribute it more readily; thus elaborate and involved schemata could be promulgated by printed word and by philosophically-minded specialists, and information retrieval was much easier than it was for the folk. Acupuncture and other specialized curing methods could flourish. No doubt the felt needs of the clientele differed also; scholar-bureaucrats and other educated people had less truck with spirit-mediumship and more interest in philosophy. The divergence of the folk and classical systems is thus caused by the different social conditions in the folk communities and in the elite community, because these different social conditions caused the people to perceive different needs, and to expect different things from a curer. Also, of course, the elite could afford to pay more, and thus draw on higher-trained personnel and more specialized personnel methods.

Proof that China did reasonably well, given its options, is found in the sheer numbers of traditional practitioners. Victor Sidel (1973:154) reports: "It is . . . probably not unreasonable to estimate the number of 'traditional' doctors in 1949 at about 500,000, or about 1 for every 1,100 of the 540 million people in China at that time." By the 1940's the traditional system was in full and rapid collapse, along with much else in China, and the proportion of traditional doctors must have been higher in dynastic times. Moreover, the number of spirit-mediums who indulged in considerable curing must have been at least as high; it is certainly far higher today in the communities we know personally, than is the number of medical practitioners. So at a conservative estimate there was one curer per 500 people in traditional China, a number which compares favorably with that in modern developed countries. The reason China in those days had worse health than the developed countries now have is to be found in the lack of basic science and technology, that could otherwise have provided the doctors with method, outlook, machinery, communication facilities, and other materials both tangible and intangible. Under the circumstances, the number and distribution of curers was maximized, while the capital per curer was minimized, so the curer had little training (usually) and little technology to draw on. This, of course, parallels the situation in the rest of the Chinese economy, where the increase in numbers of workers and the difficulty in forming more capital per worker led to the high-level equilibrium trap.

From this line of reasoning it seems that the present strategy of the PRC is in the tradition of the past. Maximize the number of medical workers, and the evenness of their distribution over the country; shorten their training; send them to do most basic and cost-effective things; back them up with specialists connected with the wider and more elaborated medical system of China and the world—this is the current strategy. Now it is done deliberately as a matter of conscious policy, and modern medicine has brought both more rational practices and more basic science and technology, so the current system is strikingly different from the traditional one. It is clear that the "Chinese medicine" in the PRC today is more a Chinese contribution to modern scientific medicine than a continuation of tradition. Acupuncture anesthesia, electrified acupuncture, insulin synthesis, limb reattachment are recent contributions to the world heritage. Outmoded and superseded are such traditional techniques as spirit-medium curing and magical rites. They had their day; they were a natural and reasonable part of feudal society; they are now superseded by techniques adapted to the new society—the spirit-medium is replaced by the community and Mao's thought (R. Sidel 1973). What has carried over from the past, as a really important heritage, is sensitivity to the cost-effective allocation of resources. Many barefoot doctors instead of a few highly trained urban doctors; herbs instead of an American-style, highly capitalized drug industry, reliance on the people instead of reliance on a few experts—these are not only in accord with Maoism, as they certainly and most explicitly are, but they are also in accord with the best traditional practice. The economic motivations we have alleged for the past are quite explicit for the present. As in so many other fields, Mao and the Chinese people have used the heritage of those same Chinese people, to the extent that it conforms to modern revolutionary social needs.

Nutrition's Fate in Modern Chinese Societies

From this disgression, which threatens to swamp the rest of the paper and take us too far from folk dietetics, we return to food. Our last point is a consideration of the fate of nutrition in modern Chinese communities.

In the two communities we studied, the traditional diet and the traditional health beliefs that supported it were breaking down. Nothing good was coming to take their place. The process was much further advanced in Kampong Mee, due to its poverty and its position in the midst of a hostile and alien social setting. Convinced of the inadequacy of their past and their traditions, the citizens of Kampong Mee were unable to adjust to their new homeland and its modernizing course; their poverty and social isolation prevented them. Thus they were substituting prestige foods, status foods, for traditional foods. Prestige means modernization, and modernization, in their eyes, meant Westernization (specifically emulation of the British, former colonial overlords of Malaysia). They adopted white bread, white sugar, soft drinks, candy, cookies, beer and brandy (if they could afford these latter, which was rarely) as the proper diet. Unfamiliar with nutritional science and unable to buy Western goods that would give them a good diet, they thus lived far too much on sugar and highly milled wheat and rice. Admittedly they had been even poorer before, and unable to buy the vegetables, meat, eggs and other items that kept them alive in 1971, but their diet was certainly worse than it might have been (Anderson and Anderson 1973b). At Castle Peak Bay, the Chinese foodways were still strong and showed few signs of weakening, but here too soft drinks and white sugar were increasing tooth decay and forcing protective foods out of the diet. Judging from observations in Taiwan and among overseas Chinese communities, these are general trends. Economic development has led to better nutrition, as more and more people become well enough off to afford adequate food, but a countertrend of switching to sugar and the like has considerably reduced the benefits of this process. Similar trends are reported for the rest of the world (György and Kline 1970; Berg 1973). In particular, the substitution of sweetened condensed milk—high in sugar, subject to contamination, and lacking vitamin C —for breast nursing is stressed by these authors and all too visible in our communities. In developed countries, there are signs that dietary quality is actually decreasing (Berg 1973; Yudkin 1972) and is inadequate for at least some members of the population (R. Williams 1971; S. Williams 1973). The same factors—shift from protective foods to sugar, milled starches, and fats—are blamed. Clearly the West is setting a bad example, especially since white sugar and the like (including soft drinks, candy, and so on) are cheaper and more widely available than many better foods. In the PRC the situation appears to be much better; gross malnutrition has apparently been completely eliminated, and nutritional science progresses, if somewhat slowly (Yeh and Chow 1973), while sugar and overmilled starches are not so easily available, and the soft drink-and-candybar diet is not yet established. Yet Yeh and Chow (1973:234) stress the lack of published materials available for training medical personnel and the many problems still to be solved. Little is known about the status of nutrition and nutritional research in China. Apparently there is no special effort to modernize and develop the folk nutrition and folk dietetics of the past, although there is a strong interest in doing so for the closely related herbal tradition. The sheer, overpowering need to get simple basic calories to everyone has had to take precedence. Now that this goal has been achieved, we can expect renewed interest in nutrition and dietetics, and in traditional and modern patterns thereof.

The world outside China, in awakening to Chinese medicine, has been particularly interested in such techniques as acupuncture. No doubt acupuncture owes some of its appeal to the fact that it is superficially more like Western medicine—it is mysterious, involves shining needles and strange technological processes, and appears to cure diseases as if by magic. Yet acupuncture too seems to act by strengthening the patient rather than by removing the insult; from the constellation of conditions for which it is recommended, it seems to us to be closely connected to the "stress syndrome" activating this system to make it react against invasion, or adjusting it so that it ceases overreacting in such conditions as allergy and rheumatism. The success of acupuncture anesthesia also informs us that it operates by manipulating and adjusting the body's own reactions, rather than by injecting some foreign anesthetic. Thus it is part of the traditional Chinese strategy of helping the patient defend himself and restoring his physiological or vital balance (Mann 1963; Palos 1971; etc.). In all the attention paid to Chinese medicine, very little has been paid to nutrition therapy. No doubt this reflects the low status of food and nutrition in so much of the contemporary medical world (Berg 1973); as we have stressed, it certainly does not reflect the Chinese picture.

We believe that the world should learn from the Chinese experience. The idea of making the best of what is available, the idea of paying maximal attention to diet in maintaining health, the idea of keeping food intake in balance, the idea of maximizing diversity and quality of diet, the idea that good food should taste good (since health involves real comfort, not just absence of serious suffering), the idea that each person has his ideal balance and that this is dynamic, fluctuating with time, necessitating dietary change—all these are in accord with the best teachings of modern nutrition. The success of the Chinese at creating varied, nutritionally good diets with absolutely minimal resources is a striking example of a cost-effective strategy. We hope the rest of the world will learn these principles of food and health, rather than allowing itself to continue the lamentable shift toward empty calories, so deplored by nutritionists and so visible at Kampong Mee. Food in Chinese society has served as a nexus, a point where the medical system, the philosophical and cosmological system, the economy, ecology and society all meet, affecting everyone's daily life. It is no wonder the beliefs about food are so elaborate, and the quality of Chinese food so famous. Whatever the merits of specific beliefs, such as the hot-cold system (to say nothing of egret soup and the like), the stress on the importance of good nutrition in all situations is worthy of more attention. Further study of the Chinese food system and its relation to the rest of society and traditional medicine is clearly worthwhile.

REFERENCES

AHERN, E.
1973 The Cult of the Dead in a Chinese Village. Stanford: Stanford University Press.

ALTSCHUL, S.
1973 Drugs and Foods from Little Known Plants. Cambridge: Harvard University Press

ANDERSON, E. N.
1969 Sacred fish. Man 4:3:443-449.
1970 The Floating World of Castle Peak Bay. Washington: American Anthropological Association.

ANDERSON, E. N and M. L. ANDERSON
1973a Mountains and Water. Taipei: Orient Cultural Service.
1973b Penang Hokkien ethnohoptology. Ethnos 1973:1-4:134-147.

BEAU, G. (tr. Lowell Blair)
1972 Chinese Medicine. New York: Avon.

BERG, A.
1973 The Nutrition Factor. Washington, D.C.: Brookings Institute.

BOULDING, K.
1973 Introduction. In Poverty and Progress, R. Wilkinson. New York: Praeger.

BURNET, M. and D. WHITE
1972 The Natural History of Infectious Diseases. Cambridge, England: Cambridge University Press.

CHAMFRAULT, A.
1969-64 Traité de Médicine Chinoise. N.p.: Editions Coquemard-Angouleme. 5 vols.

CROIZIER, R. C.
1968 Traditional Medicine in Modern China. Cambridge: Harvard University Press.

ELIADE, M.
1964 Shamanism. New York: Bollingen.

ELLIOTT, A.
1955 Chinese Spirit-Medium Cults in Singapore. London: London School of Economics.

ELVIN, M.
1972 The high level equilibrium trap: The courses of the decline of innovation in the traditional Chinese textile industry. In Economic Organization in Chinese Society. W. Willmott, ed. Stanford: Stanford University Press. Pp. 137-172.
1973 The Pattern of the Chinese Past. Stanford: Stanford University Press.

FOSTER, G.
  1953   Relationships between Spanish and Spanish-American folk
         medicine, Journal of American Folklore, 6:201-217.

FRAKE, C.
  1964   A structural description of Subanun "religious behavior." *In:*
         Explorations in Cultural Anthropology, W. Goodenough, ed.
         New York: McGraw-Hill, 1964. Pp. 111-129.

GAN, W.-S.
  1958   Manual of Medicinal Plants in Taiwan. Vol. 1. Taipei:
         National Research Institute of Chinese Medicine. (In Chinese).

GEERTZ, C.
  1963   Agricultural Involution. Chicago: University of Chicago Press.

GYÖRGY, P. and O. KLINE (eds.)
  1970   Malnutrition is a Problem of Ecology. Basel: S. Karger.

HART, D.
  1968   The Hippocratic medical system in the Philippines. Paper
         read at Annual Meeting, American Anthropological Associ-
         ation.

HAYAMI, Y. and V. RUTTAN
  1971   Agricultural Development. Baltimore: Johns Hopkins Uni-
         versity Press.

HORN, JOSHUA
  1969   Away with All Pests. New York: Monthly Review Press.

HSÜ, F. L. K.
  1943   Magic and Science in Western Yunnan. New York: Institute
         for Pacific Relations.
  n.d.   Social Change in Southwest China. "Case Study 3." Mimeo-
         graphed.
  1952   Religion, Science, and Human Crises. London: Routledge,
         Kegan Paul.
  1961   A cholera epidemic in a Chinese town. *In* Health, Culture
         and Community, B. Paul, ed. Pp. 135-154.

HUARD, P. and M. WONG (tr B. Fidding)
  1968   Chinese Medicine. New York: World University Library,
         McGraw-Hill.

HUME, E.
  1940   The Chinese Way in Medicine. Baltimore: Johns Hopkins
         University Press.

HU, S.-Y.
  1969   *Ephedra* (Ma-Huang) in the new Chinese Materia Medica.
         Economic Botany 23:4:346-351.

IBRAGIMOV, F., and V. IBRAGIMOVA
1964 Principal Remedies of Chinese Medicine. Washington, D.C.: United States Air Force (Translated from the Russian.)

KIEV, A.
1964 Magic, Faith and Healing: Studies in Primitive Psychiatry Today. New York: Free Press.
1972 Transcultural Psychiatry. New York: Free Press.

LI S.-F.
1964 Hongkong Surgeon. New York: Dutton.

LOGAN, M. H.
1973 Humoral medicine in Guatemala and peasant acceptance of modern medicine. Human Organization 32:4:385-395.

MANN, F.
1963 Acupuncture: The Ancient Chinese Art of Healing. London: William Heinemann.

MORSE, W. R.
1934 Chinese Medicine. New York: Paul Hoebner.

PALOS, S. (Tr. Translagency, Ltd.)
1971 The Chinese Art of Healing. London: Herder and Herder.

QUINN, J. R. ed.
1973 Medicine and Public Health in the People's Republic of China. Washington, D.C.: U.S. Government Printing Office.

READ, B. E.
1931-32 Chinese Materia Medica. Peking Natural History Bulletin, 6:I:1, 6:IV:1 (There were other installments of this Journal also.)
1936 Chinese medicinal plants from the *Pen Ts'ao K'ang Mu*, A.D. 1596. Peking Natural History Bulletin.

ROI, J.
1955 Traite des Plantes Medicinales Chinoises. Paris: Paul Lechevalier.

SAID, H. M.
1965 Medicine in China. Karachi: Hamdard Academy.

SASO, M.
1972 Taoism and the Rite of Cosmic Renewal. Pullman: Washington State University Press.

SIDEL, R.
1973 Mental diseases and their treatment. *In* Quinn (ed.), pp. 287-303.

SIDEL, V.
1973 Medical personnel and their training. *In* Quinn (ed.), pp 153-172.

STUART, F. P.
1911 Chinese Materia Medica: Vegetable Kingdom. Shanghai: American Presbyterian Mission.

UPHOF, J. C. Th.
1968 Dictionary of Economic Plants. Würzburg: J. Cramer.

VEITH, I.
1966 The Yellow Emperor's Classic of Internal Medicine. Berkeley: University of California Press.

WALLNÖFER, H. and A. VON ROTTAUSCHER (tr. M. Palmedo)
1965 Chinese Folk Medicine. New York: Crown.

WILLIAMS, R. J.
1971 Nutrition Against Disease. New York: Pitman.

WILLIAMS, S. R.
1973 Nutrition and Diet Therapy. St. Louis: C. V. Mosby Co. 2nd edn.

WILSON, C.
1970 Food Beliefs and Practices of Malay Fishermen. Dissertation abstract. Dept. of Nutritional Sciences, University of California, Berkeley. Mimeographed.

WONG, K. C.-M. and L. T. WU
1932 History of Chinese Medicine. Tientsin: Tientsin Press.

YEH, S. D. J. and B. F. CHOW
1973 Nutrition. In Quinn (ed.), pp. 215-239.

YUDKIN, J.
1972 Sweet and Dangerous. New York: Wyden.

CHAPTER 5

CHINESE-STYLE AND WESTERN-STYLE DOCTORS IN NORTHERN TAIWAN

EMILY M. AHERN

In Sanhsia, a township on the southern edge of the Taipei basin, there are two distinct kinds of doctors: Chinese-style doctors (*Tiong-i-siêng*) and Western-style doctors (*Se-i-siêng*).[1] Although both kinds of doctors are Taiwanese who have been educated in Taiwan or Japan, their methods of diagnosis and treatment are very different. Chinese-style doctors diagnose by feeling the pulse or studying the complexion and dispense herbs or other substances from an extensive pharmacopoeia called *tiong-iôuq*, literally, Chinese medicine. Western-style doctors diagnose with the help of instruments such as stethoscopes, thermometers, or sphygmomanometers and dispense powders, pills or injections known collectively as *se-iôuq*, literally, Western medicine. Beyond these differences, the two kinds of doctors ordinarily practice in separate settings: Chinese-style doctors in small shops that open directly on to the street and Western-style doctors in offices or hospitals with examining rooms that open on to an inside corridor to afford a greater degree of privacy.[2] (See Figure 1.)

Despite these distinctions, the separation between the two styles of medicine is not absolute: both Western medicine and Chinese medicine are often sold over the same counter in drug stores staffed by men or women knowledgeable about the uses of drugs. Neither can the two kinds of doctors always be rigidly distinguished. In my other chapter (2) in this volume it is shown that in comparison with the gods neither Chinese-style nor Western-style doctors make much effort to provide patients with explanations for the cause of their illnesses. In what follows I explore further the texture of the relationship between doctors and their patients in order to refine the conclusions reached earlier. Although in some ways the relationship between both kinds of doctors and their patients is similar, in other ways there are striking differences in the way the two kinds of doctors communicate with their patients. Some of these differences can be shown to have important implications for the system of health care as a whole.

I

The following suggestions are based on transcripts of doctor–patient interactions that took place during at least one working day in the offices of seven Western-style and two Chinese-style doctors in Sanhsia.

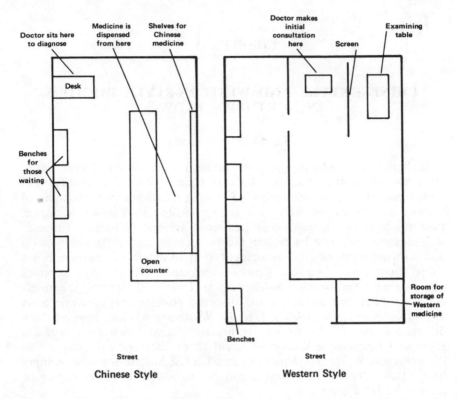

Figure 1. Floor plans of a Chinese-style doctor's shop (left) and a Western-style doctor's office (right).

Each of the doctors kindly gave permission for my assistants to record these interactions, the Chinese-style doctors allowing an assistant to sit on one of the benches facing the open counter and the Western-style doctors allowing one of them to sit in an inconspicuous corner of the examination room.[3] (See Figure 1). Thus they were able to transcribe conversations between doctors and patient, verbatim. The sample of doctors is by no means adequate to provide a definitive analysis of the population of doctors as a whole. I present this material merely to formulate initial hypotheses that might be tested more rigorously at another time.

Even without considering the evidence from the transcriptions of doctor–patient interactions, one might guess that Chinese-style doctors would be able to communicate about medical problems with their patients more easily than would Western-style doctors. Although in contrast to ordinary people Chinese-style doctors possess highly system-atic, esoteric knowledge obtained through long training as apprentices to practicing doctors, it is evident even from casual conversations that both Chinese-style doctors and ordinary people use much the same vocabulary in discussing disease. This affinity between the medical notions used by Chinese-style doctors and their patients is revealed clearly in the following excerpts from interactions in the doctors' shops.

(1) [The doctor gives an adult woman an herb.]
Doctor: Stew this herb in water for several hours. This kind of herb is good for your health. It is used to clean your uterus.

(2) [The doctor gives an adult woman an herb.]
Doctor: Now don't take any other drugs to make you stronger because they would be bad for your health. And also don't eat duck. I'll treat your liver ailment first, then your leg pain later because the drugs for the liver and those for the legs are incompatible. Both your liver and kidneys are bad and so you can't eat duck or salt.
Patient: It is said that a shot works rapidly.
Doctor: Yes, it does. But shots only relieve symptoms, and after the medicine wears off they return again. Herbs not only eradicate the symptoms, they also cure completely.

(3) [The patient, an elderly woman, and the doctor face each other across the desk.]
Doctor: What's the matter?
Patient: [She describes her symptoms in detail for about 5 minutes, saying that one-half of her body feels numb, and that she often feels dizzy.]
Doctor: How do your *kûn* [nerves] feel? [He points to the back of his neck.]
Patient: They feel very uncomfortable. I never know which one will break next.
Doctor: You know that a person usually has an equal amount of *ch'i* [vital force] on each side of her body—half on each side. Your problem is that you have lost some *ch'i* from one side of your body. That side is different and so it feels numb. [The doctor then feels her pulse and writes out a prescription for herbs.]

In these examples the Chinese-style doctors utilize concepts and employ terms that are familiar to their patients. Many of these conceptions are discussed in my other paper for this volume. In example (1) certain substances clean dirty parts of the body (p. 18); in example (2) some medicines are incompatible with each other and some diseases are incompatible with particular foods (p. 36); in example (3) the doctor mentions *ch'i* and *kûn*, two entities commonly mentioned in everyday conversations about illness. (See p. 19 in this volume for a discussion of *ch'i*.) *Kun* are small nerve-like strands that run along the back of the neck. Old people, especially those suffering from a series of strokes, mention them frequently, saying their *kûn* feels uncomfortable and are liable to break.

A detailed study of the way these notions—such as incompatibility of foods—fit into the systematic knowledge of doctors as compared to the way they fit together with other beliefs of laymen has yet to be done. The outcome of such a study might be that although doctors and patients use the same vocabulary the underlying premises they accept are often different. In a study of the relationship between other experts and laymen—geomancers and their clients—I found that this was so, and it is possible that the same pattern exists in the case of doctors and their patients (Ahern 1973:175-90). Whether or not Chinese-style doctors and their patients share the same premises, it is clear that they use similar medical vocabularies in speaking to each other.

Western-style doctors, on the other hand, not only seldom offer explanations of the sort given in example (3) above but also seem to have far more difficulty dealing with the notions their patients have about disease. The two conversations below between Western-style doctors and their patients illustrate this.

(4) [The doctor examines a 1-year-old boy and gives him a shot.]
Doctor: Don't keep him too warm.
Patient's mother: Will wind (*hông*) hurt him?
Doctor: That's not important. His temperature is nearly 40° C., so you must keep him cool.
Patient's mother: Does he have to take medicine?
Doctor: Yes, he does.
Patient's mother: Can he drink juices?
Doctor: Why don't you give him milk?
Patient's mother: He doesn't want to drink milk.
Doctor: If he's been used to drinking it, it will be all right. Be sure not to add too much sugar.

(5) [The doctor tells his patient, a young adult woman, that she has arthritis.]
Patient: It's said that arthritis is caused by wind (*hông*).
Doctor: It's literally called "wind-wet" but it's not caused by wind.
[The patient takes the medicine and leaves.]

In these examples, doctor and patient share a common vocabulary, but the patient's ideas about disease are either contradicted or ignored by the doctor. In both examples the patient brings up the notion of wind (*hông*). *Hông,* as used by laymen, sometimes refers to moving air —air that can make a baby that is inadequately covered fall sick. At other times *hông* refers to a substance that can get trapped inside the baby when a bone is broken or when arthritis is contracted. The term *hông* is also frequently used by Chinese-style doctors and they would probably have responded positively to the patients' use of it in the examples above. The Western-style doctors, however, say that *hông* is "not important" or that it does not cause arthritis. Similarly, the woman in example (4) asks whether her son can drink juice, probably out of concern that the juice will be incompatible with either the medicine or the illness. But the doctor evades her question in order to encourage her to feed the child normally. Patient and doctor talk past each other, the one bringing ideas unacceptable to the other, neither able to establish a common conceptual ground.

II

Perhaps in part because of the difficulty Western-style practitioners have in dealing with popular conceptions of diseases, there is no indication that Western medicine will supplant Chinese medicine on Taiwan. Chinese-style doctors flourish alongside Western-style doctors and are sought out by the same population. In a preliminary effort to discover whether there are different attitudes toward Western- or Chinese-style medicine among different segments of the population, I administered a questionnaire to 68 people in a village near Sanhsia [4]. Respondents represented segments of the population differentiated by sex, education and stage of life cycle as indicated in Table 1.

TABLE 1. INCLINATION TOWARD CHINESE OR WESTERN MEDICINE ACCORDING TO SEX, EDUCATION, AND STAGE OF THE LIFE CYCLE**

Approximate ages	Stage of life cycle	Education	Female	N	Male	N
<20	not yet married	≤ middle school *	0	5	—0.2	5
		> middle school	—2	6	—1	5
20–40	married; living with parents or parents-in-law	≤ elementary school	+0.8	6	+0.7	3
		> elementary school	+2	7	—0.75	4
40–60	married; living in independent household or parents deceased	≤ elementary school	+1.8	11	+2	10
		> elementary school	—0.3	3	0	3

* Middle school (grades 7-9) has been mandatory since 1969.

**Positive scores indicate inclination toward Chinese-style medicine; negative scores indicate inclination toward Western-style medicine.

The questionnaire was composed of 12 statements with which respondents were asked to agree or disagree, 6 indicating inclination toward Western-style medicine and doctors and 6 indicating inclination toward Chinese-style medicine and doctors. Examples of the former are: "Western medicine can completely cure almost all common illnesses such as colds, coughs, diarrhea"; "The Western-style doctor's stethoscope and examination are more accurate means of determining what is wrong than the Chinese doctor feeling the pulse." Examples of the latter are: "Western medicines are chemicals and hence harmful to the body"; "Shots make you feel better for only a little while." [5]

The questionnaire was then scored to give an estimate of each individual's adherence to one medical system or the other. Someone who agreed with all six statements favoring Chinese-style medicine and disagreed with all six statements favoring Western-style medicine would have a score of $+6$, indicating the strongest inclination to Chinese-style medicine; someone who agreed with all statements favoring Western-style medicine and disagreed with the rest would have a score of -6, indicating the strongest inclination to Western-style medicine. A score of 0 meant the person agreed with an equal number of pro-Chinese style and pro-Western-style statements; a score of $+2$ or -2 meant the person agreed with two more pro-Chinese style $(+2)$ or pro-Western style (-2) statements than statements favoring the other form of medicine. Averages of these scores for the 12 population segments are set out in Table 1.

Although this kind of measure (used of necessity during this short-term pilot project) is an extremely imperfect instrument with which to summarize people's attitudes about illness and curing, it does divulge several clear trends:

(1) There is considerable variation among the population, some segments inclined toward Chinese-style medicine, others toward Western-style medicine.

(2) On the whole, women, older people and less well educated people tend to be more inclined toward Chinese-style medicine.[6]

The question that arises at this point is this: Given that both Chinese-style and Western-style doctors are readily available, could it be that those segments of the population who indicate on this questionnaire that they are inclined toward one style of medicine actually make more use of doctors practicing that style of medicine? This question is particularly crucial because those people most responsible for the health of their families—married women—are also those most inclined toward Chinese-style medicine. Unfortunately, no study of differences in the use of different kinds of doctors is yet available. I can only offer evidence of another kind from a question asked of the same people represented in Table 1. They were asked what kind of professional help they thought they would seek for a variety of different kinds of ailments, from a skin rash to severe stomach pain. Despite the variation in attitudes disclosed in Table 1, practically the entire sample indicated they would make greater use of Western-style practitioners. Of course, this fact cannot be taken as evidence that most everyone actually makes more use of Western-style doctors; it is only an indication that the use of Western-style doctors is not insignificant even among those whose attitudes as described in Table 1 incline them toward Chinese-style medicine.

We have then a situation in which three conditions uneasily coexist:

(1) Many people, especially women and those in older age groups, say in one context that they find Chinese-style doctors and medicine more satisfactory than Western-style doctors and medicine (Table 1).

(2) Chinese-style doctors provide more support for laymen's notions about disease than Western-style doctors.

(3) People generally, including those strongly pro-Chinese medicine in Table 1, at least sometimes make use of Western-style doctors.

The uneasiness in this is that those who are avowedly more sympathetic to Chinese-style doctors and medicine in Table 1 (perhaps partly because they provide support for laymen's ideas about disease) are willing to confront Western-style doctors despite the difficulty in communication that we have seen exists. Similar problems in communication probably also exist—though perhaps to a lesser extent—for those in Table 1 whose inclinations are more toward Western-style medicine. Even though people may say Western-style medicine *works* better, when they talk about disease they still utilize the traditional notions so much a part of Chinese medicine.

There is little evidence that ideas about germs causing disease or antiseptics killing germs have gained general acceptance among any portion of the population—ideas that might make it easier for Western-style doctors to communicate with their patients.[7]

In this part of Taiwan, for the moment at least, a population of laymen with certain ideas about what disease is, confront one set of experts (Chinese-style doctors) with roughly similar ideas and another set of experts (Western-style doctors) with substantially different ideas.

III

One need not assume, of course, that anything will happen to bring the elements of this situation into closer fit. It may be that ideas compatible with Western-style doctors' understanding of illness will become part of ordinary people's understanding of illness, or it may not. I know of no way to make a prediction. It is interesting nonetheless to consider the opinions of the people in this situation about whether or not things are likely to change. All nine doctors (seven Western-style, two Chinese-style) interviewed thought that no change was likely in the next decade. They predicted that an uneven balance between the two forms of medicine would persist, with virtually all state funding for schools and research going toward Western-style medicine while Chinese-style doctors depend on private training. Asked what changes they thought would be desirable, all but two of the doctors said that *more* Chinese-style doctors were urgently needed, provided they were adequately trained. On the other hand, most villagers I asked about future trends said that Chinese-style medicine would surely die out in the next generation because its doctors will only pass on their knowledge to young apprentices, and young people are no longer interested in this profession.

Taken together, these responses seem to indicate that there are two possible directions for future development. Chinese-style medicine can be kept as a second-class partner to Western-style medicine in which case educated youth may be attracted to Western-style medicine. If the villagers are right, one consequence may be that Chinese-style medicine will "die," if not completely, then insofar as its development will be far inferior to that of Western-style medicine. Or, as the doctors recommend, a way could be found to increase the numbers of Chinese-style doctors and train them systematically, thus guaranteeing preservation of at least one set of medical experts who speak the same language as their patients.

The subject is too large to be pursued here, but it is interesting that the second alternative is precisely the route taken by the government of the People's Republic of China as of the mid-1950's, by providing state support for both forms of medicine (Croizier 1968:157-209). One reason for this, in addition to the many practical and political ones, may have been that this was one more way of assuring a link between those who are trained to administer medical services and those whom they serve. One need only assume that the pattern described here for Taiwan existed on the mainland before 1949—such that patients' understanding of disease was closer to Chinese-style doctors' than to Western-style doctors'; the link in question would be a closer conceptual fit between popular and expert ideas about the causes and mechanisms of disease.

NOTES

1. Taiwanese words are spelled according to the system outlined in Nicholas C. Bodman's *Spoken Amoy Hokkien* (1955). They are italicized, and marked for tone on first occurrence only. Mandarin is used for place names and for words that commonly appear in their Mandarin forms.

2. See Katherine Martin's chapter in this volume (Chapter 9) for a discussion of some of the social differences between the two kinds of doctors.

3. I would like to express my deep appreciation for the cooperation of the nine doctors, who shall remain anonymous, and the labors of my two assistants, Liu Hsiou-yüan and Chou Pi-se.

4. There was no attempt made to choose a random sample of respondents. The questionnaire was simply administered during the course of other interviewing as people were willing to fill it out. Consequently these results cannot be taken as representative of the population.

5. An English version of the complete questionnaire is as follows. Agreement with statements (1), (2), (7), (8), (10) and (11) indicates inclination toward Chinese-style medicine; agreement with statements (3), (4), (5), (6), (9) and (12) indicates inclination toward Western-style medicine.

   (1) If a young person doesn't take tonic medicine [a "hot," strengthening potion] at puberty, he won't grow up properly.

   (2) Only Chinese-style medicine can really cure the root cause of illness.

   (3) The substances used in Western-style medicines are the same as those found in herbal medicine, only more refined. One might as well take Western-style medicine.

   (4) Western-style medicine can completely cure almost all common illnesses such as colds, coughs, diarrhea.

   (5) Nowadays we don't need Chinese-style medicine anymore.

   (6) The Western-style doctor says we must operate for appendicitis to save a boy's life but the Chinese-style doctor says it's not necessary to operate because herbal medicine will heal him slowly but surely. In this situation we should definitely operate.

   (7) There are some illnesses such as *phà:kia:tiôuq* [literally "fright"; a childhood malady] that no Western-medicine can cure.

   (8) The best cure for *tiôuq–káu* [literally "hit by a monkey"; a childhood malady] is to banish the monkey by burning chicken feathers and feces.

   (9) Measles vaccine is effective and good for children. Therefore, every child should have it.

(10) Shots make you feel better for only a little while.

(11) Western-style medicines are chemicals and hence harmful to the body.

(12) The Western-style doctor's stethoscope and examination are more accurate means of determining what is wrong than the Chinese-style doctor feeling the pulse.

6. The one figure that contradicts the statement that more educated people are more inclined to Western medicine is the score of $+2$ for married women living with their parents or parents-in-law who have more than an elementary school education. This may be a result of influence from the mothers-in-law who are living under the same roof. For one thing, much readily available advice about illness comes from a woman's mother-in-law. For another, the more a young woman cooperates with her mother-in-law the smoother her relationship with the rest of the family will be.

7. This is a subject that needs further study, especially because elementary and middle-school texts on health and hygiene make use of ideas about germs in their discussions of disease.

REFERENCES

AHERN, E. M.
   1973   The Cult of the Dead in a Chinese Village. Stanford: Stanford University Press.

BODMAN, N. C.
   1955   Spoken Amoy Hokkien. Kuala Lumpur: Charles Grenier and Son, Ltd.

CROIZIER, R. C.
   1968   Traditional Medicine in Modern China. Cambridge: Harvard University Press.

CHAPTER 6

CHINESE AND WESTERN MEDICINE IN HONGKONG: SOME SOCIAL AND CULTURAL DETERMINANTS OF VARIATION, INTERACTION AND CHANGE

MARJORIE TOPLEY

Hongkong is a British Crown Colony lying just inside the tropics, to the South-east of China adjoining the province of Kwangtung. Its 400 square miles includes the island of "Hongkong," and the peninsular, Kowloon, ceded to Great Britain in 1841 and 1860 respectively; and the New Territories, a settled rural area, added by a 99-year lease in 1898.

Both traditional and modern, or "Chinese" and "Western" medicine, as they are commonly called, are officially recognized; they have always been officially regarded and administered as separate systems. Since the end of the Japanese Occupation however, although they continue to be clearly distinguished by legal and other officially sanctioned rules, changes have taken place. Western and Chinese therapy or drugs are combined; new categories of "Western" and "Chinese" practitioners have emerged, and they interact with each other. Many new practices and practitioners are illegal, but the innovations, legal and otherwise, add to the range of choice people exercise in seeking out and providing health care.

Anthropologists studying traditional medicine and assessing its role in health care, often focus on a particular set of beliefs and practices. But it is also important in modernizing societies, particularly when governed by a people culturally different from the majority, to understand the whole context within which traditional institutions operate—how far traditional, and traditional and modern, institutions, compete, complement, or interact with one another; what their official statuses are; and how different people use and evaluate the alternative services. Hongkong is a modernizing industrial society where 98 percent of the population is Chinese, and the government consists of British expatriates and Westernized Chinese. It may be some time before we have detailed data on all its medical institutions; study of popular beliefs and practices is just beginning. Nevertheless it is possible to present a general picture on the basis of existing information, and in this essay I examine what I know of the medical system; the changes that have taken place, some major reasons for these changes, and their importance for the people. My material for analysis is derived from documentary and field research.[1]

I use the term "system," which is a natural science metaphor commonly used by social scientists in the analysis of social and cultural behavior. Here I take it to mean a set or assembly of phenomena connected,

111

associated, or interdependent so as to form a complex unity (Onions 1955). Systems are governed by norms—rules and laws. They are the statics of the system, setting a precedent and representing the principle of continuity. But as the anthropologist Raymond Firth points out, the observer is faced with the problem of accounting not only for continuity but also change (Firth 1951: 35–40). Firth locates the principle of change in the dynamics of the system—the variety of ways relationships are ordered and events put together and which depend upon decisions and choice. "Structure" and "organization" are terms often used synonymously to describe the continuous aspect of a system; but Firth used "structure" for norms, reserving "organization" for this dynamic activity. He points out that while structural forms limit the range of alternatives possible, it is the possibility of alternatives that makes for variability.

I have adapted this conceptual framework for my analysis. Firth uses it for the analysis of social behavior; but decisions and choices are cognitive events. People may be influenced in their decisions and choices by their perceptions of conditions outside the system, but they are also influenced by their conceptions and evaluations of the system itself. One might also talk of a cognitive system, and of cognitive structure and organization: the norms people use in classifying and ordering concepts, and the ideas they are able to form on the basis of these norms—the variations possible. I will look at some of these norms and variations in order to understand some aspects of social change and the importance of this change.

I begin my analysis by examining the official social structures devised for Chinese and Western medicine. Described in outline are the forms of social organization we find, pointing up the divergence between intended and actual. In the rest of the essay I will examine the main social and cultural factors which appear to have determined this divergence, and its significance for the people.

Social Structure and Organization of Medicine in Hongkong

Statutory provisions are made in the Medical Registration Ordinance for anybody of "Chinese race" to practice traditional medicine professionally, i.e. for gain (Hongkong Government 1966a:15). No qualifications or registration are necessary. Although traditional practitioners' associations exist, none has ever been given the legal right to define standards or scales of efficiency, or to discipline members of the profession. Chinese medicine is not defined in law; it is any technique or belief that is "customary."

Variations in Chinese medicine have always existed on the basis of the subcultural differences of dialect groups. Over 75 percent of Hongkong's Chinese originate from parts of Kwangtung where Cantonese is spoken; and some 90 percent (including the children of non-Cantonese speakers) at the census returned Cantonese as their usual language (Census and Statistics Department 1972: 9–17). Traditional practitioners' associations, to which most of the physicians belong, list places of origin of their members. From them it would appear that Cantonese forms of medicine predominate.

Administratively, Chinese medicine comes under the Secretariat for Home (formerly "Chinese") Affairs which deals with problems in the interpretation and protection of custom. Chinese traditional practitioners may be prosecuted for infringement of laws forbidding them the right to certain practices. Some medical customs, for example, are regarded as dangerous. Thus no traditional practitioner may treat eye diseases, although traditional treatments exist for such diseases (Hongkong Government 1966a:15), and no such practitioner may use opium—which is a traditional medicament (Hongkong Government 1968a:14f.). All other medicaments in the Chinese pharmacopoeia are allowed.

No traditional practitioner may call himself "doctor" *(i-shaang)* [2]; this privilege is restricted to qualified, registrable Western-trained physicians. He may call himself *chung-i* in Chinese, which means "Chinese doctor," but in its English translation, or the translation of any other Chinese term he uses, he must include the term "herbalist." This is not to distinguish his speciality but to ensure that no member of the public is induced to believe he is a "Chinese person trained in Western medicine" (Hongkong Government 1966a:15). All traditional practitioners are thus "herbalists."

No herbalist may do anything restricted as a privilege to qualified registrable Western-trained doctors or auxiliaries. Thus he may not issue birth, death, or international inoculation certificates; use drugs on the Part I list of the Pharmacy and Poisons Ordinance (Hongkong Government 1969a:19); use antibiotics (Hongkong Government 1966b) or other medicines which, like opium, are on the Part I list of the Dangerous Drugs Ordinance (Hongkong Government 1968a:14f.). He may not perform Western-type surgery or use X-ray equipment. And an herbalist may not do anything forbidden to a legally recognized Western-trained doctor. Thus he may not advertise to the public (Hongkong Government 1968b:1f.), or perform abortions, which evidence suggests was a traditional activity.

Herbalists are not required to report infectious diseases. Although the government permits Chinese medicine, it has always believed that ". . . traditional beliefs . . . as to the cause of diseases, the means of spread and factors affecting its course are so at variance with modern teaching that there is little chance of promoting voluntary cooperation . . . in . . . prevention and control . . ." (Directory of Medicine 1928:6).

The government protects Chinese medicine, but promotes Western medicine. It is concerned with its own medical services' development, organized through a Department of Medicine and Health, and the provision of doctors in the private sector. Thus it subsidizes medical education at the colony's only medical school in the University of Hongkong. Because of increased medical costs due to advances in diagnoses and cure, and because Hongkong's industrial economy is vulnerable to foreign markets—depending on them for raw materials and sale of manufactured goods—it was considered unrealistic, in the post-World War II period, to plan services to standards equivalent to those of developed countries (Hongkong Government 1964:9ff.). Estimates of requirements for doctors have been based on arbitrary ratios of 1:3000; 1:2500; or 1:2000, implying the colony lies between developed and undeveloped countries (Committee Appointed to Review the Doctor Problem 1969:56f.). The government gives high priority in its own services to health education and preventive measures, seeking to meet the "most urgent needs" in therapy and directing low-cost services at the poor (Medical Plan Standing Committee 1970:1).

The government thus has an important stake in Western medicine, but it recognizes the right of the profession to set its own standards and measure efficiency against scales it devises itself. This right is exercised by a Medical Council of which the Director of Medicine and Health, himself a doctor, is *ex officio* chairman (Hongkong Government 1966a:4f.). The Council registers Western-trained doctors for private practice, issuing them with a code of practice. Qualifications for registration are those accepted by the General Medical Council of Great Britain and obtained from schools in the United Kingdom and parts of the Commonwealth, including Hongkong, where instruction is in English.

All registered doctors must be experienced, and new graduates of Hongkong's medical faculty work as interns for 12 months in government hospitals and clinics, being provisionally-registered while gaining this experience (Hongkong Government 1953). Some persons are exempted from registration and are legally entitled to call themselves "Western doctor" (*sai-i*) along with the registered. They work on ships, in the British Forces, for foreign governments, in university teaching and government service (Hongkong Government 1966:14). Exempted doctors in government are unregistrable, and unregistrable doctors may not practice privately. The two major professional associations, the local British Medical Association (B.M.A.) and the Hongkong Medical Association (H.K.M.A.) (formerly Hongkong Chinese Medical Association (H.K.C.M.A.)), do not accept unregisterable doctors for membership One other class of unregistrable practitioners is legally recognized but may not take the title "Western doctor," practice privately, or join the major associations—they work in charity clinics, themselves exempted from registration (Hongkong Government 1966b:6). Unlike the exempted and provisionally-registered doctors, they may not use dangerous drugs, or issue birth, death and international inoculation certificates (Hongkong Government 1963). Whereas the Medical Council disciplines private doctors, those in government services or the charity clinics are usually disciplined by the government itself.

Registered private doctors have the right to dispense medicines (Hongkong Government 1969a). This is not favored by the Pharmaceutical Society but considered necessary because there is no local training for registrable pharmacy qualifications, and a shortage of trained personnel (H.K.R.S. No. 49 D&S 1/15). While the Registration Ordinance states who may practice Chinese medicine (anyone of "Chinese race") it does not state who may not. To clarify the situation and because of growing interest among Western-trained doctors as a result of developments in China, the Medical Council issued a letter to the two major associations advising them that acupuncture therapy might be practiced by doctors of any ethnic affinity on their own responsibility. It did not advise acupuncture anesthesia, considering it "still in the experimental stages" (Chairman, Medical Council 1973).

For a population of about 4 million in 1971 there were 2,585 officially recognized Western-trained medical practitioners in Hongkong. There were 2,041 registered doctors (although some with names on the register may have retired); 116 provisionally registered; 108 unregistrable and in government service; and 320 practitioners in exempted charity clinics (personal communication, Director of Medicine and Health Services). There were some 20 medical associations based on common specialities, ethnic identities or religious affiliations. Most belonged to a federation of societies formed by the two major associations to represent mutual interests. There were also two associations for Chinese working as recognized unregistrable doctors. At the end of 1972 the B.M.A. had 500 members, mostly non-Chinese, and the H.K.M.A. 1087 members, 90 percent of whom were Chinese.

Very few private doctors, and no government doctors so far, practice acupuncture. Those who do train with local acupuncturists, preferably those trained in both Western and Chinese medicine who came to Hongkong as refugees in 1972 and 1973 and cannot return to their Southeast Asian countries of birth (South China Morning Post, November 11, 1972). There were estimated to be some 200 in 1972, and they cannot be registered as Western doctors (China Mail, May 29, 1973). Apart from this training there is little contact between recognized Western-trained doctors and practitioners of traditional medicine on the professional level, and they do not refer patients to one another (see Lee, Chapter 15 of this book). More than two-thirds of the registrable doctors were in private practice in 1974, and 100 vacancies existed in government hospitals and clinics. It is estimated that about 30 percent of the newly-qualifying doctors emigrate (Hongkong Standard, April 14, 1974). Most doctors dispense their own medicines and insist patients use them. They often require payment of additional consultation fees when prescriptions are refilled.

In addition to the number of recognized doctors listed, the police estimated there to be more than one thousand unqualified and unregistered people illegally practicing Western medicine exclusively in 1974. They said that these people freely dispense controlled medicines and poisonous drugs, and conduct surgical operations in their homes. Most of their clinics are well advertised by signboards and in the Chinese Press, and many specialize in gynecology, abortion, and plastic surgery (The Star, April 4, 1974). Some "black-market doctors," as they are known, include recent refugees, qualified and trained in Western and

Chinese medicine but preferring to practice the former. Some have older qualifications and some no qualifications at all.

It would appear from a signboard count by the H.K.C.M.A. that in 1969 there were some 4,000 herbalists practicing Chinese medicine. In fact there were probably more. Not all traditional therapists announce themselves on signboards—some own or work in pharmacies, in temples, and traditional charity organizations. Since 1973 they have been joined by some of the refugee doctors who usually practice acupuncture (*South China Morning Post,* November 19, 1973).

One finds in Hongkong a variety of practices falling within the legal framework of Chinese customary medicine. There are spirit-healers, secular healers, those performing both types of healing; and there are people curing by secular means but diagnosing according to non-secular beliefs and vice versa. Traditional practitioners are commonly listed in association handbooks according to their therapeutic speciality or the particular diseases they treat. Thus there are, besides acupuncturists, "general" therapists using medicines derived from herbal, animal, and mineral compounds, and there are bone-setters. There are physicians specializing in the diseases of the sexes, and in pediatrics and gerontology. They include, although it is not mentioned in the handbooks, those using non-secular ideas and ritual cures. Some of the physicians are highly qualified, and although their qualifications are not legally recognized, they have degrees from Chinese universities and diplomas from schools of traditional medicine in China and Taiwan. Some have qualifications from locally run schools. Others—some authorities believe the majority —have no qualifications or training at all, although their practices are equally legal.

One also finds that despite restrictions placed on the traditional practitioner, many "herbalists" combine Chinese medicaments with antibiotics and other forbidden drugs, although usually diagnosing according to Chinese methods. There are bone-setters performing plastic surgery and using X-ray equipment, and "general" therapists performing abortions by both traditional and modern methods. Like illegal Western practitioners they charge their patients and get paid; and they advertise in the Chinese press.

All these practitioners—illegal Western doctors, qualified and unqualified practitioners of Chinese medicine, and traditional practitioners combining Western and Chinese therapy (and who may also use ritual remedies)—align themselves together through membership in a network of associations. Illegal Western doctors who, to add to the complexity, also call themselves "herbalists," associate with their fellows in some associations, but in others they associate with traditional physicians combining medicines; qualified and unqualified traditional practitioners associate together despite the formers' occasional public attack on the latter (*South China Morning Post,* October 8, 1973; October 2, 1973; October 8, 1973). Secular and non-secular practitioners sometimes associate together; those combining medicines associate with strictly traditional practitioners (who are rare), and many of their associations are federated together.

So there is a recognizable system of official Western medicine in which physicians organize activities and form alignments in ways permitted by the official structural norms. Recognized Western doctors practicing acupuncture do not form a new category for they act "on their own responsibility" which means they are judged by the standards and scales of the Western profession. But there is no clearly recognizable system of Chinese medicine. Rather, there is a new system in which Western and Chinese activities combine—and new alignments are formed among a number of legal, illegal, qualified, and unqualified categories.

Several contributory factors have been suggested for this situation by government and community bodies—heavy demand for medical services; lack of a "realistic" policy in Western medicine; government indifference to controls over Chinese medicine; lack of integrity and the influence of economic factors tempting traditional practitioners to use Western therapy; the need for new alignments for mutual aid in the face of bureaucratic procedures, "protection" rackets, and legal restrictions; and public "ignorance, superstition and apathy" in participating in this unofficial system (*South China Morning Post,* January 27, 1972). I want to examine these social and cultural factors in terms of my conceptual framework.

Demand For Medical Services

The emergence of illegal practitioners and the continued existence of traditional doctors, including those with no qualifications, are often linked with heavy demand for medical services. This demand is usually explained in demographic terms, so I will consider demography first.

The population first began to expand as those leaving at the fall of the colony began to return. But around 1949 Hongkong experienced the largest influx of people in its history. There was another significant influx in 1962 (Hongkong Government Annual Reports 1949–1963); and the influx of 1972–73, bringing in refugee doctors, also brought in many young people, and disabled and elderly persons.

Before the Occupation people were relatively mobile; many returned to China when seriously ill or when epidemics occurred. The age and sex pattern was that of a typical immigrant community, strongly influenced by young single men. In contrast, the age and sex pattern in 1971 was that of a settled population. Few newcomers left, and more than 50 percent of the population were returned at the last census as born in the colony (Census and Statistics Department 1972:9–17).

Hongkong does not have particularly bad health. There have been consistently falling levels in the overall death rate, in infant and maternal mortality, and the incidence of infectious diseases (Maclehose 1973:6). But the climate, geography, distribution of income groups, and population densities, make it vulnerable to epidemics and diseases associated with crowding and poverty, especially tuberculosis, which is a major problem.

And changing, Westernizing, life-styles, make it vulnerable to hypertension, cerebrovascular lesions and other "modern" diseases.

Some people have become rich as a result of post-war industrialization, but many are relatively poor. The 1971 census indicated that 42.5 percent of all households earned under 600 Hongkong dollars (approximately US$98) (Hongkong Government 1971:2). In 1972 densities were high; in one part of Kowloon there were over 160,340 persons per square kilometer. More than 180,000 households shared accommodation with others at the end of 1971, and 275,000 persons were estimated to live in squatter structures. Large redistributions in population have taken place. Today 90 percent—not only people from China but also from the rural New Territories—are concentrated in urban areas (Census and Statistics Department 1972:11ff.). The New Territories area, much of which is mountainous and cannot be developed, occupies about 90 percent of the total land, and little space is available for further urban expansion. Because of high rents in the private sector and the need to clear older buildings for improvements, vast "resettlement" and low-cost housing estates, some virtually townships, have been built, and the government has become landlord to nearly 43 percent of the population. It does not follow that only the poor live as squatters or in resettlement and low-cost housing. Chinese in Hongkong tend to allocate less resources to superior housing as their incomes improve than do people in modern Western societies (Topley 1969:195f.), but certainly few wealthy persons are found in some residential areas and few poor in others.

In 1971, 74.55 percent of those over the age of 10, and whose usual language was not English, were unable to speak any English at all (Census and Statistics Department 1972:72). Many people demanding medical services must do so through speakers of their own language. Women, moreover, tend to make major decisions about family health, and many are without any education. In 1971, of the 42 percent people aged 5 and over with no schooling, 30.5 percent were women (Census and Statistics Department 1972:63). Probably the majority of people without English, and without education, have ideas about constitutional disorder and the values of health care having their roots in traditional theories of health and morality. It does not follow however that those *with* education, who speak English, and who are men, do not have such ideas as well. But they tend to have a more secular approach, going to spiritual beliefs when secular therapy fails. I do not examine here the attitudes towards medical services these ideas and values engendered; this is taken up later. But I must write something about the ideas themselves because they tend to encourage heavy uses of medical services.

Concern for the health of the family is seen as a prime duty of mothers and filial sons, although just as mothers care for the health of their children, daughters-in-law usually care for the health of their husband's parents, even if they live separately as is common in modernizing Hongkong. In a 1969 child-rearing study conducted with 20 non-English speaking, illiterate and semiliterate mothers,[1] I found informants tended to use the evidence of money and time spent on children's health as a sign of their love and affection. But they spent much time and money because they held certain ideas of ill-health.

It is widely believed that the old and the young, and certain other classes of people, have constitutions particularly prone to minor illnesses and that these are not self-limiting—they must be cured to prevent serious disease. Some informants, comparing the attitudes of Western and Chinese mothers, remarked that the former, who do not take children to doctors for minor symptoms like cough or cold, showed a disregard both for their duties and their children's health. There is a further belief that the serious diseases which may follow are caused by additional external agents.

Man as an individual—and I distinguish individual from "social person" for reasons we will see—is conceptualized as a psycho-physical entity. The constitution is *huèt-heì*: "blood and ether." These flow continuously between various vital organs of the body. Some additionally believe the flow to be regulated by "five elements" *(nğ-hōng)* and/or two souls, which, in the life of the individual, interact with the five elements—which in turn interact with one another—to control balance. The constitution may be imbalanced because of natural conditions, and this manifests itself in humors: "hot air" *(ît-heì)*, "cold" *(leŭng)*—also associated with "emptiness"—"dryness" *(ts'ò)*, "wetness" *(shap)*, "fire" *(fóh)*, and "wind" *(fung)*. Many believe that the young are not yet emotionally or physically stabilized. They are prone to "hot air" and "dryness," and physical symptoms like fever, rashes, coughs and colds (in the Western sense of "colds"). They also are prone to emotional disturbance indicating "wetness" manifest in "chestiness," insomnia. trembling and crying. Old people have weakened constitutions. They are subject to "cold," "wetness" and "wind," and "not enough blood" *(m̄-kaù huet)*, with physical symptoms such as dizziness, rheumatism, and general weakness; and emotional symptoms such as "strange talk." Menstruating women are prone to "cold" and "not enough blood." People with certain horoscopes, which indicate the constitutional pattern, may also be inclined to some particular imbalance. Those over-indulgent in food and drink are prone to "hot air," while those over-indulgent in sex are "cold" with "not nough blood." Those emotionally over-indulgent are prone to imbalances relating to different emotions, for example fear and grief are "wet" and "cold"; anger is "fire" and happiness "hot."

Prevention of imbalance symptoms is brought about by living a regular life, and for children, a quiet environment; and by taking regular brews appropriate to the constitution—for example, "purifying-cool" teas *(ts'ing-leūng)* for "hot" constitutions and tonics to build the blood *(pó-huèt)*, or strengthen the ether *(pó-heì)*. Many people, irrespective of their backgrounds, know of these remedies and use them regularly. If symptoms do arise the more traditional person will usually treat them himself; this was common custom. But in Hongkong they may use traditional or modern medicines—including antibiotics for fevers (bought from illegal pharmacists), and Western as well as Chinese tranquilizers. Others visit therapists and expect some sort of treatment (not merely to be told to go home and rest).

Various external agents may exacerbate the situation in those suffering humoral conditions. These are imbalanced phenomena: foods—which are also "hot," "cold" and so forth—malevolent spirits (*kwaí; ιu-kwaaì; ts'ē-shān*); miasmata (*ts'ē-neì; ts'ē-fung*); and weather conditions, literally hot, cold, damp or humid, and windy. If the agent has an imbalance similar to that of the sufferer, an imbalanced disease will result—"hot" "cold," etc. If it has the opposite imbalance however, there is a sort of catalytic effect: "blood" and "ether" rush together to form "poison" (*tûk*)—for example, pus or phlegm. Many incurable diseases or very serious diseases are "poisonous"—cancer, leprosy, and tuberculosis. Sex with an "imbalanced" person gives a disease; for example, an elderly man having intercourse with a young woman may become very ill; as may a man having sex with a woman in the puerperal period when she is regarded as polluted.

Disease may also be "caught" from particular social categories of people. If the horoscope is at odds, for example, with a yearly cycle (detectable by a diviner) a person must avoid brides (socially "hot") and mourners (socially "cold"). Immoral persons weaken their constitutions and are prone to "infection" from agitated spirits, for example an ancestor whose worship has been neglected.

Thus a person may be predisposed to disease by his constitution and get minor symptoms. He may then get a serious disease through the action of external agents. Western-trained doctors (especially those who are Westerners) often say the Chinese are hypochondriacs. Certainly, people may be very anxious about disease if they see themselves as in a state engendering imbalance; or if they think they might have been in contact with some external disease-causing agent. And for similar reasons they may worry about their children or parents; they may frequently visit health specialists.

Western Medical Policy

Those talking of an "unrealistic" policy in Western medicine commonly complain of two things; one is the permissiveness of the structure, the other its restrictiveness—and they blame the government for not exercising more control over the profession which largely determines this structure.

By permissiveness they mean lack of control over where registered doctors may work, and how much they may charge. Complaints about the cost of private medicine are common in Hongkong (*South China Morning Post,* December 26, 1971; November 1, 1972).

Doctors tend to cluster in the central areas more accessible to the rich; and they charge what the market will bear. Private practice has been condemned by a group of concerned medical students. In their official publication *Caduceus* one student claimed that "building one's fortune on the physical mishaps of others permits greater scope of malpractice . . " (Ng 1973:1f.). It was claimed there should be fixed scales of charges and compulsory refresher courses on new medical developments. Some Western-trained and recognized doctors also complain of actual malpractice and insufficient vigilance on the part of the Medical Council, which spends most of its time on the more easily detected advertising offenses. In malpractice these doctors include wrong diagnosis, abortion, and conspiring with pharmacists to provide forbidden drugs to illegal practitioners, (signing the poisons book for more than they require—for a financial consideration). They complain that "Western ethics" are not learned along with Western "science" (one wonders if they always are in the West), and that such behavior makes it difficult for the public to distinguish the legal from the illegal doctor.

One prominent Western-trained registered doctor, who is Chinese, claims there is not really a shortage of doctors, only bad distribution between private and public sectors (*Hongkong Standard* (Sunday ed.) October 21, 1973). Public service salaries cannot compete with private practice (Committee Appointed to Review the Doctor Problem 1969:16). A British Medical Association spokesman, responding to the *Caduceus* articles, said a ban on private practice would lead to "wholesale migration of doctors . . ." (*China Mail,* October 9, 1973). The government finds it difficult not only to get recruits, but to keep them. Nevertheless, the Director of Medical and Health Services defended doctors leaving government to work in private practice as "benefiting the community" (*South China Morning Post,* November 30, 1973). The government's own registrable doctors are disinclined to work in the poorer, more remote areas, and it is notable that it is there that its unregistrable recruits (who cannot go into private practice) are usually found. Besides the government's own unregistrable doctors, most of the "practitioners in charge" of exempted clinics are in the poorer areas, as are also the illegal Western doctors and unqualified traditional doctors, and those combining medicines. For example, a survey of Kwun Tong, a new industrial town, made in connection with building a United Christian Hospital, revealed that with a total population of almost half a million there were in 1970 only 53 registered doctors and 16 unregistrable recognized physicians. There also were some 230 unregistered doctors, of which about 31 manifestly were illegal Western practitioners, the rest describing themselves as some sort of "Chinese practitioner" (Sub-Committee of Task Force on Community Health, 1970).

A newspaper article stated that "A hungry man finds a bowl of rice but refuses to eat. He wants to plant own (sic) paddy field." The hungry man is the Medical and Health Department, "diseased" by a shortage of doctors; the "rice bowl" is the supply of unregistrable doctors from China it cannot use (*Hongkong Standard,* April 14, 1974). It cannot use them because it does not control registration.

After the Occupation, when the population began to expand, registrable doctors were in short supply. Numbers could not easily be made up by enlisting doctors from overseas, because necessary in Hongkong are doctors speaking Chinese. Qualifications from China and Taiwan do not render their holders registrable because either they are from unknown schools, or the schools teach in Chinese. The main criterion for recognition is that the school should be open to inspection by the General Medical Council in Great Britain, and this means that it should have right of access to the school, and that the school should teach in a language the council understands.

The year 1949 brought a large influx of people to Hongkong, but many persons entering claimed to be trained in Western medicine in China. In his annual report the Director of Medical Services (as he was then called) remarked that it was " . . . an ill wind that blows nobody any good." The government began to take on numbers of these physicians when they had evidence of qualifications, commenting that many were "leaders in their profession." They were accommodated within the "exempted" category. The two major professional associations viewed this policy with dismay, but recognized that the government could not have met its commitments without drawing on this "reserve."

To sort out problems of status, the government proposed amendments to the law; but at a meeting with the associations "many cogent arguments were brought forward why . . . (they) . . . should not be admitted to the Register." The associations proposed an alternative scheme for private doctors to help out in government clinics; but it was not successful. In 1958–60 the Society of Apothecaries—the oldest examining body in Britain—sent out examiners to help refugee doctors obtain registrable qualifications. But only graduates from 12 known Chinese medical schools, qualifying before 1953, were accepted. Although many claimed to be qualified doctors, only 177 sat the examinations and only 126 passed (Advisory Committee on Clinics 1966:40).

However, owing to a legal loophole many unregistrable doctors not in government service were beginning to practice in "charity" clinics. The law said they could not practice for gain, but that anyone could practice without gain. It was not said, for example, that such physicians could not receive a "donation"—a method of payment sanctioned by custom. During the 1950's charity clinics mushroomed, and since, as the Director of Medicine and Health stated in his annual report (1957:7), "hundreds of patients . . . (had) . . . literally to be turned away daily from Government outpatient clinics in the urban areas," there clearly was a need for this type of clinic.

In 1958 the government attempted to introduce a Roll of Licensed Medical Practitioners to control these doctors (Advisory Committee on Clinics 1966:41). A Board would hold examinations for admission and once completed the roll would be closed. The professional associations objected to the scheme although it was not proposed to admit the "licensees" to private practice; so did unregistrable practitioners, who had started their own associations.

For a short time the problem was shelved; but in 1962 a second influx of people exacerbated the situation. An investigation in 1964 showed that 60 percent of practitioners in charity clinics had been practicing for 2 years or less (Advisory Committee on Clinics 1966:41). The qualified profession demanded control, and an ordinance was enacted, coming into effect in 1964, which in essence required all clinics to apply for registration, and enabled the Director of Medical and Health Services to reject them if the clinic, or its services or practitioners, were unacceptable. Clinics already in existence might continue to employ unregistrable doctors if they passed an interview and could be classified as "exempted," but new ones had to employ registered doctors. The legal loop-hole was also closed.

Launching the new legislation was a delicate matter. Many physicians were interviewed and charities investigated. Eight-hundred-and-twelve persons claimed to be unregistrable qualified practitioners but only 482 were reckoned sufficiently competent to practice (Advisory Committee on Clinics 1966:6). Seven-hundred-and-eleven clinics applied for registration but only 387 were granted exemption and only 79 employing registered medical practitioners were fully registered (Advisory Committee on Clinics 1966:7f.). The interviewing panel claimed standards set were low: " . . . medical students, and . . . nurses and dressers, could quite easily have passed . . . " Many instances were claimed of candidates being "without any knowledge . . . of medicine . . . " and some had forged diplomas (Advisory Committee on Clinics 1966:6).

Several clinics were discovered to be run by pseudo "charities"—bodies claiming to be community or church organizations but having nothing to do with either. The practice was for physicians to pay for the use of the clinics' names and to give them a percentage of "donations." In fact the clinics were usually family businesses run by a man and his wife in their home. A few pseudo-charities ran large chains of clinics, some specializing in clinic-vans, unroadworthy but set-up permanently in resettlement estates to avoid high rents (Advisory Committee on Clinics 1966:8; also personal communication from government officials).

The Medical and Health Department had to convince the two associations of the need to retain some clinics, even if they were not up to standard; and the Secretariat for Chinese Affairs had to convince the public that some must be closed. The sponsoring bodies and unregistrable doctors' associations vehemently opposed the legislation, organizing protest meetings and press conferences in which they tried to involve trade unions, clan associations and other community institutions. They complained that in the prior 8 years nothing had been heard of "mistakes done to patients," nor were the clinics criticized by the public (*Wah Kiu Yat Po* (Chinese): January 22, 1964).

The legislation was not withdrawn, however. The Director's power of exemption was to end in 1966 and a Committee was set up to look into the workings of the ordinance. It showed that exempted clinics accounted for some 37 percent of all clinic attendances (Advisory Committee on Clinics 1966:27); but it also showed that some clinics did not come up to professional standards—they were short on space and privacy, and attendances were low. Some saw as few as 10 people a day and rarely as many as 40 (Advisory Committee on Clinics 1966:36), but a small clientele is traditional. Medical professionals often have additional jobs. The author's investigations of traditional physicians show that many have as few as five or six patients a day. This means that one has to be cautious in placing too much significance on numbers, but it also means that if some practitioners are eliminated, others in exempted clinics would not necessarily want to increase their scale of operations.

The law was tightened further. Exempted clinics were required to register annually, and new clinics were required to be managed by registered doctors only. Mobile clinics were outlawed; and a further recommendation was that unregistrable doctors be placed on a Roll, if they wished, after a compulsory examination (which also covered exempted unregistrable doctors in government). They would then have the status of Medical Assistant Practitioner (Advisory Committee on Clinics 1966:47–55). This was opposed by the two major professional associations and the two associations of unregistrable doctors. The former were against a "double register" for rich and poor; the latter claimed holding examinations of a high standard (that of medical students taking finals) would be discriminatory. They accused the committee of wanting to keep them in poorer areas—which undoubtedly was true. The recommendation was dropped and the unregistrable physician in a limited number of charity clinics remains to this day.

The government then attempted to meet the problems of shortages, in its own services and in private services aimed at the poor, by accommodating unregistrable doctors in the medical structure. The profession, judging these practitioners and their charity clinics according to standards and scales developed in the West, thwarted any attempt to allow a person or clinics not complying with them to practice and offer services privately. But it was not able to prevent the government from taking on some unregistrable practitioners itself, or force them to be examined by the profession.

After the clinics legislation, numbers of illegal Western practitioners began to appear. We saw that they call themselves "herbalists." One reason is that traditional doctors are relatively free from control—there is no regular system of inspection; there is a shortage of pharmacy inspectors; the Medical Council has no jurisdiction over them; they themselves are unlikely to inform the authorities of their "colleagues' " activities, particularly if they are combining medicine; and, as will be seen, they are "protected" by racketeers. This leads to the question of government "indifference" and traditional medicine.

Lack of Control Over Chinese Medicine

When Hongkong was founded the British announced to the population that they would not interfere with Chinese customs unless they were unjust or dangerous (Committee Appointed by the Governor 1948:96; 121). From time to time there has been debate as to what precisely this meant: whether customs should apply in some interim period, until full colonial government was established; or whether British law should be inapplicable to institutions that had their own customary rules. Essentially the latter explanation has been favored, and the general rule is to allow Chinese institutions to operate according to custom as long as that custom exists; but to introduce legislation when it is found no longer to apply.

One question sometimes besetting the authorities is precisely what customs should be followed: those of the Ch'ing Dynasty during which Hongkong was founded, or some possible modifications emerging in the changing and developing climate of the colony? This issue has not thus far been raised directly in respect of customary medicine, although certainly the view is taken that modern scientific medicine is *not* traditional custom. An additional question, however, concerns the possible dangers of customary practice.

The authorities appear reluctant to legislate against customs the Western profession may regard as dangerous—if they have a long history and are accepted by a majority. We saw that they *did* legislate (in the post-war period) against treatment of eye diseases and uses of opium— where there had been considerable evidence of dangers—but in fact the practices were forbidden to all *unregistrable,* non-exempted practitioners, of which traditional physicians were only one category. Indeed, in 1949 a committee set up to investigate infant mortality mentioned the "belief in aged and harmful customs . . . and Chinese medicine" as contributory factors. But it did not think it "advisable, at this stage, to speak directly of the errors of . . . belief . . . ", adding: ". . . we could achieve our aim by making known to the Chinese . . . the recent advances of Western medicine" (Director of Medicine 1949:76). Essentially the aim has been to entice people away from traditional medicine by education, including health education. Along with this is a reluctance to give publicity to Chinese medicine: by talking publicly about "errors" people might be induced to think there are "accuracies." It is this policy which is attacked as "indifferent."

Some argue that even if customary medicine itself remains officially undefined, those practicing should be qualified and/or registered. In 1970 one writer to the editor of a major local newspaper said ". . . there is no control board, it is not possible for the public to distinguish the true herbalists from the charlatans. It is a discredit to the herbalists to be grouped together with . . . (charlatans) . . ." (*South China Morning Post,* March 3, 1970). A leader in another paper states that "the astonishing lack of proper safeguards and controls . . . (is) . . . a serious flaw in the Colony's laws . . . any Chinese, trained or untrained, ethical or unethical . . . (can) . . . practice . . ." (*Hongkong Standard,* April 11, 1974). The local Reform Club argued, ". . . in officially recognizing herbalists, the authorities should . . . establish an official register of all . . . now practicing to give better control in future . . . new recruits . . . should undergo a recognized apprenticeship . . ." (*China Mail,* March 12, 1974).

But who will sit on the control board, who will recognize the apprenticeship? One official said to me: The first step is for the profession to separate the "sheep" from the "goats." The Western profession can do this because it has uniform standards and scales of measurement and monopolies over knowledge. How far is this so in the Chinese case?

It is generally agreed that ethical standards are important. A therapist must be virtuous before his therapy can work: as with the Greeks, virtue is power, but "virtue" itself is vaguely defined. Certainly it includes personal restraints—the therapist's character should be without taint; some say he should not demand payment—it is up to the patient to decide what he will "donate"—although standard payments are now more common in Hongkong. Others include a courteous and attentive manner and willingness to listen to the patient's description of his symptoms.

There is no agreement on qualifications because there is such a variety of theoretical approaches, and all, as we will see, may be considered equally valid. Ritual specialists say certain powers are needed, but are not necessary for the secular doctor. They usually are derived from a special fate determined by complex conditions and often revealed to the possessor in dreams along with specialist knowledge. However, it is not that people without such powers should not practice; it is simply that it would be dangerous for them to do so and their practice would be non-efficacious. Taoist priests practicing therapy also have qualifications, a hierarchy of ranks determines what they may do, and they have esoteric texts. But Taoist priests view ill-health as only one category of individual "imbalance"—the same conditions causing ill-health may cause other misfortunes (see p. 129). Thus both the qualifications and the texts relate to matters other than medicine. Qualifications for healing are necessary in China and Taiwan but apply only to secular medicine, and they rarely are exclusive requirements for membership of an "herbalist" association, as we will see. Qualifications are also obtained from local "schools" usually consisting of a master and his medical disciples. Some of their texts are exoteric, but attempts are made at exclusion by special interpretations within the school and by using additional texts based on the clinical experiences of the line of masters. This works against the development of a uniform body of knowledge in the profession, and because basic texts are exoteric they are open to all who can read and comprehend them. This would not prevent any literate person using them for practice, indeed if he is virtuous he would likely be successful.

Counter to the trend of exclusiveness is a trend towards inclusiveness —a virtue to make medical knowledge widely known. Some doctors publish glosses on difficult texts and books of prescriptions describing disease symptoms and etiology. Aimed at the masses, who also have an oral tradition, they give depth to the basis of practice of ordinary people treating their families, and to the basis of practice of unqualified persons who also share an oral tradition.

If scholarly and ordinary people can share knowledge, and the latter also have an oral tradition, one might suppose some common theoretical ground. But sinologists usually study scholarly texts, not popular "folk" ideas; and anthropologists usually study popular ideas, and not scholarly texts; and their respective writings have suggested more differences than similarities. A conceptual framework was developed for studying all folk and scholarly thinking as separate traditions. Scholarly ideas formed the "great tradition"—that of the reflective minority, consciously cultivated and handed down. Popular or "folk" ideas formed the "little tradition"—that of the majority who take it for granted, making no conscious effort to analyse or refine (Hui-chen Wang Liu 1959:95). Croizier (1970), influenced by this dichotomy, talks of a great tradition in medicine as a theoretically articulated body of ideas; and the little tradition as a generally empirical set of remedies. Although he warns against thinking of folk medicine as a grab bag, without any system, he says that the first requirement in sketching-in the main features of traditional medicine is "to distinguish traditional . . . medicine from the 'folk' . . ." Traditional medicine thus *is* the great tradition. Such a narrow definition would take us but a little way in understanding traditional medicine in Hongkong, and would tend to thwart our attempts to look for connections.

In fact, Croizier himself suggests that the great tradition may be *influenced* by cosmological ideas *shared* by folk medicine—cosmology here being used as one of the intermediaries of communication sought by the "great/little" adherents to explain why China did not fall apart culturally with such differing traditions (for further differences are supposed between secular and non-secular, equated with the "scholarly" and "folk" as we will see). The author's experience, however, suggests something more: scholarly and folk are *united* by a common cosmology providing them *both* with their concepts of medicine. The situation is very different from the West where a more-or-less broken tradition exists —folk medicine being based on Galenical ideas, and scholarly on modern scientific theory.

Outside the study of medicine, and in other aspects of Chinese thought, the great/little dichotomy is being abandoned as more evidence is unturned that scholarly and folk are transformations of each other. The writer's own work suggests a similar state of affairs for medicine. More precisely, that there is a series of transformations, a conceptual continuum rather than a dichotomy, and at the level of social reality a continuum of practitioners using similar categories but with different terms for root concepts; working with overt and covert root concepts; or exploring different categories in terms of an identical concept. A great number of accommodations appear possible. The author's studies are not yet at a stage at which a comprehensive account can be given but a few examples are here included.

All doctors and most people use the categories "hot," "cold," and suchlike, but scholarly physicians subsume them under the concepts *yang* (*yeūng*) and *yin* (*yam*)—the binary principles of polarization accounting for entire existence. Many ordinary people either do not know these terms, or how to use them in medicine. Some have no generic term at all for these humors, while other use a single term: *kwaaì* which means "extreme" (i.e. polarized state) or "strange." And the connotation "strangeness" allows further categories to be explored. Again, ordinary people use the concepts *shān* and *kwaì* to represent spiritual beings or human souls after death. Secular scholarly professionals use them to represent abstract principles of "spirituality," aspects of *yang* and *yin,* respectively. Physicians practicing both secular and non-secular medicine may use them in both senses at different times. Explanations of the efficacy of drugs may also involve transformations. Thus the rationale for avoiding chicken in diet while taking a medicine made from scorpions for cancer, a "poisonous" disease, is, according to one scholarly physician, that poisonous diseases are driven out by "poisonous" medicines (*i-tûk kung-tûk*) and scorpions are "poisonous." But chicken is a *yang* substance and *yang* phenomena neutralize poisons—the medicine would be ineffective. The popular explanation is that "as everybody knows" chickens and scorpions are antipathetic; chickens may frequently be observed attacking and killing scorpions. Chinese scholarly practitioners, popular practitioners and also ordinary patients use, then, variant forms of the same theoretical language. This is why they may communicate with each other. Why they should *associate* together is taken up below.

Secular and non-secular physicians are also able to communicate, and able to view each other's services as complementary. This does not accord with what we learn of the great and little traditions in medicine, for "great" is usually defined as secular and rational (Croizier 1970:4f.); "little" as non-rational, religious or magical. Both the Kuomintang and the PRC have made similar distinctions—scholarly secular medicine *is* Chinese medicine, and this is the common view of Western-trained doctors (although not necessarily all Westernized people) in Hongkong.

Governments in China have been guided by the existence of a self-conscious full-time practicing group of physicians who use only secular texts and would disassociate themselves from non-secular "folk" practices (Croizier 1968). And this in turn, at least partly, was because of a self-conscious effort by those doctors to have Chinese medicine seen as "modern" in the eyes of the world. But what about situations where such sentiments did not, or do not, exist? In the Ch'ing Dynasty, or modern Hongkong?

Certain assumptions implicit in the great/little dichotomy are that rational secular beliefs about sickness are incompatible with non-secular beliefs, and that since the latter are "folk," and folk as a social category are illiterate and semiliterate people, they cannot be believed by a scholar. But first, non-secular beliefs are not necessarily "folk"—some

Taoist priests are scholars using scholarly texts. And secondly, if we look at the theoretical structure—the cosmology within which the concepts and categories referred to developed—we see that secular and non-secular are compatible. There need be no competition between them because they relate to universes which are not only homologous—identical in structure, obeying the same laws—but also intersecting. To use Chinese concepts: the phenomena of "Heaven" (the universe of spiritual beings, invisible vapors, stars and plants); the phenomena of "Earth" (the universe of physical tangible things); and the phenomena of "Man" (the universe of social entities, individuals, part spirit, and part physical), all have similar properties of balance and propensities to imbalance and disturbance. And because the universes intersect, imbalance and disturbance in one may cause similar conditions in another. Thus it is possible to believe that an immoral or emotional man may not only weaken his own constitution, predisposing himself to disease, he may weaken the "constitutions" of other phenomena with which he shares Heaven or Earth characteristics. This may cause disturbances or imbalances in nature, or in the realm of the spirits; external agents arise to cause serious disease to all those who are predisposed. This is how ideas were organized in Hongkong to explain the bubonic plague epidemic of 1894 (Col. Surgeon 1896:55–58).

So, "religion," "chemistry," "geography" and so on, to use Western concepts, may be regarded as complementary disciplines. Different in kind but not order, they all contribute to the understanding of imbalanced conditions and their treatment. To the Taoist who engages in therapy, illness is just one type of imbalance or disturbance resulting from human and universal processes. It has to be treated, as does all misfortune, by rebalancing activities. Therapy may include ritual to rebalance the external agents, for example; charms to rebalance spiritual beings, and medicine and diet to deal with the constitution. Secular doctors focus on the individual's symptoms and internal state of balance, using therapy relating to "Earth"—medicine and diet, acupuncture and bone-setting. But they may not deny the value of the non-secular approach if the illness persists and the predisposing cause cannot be found. A few secular physicians trained in China may discount the value of priests and ritual specialists, but the author has interviewed some who started their careers with ritual healing, moving later to secular medicine because they felt they had no real calling for the former. There are also members of what one might term "paramedics" and "auxiliaries": persons who deal only with emotional disturbance; persons who deal only with socially caused diseases, for example breaking moral proscriptions; persons specializing in diagnosis from the horoscope; and geomancers diagnosing in terms of miasmata — environmental disturbance — and performing activities aimed at rebalancing the external features causing the patient's disease.

Thus a variety of persons concerned with therapy speak "the same language" and share the same knowledge. The Chinese profession does not fix its own standards, decide its own criteria for skills, or have a monopoly over knowledge in Hongkong; it also does not, in the majority of cases, regard with hostility the existing wide variety of practitioners. Whether one can call them all "professionals," of course, depends on one's definitions. Certainly many traditional therapists do not practice full-time, or wish to do so—and this must add to their acceptance of many "competitors." While the many kinds of therapists in Chinese medicine accept one another, how are traditional physicians able to accept Western medicine, and why should they do so?

Traditional Physicians and Western Medicine

Explanations commonly given for traditional physicians combining medicine are as we saw, lack of integrity and economic necessity. I start with "integrity." Those claiming lack of integrity usually suppose that Western medicine is inconsistent with the theories of the traditional physician (one may of course ask whether acupuncture is consistent with the theoretical premises of modern scientific medicine). They also argue that traditional physicians do not understand the properties of the Western medicines they use, and are unscrupulous to use them.

Traditional physicians argue that Western medicine is not inconsistent with Chinese theory. There is only one natural law of the universe, and if Western medicines work, they are "true." Even in the nineteenth century, when a hospital for traditional medicine was flourishing (now fully Westernized), the directors stated that "Chinese and European medicines each have their own use, and we should not have different views of . . . (them) . . . if a cure can be effected all the same" (Board of Director's Tung Wah Group of Hospitals 1970:27). At the time the hospital hoped its physicians might be trained in Western medicine by the government, but they did not come up to the standards required for medical students and it was felt by the authorities their existing ideas about medicine would prevent them from absorbing Western knowledge.

If Western medicine works according to the basic law of the universe, it follows that medicaments can be classified by Chinese methods. Some Chinese drugs are "noble"—they are *yin* and *yang* in property; some are perfectly balanced *(tsîng-heì)*; some are "poisonous"; and others are *pó*: "tonic" in property (what Martin in this volume (Chapter 3) calls "patching"). Western medicines began to be similarly classified. Antibiotics, for example, are generally regarded as "poisonous" although some say they "scatter the vital forces." When taking them diets are needed to prevent side-effects. Some traditional physicians claim that Western science has discovered important and powerful medicines, but that it does not understand their true properties, and how to prescribe them with other medicines and diet to offset their unwanted effects. Western-trained doctors claim that physicians do not understand the importance of limiting antibiotics to serious conditions, and not prescribing them for undue lengths of time.

After the war and with the increasing popularity of Western medicines among the Chinese, traditional doctors started to experiment, combining all sorts of medicines for "greater efficacy." Bone-setters started to use X-rays to improve their diagnosis. They claimed they were "no longer identifiable with Western medicine alone," but with "the science of bone-setting" (personal communication on letter sent to Radiation Board by 40 bone-setters). Abortions traditionally performed by the use of "poisons" to drive out "poisons" (pregnancy is a "poisonous" state), began to be performed also with modern scientific instruments. (People are wanting to limit their families but family planning does not yet affeċt all people in all circumstances.) The demand for plastic surgery to which bone-setters also turned, is comparatively new. It seems connected with the greater preoccupation people have with their image as individuals in Hongkong's individualizing society, and the requirements of women servicing the "entertainment" industry, itself in great demand.

A demand for certain services then tempted traditional practitioners to some innovations, and existing ideas and attitudes in many cases justified innovations in their eyes—but what about "economic necessity"? In 1962 the Secretariat for Chinese Affairs, the protector of Chinese customs, said that while there was still an enormous demand for "herbal" treatment, the herbalists were up aga`ıst (1) increased costs of herbs and other traditional ingredients, most of which have to be imported; (2) sharpening competition as the result of the influx of immigrants including people ready, if not experienced, to try to make a living by traditional medicine; (3) a growing belief in the unbounded efficacy of Western antibiotics and the "miracle" of the "inoculating needle"; and (4) hard-selling techniques by commercial interests relating to Western patent medicines (personal communication). Another factor may now be added: the combining of Western and Chinese ingredients in relatively-cheap Chinese patent medicines imported into the colony. These are heavily advertised and in demand by both physicians and people for their relative convenience over herbal concoctions, which often have to be distilled or brewed. Some physicians and people are unaware that these medicines often contain poisons listed in Part I.

Professional Alignments

Various kinds of traditional doctors have always associated together for mutual advantage, some social, some professional. If one looks at the records of registered societies (kept by the Registrars of Societies, and of Companies) it is seen that some societies of herbalists demand qualifications for entrance, such as diplomas from local or outside schools. ne society claims to have been accepted by the Kuomintang as the "sole legal Chinese doctors' association in Hongkong" (established 1928); but most associations also accept anybody who is "experienced," introduced, or willing to pay for life membership. Such groups often run funeral-benefit clubs like other traditional Chinese associations; many offer assistance to members dealing with the government, even a translation service; and they provide members with very official-looking certificates to hang in their surgeries.

Secular doctors such as acupuncturists and bone-setters also belong to specialist associations. Bone-setters' societies are sometimes interwoven with secret societies, the link being Chinese *kung fu* (martial arts) which the latter often control. Bone-setters get their knowledge of anatomy from practicing *kung fu,* for part of the instruction is in how the bones and muscles work. Secular and non-secular physicians join charity associations providing medicine and ritual therapy to the poor. Membership is seen as an act of merit, part of the physician's "virtue." But for some associations herbal mutual aid has a special meaning. It is also traditional in Hongkong for anybody acting illegally to seek "protection" from prosecution. Two groups provide this protection: one is the secret society of the "triad" variety: "Heaven, Earth and Man" (Morgan 1960); another, allegedly, is corrupt policemen. Illegal practitioners may be required to join a secret society for their protection, and for payment of protection "fees." If one examines the prosecutions for triad society membership one sometimes finds people who are members of herbalist associations, or even association office-bearers. Other societies of illegal doctors, I am told, are formed to pay one another's fines when they are prosecuted.

One factor bringing many practitioners together was the common threat of tightening legislation after the war, which began with the forbidding of eye treatments in the late 'fifties. Through their associations they mobilized public opinion and held press interviews (as did charity associations when the Clinics Ordinance was introduced). They were unable to prevent the new law, but on the day it was passed they formed a federation, declaring it "Integration Festival Day" (1958). "Herbalists' " associations also combined to face another threat—the banning of Chinese medicines containing Part I poisons. This was in the late 'fifties and early 'sixties, before the new patent medicines appeared in large quantities, and related to traditional ingredients which sometimes contain natural traces of such poisons.

The cause of the threat was the death of children with diphtheria who had had a traditional medicine, *hūng-wōng,* blown down their throats. It was found to contain arsenic disulphide, normally inert but when in contact with air, especially when breathed down the throat, capable of turning into white arsenic. Soon afterward a Western-trained registered doctor was censored by a coroner, after a child who had ingested cinna mon oil (a traditional medicine meant to be used externally) before visiting his surgery, died under his subsequent treatment. The oil was found to contain a dangerous proportion of eugenol. The H.K.C.M.A. took up the case, demanding a complete list of Chinese medicaments with their components and antidotes in the case of poisons. The Secretariat of Chinese Affairs retorted that this was an impossible task, and the H.K.C.M.A. then called for a ban upon all Chinese preparations (personal communication based on correspondence).

The Secretariat of Chinese Affairs also argued that it was unrealistic and unwise to control herbal medicines; and the herbalists' associations argued that Chinese prescriptions—which according to the British Pharmacopoeia would prove fatal—had been used for thousands of years without killing off the race. The process of combination in prescription techniques, they argued, eliminates fatalities (personal communication, secretaries of herbalists' association). The outcome was that arsenic disulphide was put on the Part II poisons list (permitted to traditional practitioners) and other Chinese medicaments were exempted by the Pharmacy and Poisons Ordinance.

Chinese medical associations originally emerged, then, to deal with common social and professional matters; but further alignments emerged, as did further associations, to deal with protection rackets controlling illegal activities and new legal controls from the government.

Public Support for the "New System" of Medicine

We saw it suggested that "ignorance, apathy and superstition" made people use the services outside the official Western system; and that people commonly move about between Chinese and Western medicine is well known to the medical authorities. In 1970 it was stated in a Government Information Service handout that "although Western medicine . . . is entirely acceptable . . . many still consult practitioners of Chinese . . . medicine . . . That . . . (it) . . . still retains a popular appeal is evidenced by the fact that 74 percent of patients other than emergencies, admitted to . . . (a government hospital) . . . had been treated at some stage of their illness by practitioners of traditional medicine." (Govern-Information Services 1970). The author has tried in vain to trace the source of this apparent survey.

Personal investigations have shown that Westernized Chinese also use Chinese medicine. In a small survey that the author conducted among the more cooperative medical students in Hongkong University in 1973, it was discovered that 150 out of a total 241 respondents (the full force of medical students was 722) said that they consulted Chinese physicians at some time or other. Sixty-five did not specify the complaint, but out of 85 who did, 31 went to traditional practitioners for fever; 22 for "colds"; 12 for cough; 10 for dislocation and fracture; 9 for influenza; 6 for headache; and 43 for miscellaneous complaints including insomnia, "nerves" and measles.

In the above cited handout the medical authorities also stated that the "most frequent practice . . . is to have recourse to traditional medicine first and then if . . . ineffective . . . to turn to Western medicine. Sometimes . . . (it) . . . works in reverse." In fact, however, the situation might be much more complex. Some diseases are not classified according to Western taxonomy, and those that are may be given a different etiology. Thus there are "culture-bound" syndromes—conditions from which people suffer because they believe certain things about health—predisposition, external agents and so forth. One of these, "injury by fear," I have described elsewhere (Topley 1970:429–435); and diseases with different etiologies includes measles (Topley 1970:425–529), tuberculosis, leprosy, influenza, insomnia and various psychoses. In organizing their diseases people may therefore sometimes ignore as irrelevant certain important symptoms. By the time their condition is diagnosed by modern scientific methods their condition may be very serious, if not terminal. Then a Chinese "miracle" cure will be tried, and stories abound in Hongkong concerning remarkable cures of cancer through traditional medicines.

In organizing his disease and his treatment, a Chinese patient has an enormous variety of choices (Topley 1971). He may choose to see only a simple malaise, ignoring the possibility of a predisposition. He may then try some traditional or modern remedy himself. If this fails he may visit a Chinese or Western type physician, and by now he may consider also the question of predisposition and visit a horoscope reader, or priest, for a full explanation of what is happening to him. At the same time he may go again to a Chinese or Western type doctor or, as a result of his interview with the priest, to an "auxiliary" such as a geomancer. If he gets as far as a "miracle" cure and it does not work, this does not necessarily mean others lose faith in the cure. One example the writer was given was of a man taking the scorpion remedy, who died. It was explained that he stopped taking it at Chinese New Year, which is a time when popular tradition says one should not take medicines. The doctor had told him not to stop until the prescribed 10-day treatment was over. The doctor explained that he had omitted to tell him that "poisonous" medicines *could* be taken at Chinese New Year; it was only "noble" medicines that one must stop. The doctor was in error, but not the medicine.

A person's decision about what to do when he is ill is influenced also by a variety of external factors: how much doctors charge; where they live; what their mothers or neighbors recommend; what they have read in the papers, or heard on the television; whether or not a doctor has a reputation for honesty; and whether or not one can expect an explanation from him as to why the particular person is ill. Registered doctors sometimes complain that in Hongkong there are "4 million people and 4 million doctors"—people are always telling one what they think is the cause of their disease. People argue that many Western doctors do not listen to their explanations concerning their predispositions, what external agent they may have encountered, and so on—factors *they* consider important in describing their symptoms. They are not content with an explanation that they have something "going around," and if they are told they have some germ or virus they want to know why *they* in particular. Many people have learned to accept the existence of germs and viruses, but many also do not think they will get them unless predisposed. Perhaps for this reason they do not overly worry about the cleanliness of clinics. If they want an explanation they prefer to go to physicians who have plenty of time to explain. Thus they prefer one of the physicians who takes only a few patients a day. Many people use several doctors, for each member of the family, because they believe one may be good for one person and one for another—they have an affinity. Others prefer doctors combining medicines (few know this is illegal) because they can then treat different members of the family. Some people believe that a young person, being stronger, can take anti-biotics, but an older person needs Chinese medicine. Some people know their doctor is illegal and even defend him on the grounds that he is less arrogant, has more time, and is more inclined to give explanations. Many do not understand the subtle distinctions between titles, however, or they do not understand why a physician claiming to be qualified in China, and sometimes having a diploma hung on the wall of his surgery to prove it, should be considered "unqualified" to practice.

People, then, are often "superstitious" and sometimes "ignorant," but they are seldom "apathetic." They do have standards and scales of measurement and can recognize if a therapist has "knowledge," but their standard, scales, and notions of knowledge, are not the same as those of the Western medical profession.

Discussion

Some sectors of the community would like to see the "new system" of medicine dissolved. They suggest different ways of achieving this aim. The government relies on general and health education on the one hand, and the economic laws of supply and demand on the other.

The government anticipates that education will make people accept Western standards enabling them at the same time to differentiate by title the legal from illegal Western practitioner. Although it is hoped that education will also entice people away from Chinese medicine it is beginning to be recognized that new developments in China are complicating the situation—registered doctors react to them positively. In a way, the government would like to keep traditional medicine alive, because it is recognized that traditional physicians take some of the strain off Western doctors in dealing with self-limiting diseases (Committee Appointed to Review the Doctor Problem 1969:7). But the government is concerned by the fact that they also treat more serious diseases.

People outside the government, including Western-trained registered doctors interested in developments in China, would like to see Chinese medicine absorbed in the officially recognized Western system. But so far such doctors are only interested in acupuncture, which incidentally does not enjoy such popularity with ordinary people. Most people want medicine. But it is difficult to envisage registered doctors learning the art of combination in Chinese prescriptions, which, I am told, needs long training and a knowledge of Chinese theory. Acupuncture is accepted as a technique which somehow or other works; other Chinese therapeutic measures cannot be accepted as readily; certainly not the religious therapy given for emotional disturbances. There is a shortage of psychiatrists in Hongkong; many parents of qualifying doctors do not like to see them enter this field, considering it "not very nice." And many people do not agree with modern diagnoses of mental afflictions, (see Yap 1967:73–85 on popular notions of mental affliction).

The other reliance of the government, on the economic laws of supply and demand, is linked with a new policy to supply more qualified doctors. The idea is that more doctors will mean that they will be driven into the poorer areas by competition, where they will perforce have to charge lower fees. In a recent speech by the Governor it was said that by the end of the decade Hongkong will need 100 more doctors a year than currently are being supplied (Maclehose 1974), and there is talk of a second medical school. However, it takes 6 years to train doctors, and there is no guarantee that they would stay in Hongkong if competition sharpens, and there is no control over the number of patients a recognized doctor sees. Doctors may prefer to take fewer patients and stay in the richer areas.

Other people want the China-trained doctors to be recognized and brought into the official system (*China Mail,* December 24, 1973; *South China Morning Post,* April 17, 1974). Experience, however, suggests that many "China-trained" doctors are in fact unqualified and untrained, and therefore unacceptable to the profession. Qualifications are based on what is accepted in Great Britain, where the public has learned to accept professional standards.

There are those wanting herbalists to continue, but to be controlled. One suggestion made by a prominent doctor (a Chinese), is to have a school of traditional medicine similar to those in Taiwan (Ding 1972: 1ff.). Such training would undoubtedly be based on secular theories and methods. Where would other specialists stand; filling as they do a demand for "spiritual" therapy? Another suggestion is to tighten the laws governing uses and the import of pharmaceutical products (*South China Morning Post,* February 16, 1974). But one wonders what would happen if all Chinese patent medicines were banned, as is currently suggested.

At present there is a system, illegal from one point of view, useful from another. It does not accord with Western ideals concerning justice, standards of efficiency and competence, or morality; but it works reasonably well. A stronger arm of the law might bring problems of social and political disturbance, and deny people the services they have come to accept. This system allows people, who are changing and accommodating to new ideas, a flexibility of choice. As one lawyer remarked to the author, the more one legislates to create either "fairer" or more efficient conditions, the more one creates illegalities, and helps to further support those in Hongkong who have traditionally profited by the distances between Western and Chinese viewpoints and theories.

NOTES

1. Data for this essay come principally from a study of the development and functioning of the Hongkong medical system sponsored by the Centre of Asian Studies (University of Hongkong). It began in 1971 and will be completed in 1974. In-depth interviews were conducted either in Cantonese by myself, or in Cantonese and Mandarin by my parttime research assistant. Additional data comes from a child-rearing study conducted by me personally in 1969 in resettlement and low-cost housing estates, and sponsored by a project on development and rearing of Chinese children in Hongkong, undertaken by the Pediatric Department of the University of Hongkong with a grant from the Nuffield Foundation and other organizations.

2. All terms connected with medicine in Hongkong are usually romanized in official documents in Cantonese. Here I follow this practice, using the romanization method of Myer and Wempe (1947).

REFERENCES

ADVISORY COMMITTEE ON CLINICS
  1966   Report. Hongkong: Government Printer.

BOARD OF DIRECTORS, TUNG WAH GROUP OF HOSPITALS
  (1970)   One hundred years of the Tung Wah Group of Hospitals 1870–
           1970. Vol. 2 Hongkong: "United China Publishing Co."
           (Chinese and English).

CENSUS AND STATISTICS DEPARTMENT
  (1972)   Hongkong Population and Housing Census: 1971 Main Report.
           Hongkong: Government Printer.

CHAIRMAN, MEDICAL COUNCIL
  1973   Letter to the Medical Associations. M.C. 1/AG.

CHINA MAIL
  1973   If you're an alien it's bad medicine. May 28. BMA defends
         private practice. October 9. Why not solve the doctors' dilemma?
         December 24.
  1974   Recognize herb doctors—reformers. March 12.

COMMITTEE APPOINTED BY THE GOVERNOR
  1948   Chinese Law and Custom in Hongkong. Hongkong: Govern-
         ment Printer.

COMMITTEE APPOINTED TO REVIEW THE DOCTOR PROBLEM
IN THE HONGKONG GOVERNMENT
  1969   Report. Hongkong: Government Printer.

CORRESPONDENCE AND PAPERS RELATING TO THE PHAR-
MACY BOARD
  1957–
  1967   H.K.R.S. No. 49. N & S No. 1/15.

CROIZIER, R.
  1968   Traditional Medicine in Modern China: Science, Nationalism
         and the Tensions of Cultural Change. Cambridge: Harvard
         University Press.
  1970   Traditional medicine as a basis for Chinese medical practices.
         In Medicine and Public Health in the People's Republic of
         China, ed. Joseph R. Quinn. Washington: U.S. Department of
         Health, Education, and Welfare, Public Health Service, Fogarty
         International Center, National Institutes of Health.

DING, L. K.
  1972   Is a Second Medical School Needed in Hongkong? Caduceus
         4:1–2

DIRECTOR OF MEDICINE (AND HEALTH SERVICES)
1928 Annual Report. Hongkong: Government Printer.
1949–
1973 Annual Reports. Hongkong: Government Printer.
1964 Development of Medical Services in Hongkong. Hongkong: Government Printer.

FIRTH, R.
1951 Elements of Social Organization. London: Watts & Co.

GOVERNMENT INFORMATION SERVICES, HONGKONG
1970 Hongkong's Medical & Health Services. July.

HONGKONG CHINESE MEDICAL ASSOCIATION
1969 Expansion of the Result of the Survey on Medical & Paramedical Services in Hongkong. August. (mimeo.).

HONGKONG GOVERNMENT
1896 Medical Report on the Epidemic of Bubonic Plague in 1894. A Chinese View of the Plague. Hongkong: Government Printers.
1948–
1973 Annual Reports. Hongkong: Government Printer.
1953 Medical Registration (Amendment) No. 2. Ordinance. Hongkong: Government Printer.
1963 Medical Clinics Ordinance (Section 8(7)). Code of Practice for Unregistrable Medical Practitioners. Hongkong: Government Printer.
1966a Medical Registration Ordinance. Hongkong: Government Printer.
1966b Medical Clinics Ordinance. Hongkong: Government Printer.
1968a Dangerous Drugs Ordinance. Hongkong: Government Printer.
1968b Undesirable Medical Advertisements Ordinance. Hongkong: Government Printer.
1969a Pharmacy and Poisons Ordinance. Hongkong: Government Printer.
1969b Antibiotics Ordinance. Hongkong: Government Printer.

HONGKONG STANDARD
1973 Medical plan slammed by Hongkong doctor. October 21.
1974 The herbalists and the law. March 10.
The doctor's wife weeps every night. April 14.

HUI-CHEN WANG LIU
1959 An analysis of Chinese clan rules: Confucian theories in action. In Confucianism in Action, eds. David S. Nivison and Arthur F. Wright. Stanford: Stanford University Press.

MEDICAL PLAN STANDING COMMITTEE
1970 Annual Report, April 1969–March 1970. Hongkong: Government Printer.

MEYER, B. F. and T. F. WEMPE
1947 The Student's Cantonese-English Dictionary, New York: Field Afar Press.

MORGAN, W. P.
1960 Triad Societies in Hongkong. Hongkong: Government Printer.

MACLEHOSE, MURRAY, K. C. M. G., M.B.E.
(1974) Speech to the Legislative Council. October 17.

NG, B.
1973 Private Practice in Hongkong: The Doctor in Pinstripe? Caduceus 5:1–2.

ONIONS, C. T., ed.
1955 The Shorter Oxford English Dictionary. Oxford: Clarendon Press.

SOUTH CHINA MORNING POST
1970 Charlatans in the medical profession. March 3.
1971 Fees charged by physicians absurd. December 26.
1972 Fees rise not a free market concept. January 11.
Good health but there are some scars. January 27.
Top Chinese doctors in colony. November 30.
1973 Danger in superficial study of acupuncture. October 8.
Controls on acupuncture practices. October 12.
Chou flooded with pleas for exit permits. November 19.
Doctors who leave department defended. November 30.
1974 Doctors as pharmacists. February 16.
Making more use of China-trained doctors. April 17.

SUB-COMMITTEE OF TASK FORCE ON COMMUNITY HEALTH COMMITTEE
1970 Survey of Kwun Tong Medical and Health Services. September 11 (mimeo).

THE STAR
1972 Tighten up on drugs. March 20.
1974 1,000 quacks in Hongkong: April 4.

TOPLEY, M.
1969 The role of savings and wealth among Hongkong Chinese. In Hongkong: A Society in Transition—Contributions to the Study of Hongkong Society, I. C. Jarvie, ed. London: Routledge & Kegan Paul.
1970 Chinese Traditional Ideas and the Treatment of Disease: Two Examples from Hongkong. Man (N/S.) 5:421–437.
1971 Chinese Traditional Etiology and Methods of Cure in Contemporary Hongkong. New York: Wenner-Gren Foundation for Anthropological Research (mimeo). (Published in Asian Medical Systems, C. Leslie, ed., Berkeley: University of California Press, 1976.)

WAH KIU YAT PO (in Chinese)
  1964   Section 2. October 22.

YAP, P. M.
  1967   Ideas of mental disorder in Hongkong and their practical influence. *In* Some Traditional Chinese Ideas and Conceptions in Hongkong Social Life Today, M. Topley, ed. Hongkong: Hongkong Branch, Royal Asiatic Society.

CHAPTER 7

MEDICAL CARE IN THE CHINESE COMMUNITIES OF PENINSULAR MALAYSIA

FREDERICK L. DUNN

Introduction

The federation of Malaysia, at the heart of modern Southeast Asia, links the two Bornean States of Sarawak and Sabah with 11 states in the southern two-fifths of the Malay Peninsula. Until 1963 the latter states comprised the Federation of Malaya, and today they are collectively designated Peninsular Malaysia. With the creation of Malaysia on August 31, 1963, Singapore entered the federation as a 14th state, but this relationship ended 2 years later as Singapore became an independent republic. In pre-1965 publications concerning Singapore the island state was customarily described as part of Malaya, or Malaysia.

The scope of this contribution is limited to the 11 States of Peninsular Malaysia, but some reference to studies in Singapore is also necessary. Very little has been published about the health and medical behavior of Chinese communities in Malaysian Borneo and the writer has not had the opportunity to carry out any personal investigations of Chinese medical care in Sabah or Sarawak.

Peninsular Malaysia is a land of considerable ecological and cultural diversity. In its ethnic heterogeneity, and in the history of immigration that has led to this modern diversity, there are many resemblances to the American experience and to modern American heterogeneity, although, of course, ethnic composition is very different in the two nations. Malaysian ethnic diversity has led to some of the same problems and challenges that face the United States; this applies with special force to the delivery of health care. Although there are obvious medical ecological differences between tropical Malaysia and the largely temperate United States, the distribution of diseases and disorders in Malaysia's population is coming to resemble that of the United States more closely every year, and the problems of health-care delivery, especially to rural and to economically-deprived segments of the population, are broadly similar.

As a reflection of ethnic diversity Malaysia has acquired a range of traditional approaches to medical care (traditional medical systems) at least as broad as that in the United States. In Malaysia, as in the United States, research on traditional medical behavior has thus far been very limited. It is generally true that American medical students and young physicians complete their formal training with little appreciation of the alternative modes of medical practice that exist in their own communities in parallel with the cosmopolitan (Western) medical system into which they have become enculturated.[1] The same can be said for the students and graduates of cosmopolitan medical schools in other parts of the world, including the countries of Southeast Asia. In the absence of knowledge and understanding of each other's approaches, both on the part of Western-trained and traditional practitioners, there is inevitable suspicion, unnecessary competition, and an absence of cooperative action toward the general goal of increase in human health levels.

This paper is focused on medical care in the Chinese communities of Peninsular Malaysia, and especially on a preliminary view of what is known of Chinese traditional medical behavior, in all its variety. The account that follows is based upon a very limited literature (even in the Chinese language) for Malaysia and Singapore, and upon observations and interviews in the Chinese communities of Kuala Lumpur and its environs in the State of Selangor. It is added that the literature on traditional medicine in Malaysia is limited only with respect to the Chinese (and Indian) communities. Malay medicine has been the object of extensive research, at intervals over a span of at least 80 years (e.g. Skeat 1900).

The Chinese Communities in Peninsular Malaysia

The 1970 census of Malaysia employs the term "community" (masharakat) defined as follows:

> The term "community" has been used in preference to the term "race." This follows the practice adopted in earlier Malayan Censuses. . . . The term race would be confined to groups of persons exhibiting common physical characteristics. "Community" on the other hand is more appropriate in describing a group of persons who are bound together by common interests, that is to say language or dialect, religion and customs (Chander 1972:22).

Data were collected in 1970 for 32 separate "community groups" in Peninsular Malaysia, including 10 under the general heading Chinese, 9 under the heading Malay, 8 under Indian, and 5 other groups including Thai, European, and Eurasian (Chander 1972:291). The Chinese community groups, based on dialect, and transliterated as for the census, are Hokkien, Cantonese, Khek (Hakka), Teochew, Hainanese, Kwongsai, Hokchiu (Foochow), Henghua, Hokchia, and Other Chinese.

The 1970 census enumerated 8,810,348 persons in Peninsular Malaysia, including 4,685,838 Malays (53.2 percent of the population), 932,629 Indians (10.6 percent), 69,531 others (0.8 percent), and 3,122,350 Chinese (35.4 percent). The Peninsular Chinese populations for each community (dialect) group are set out in Table 1.

The census analysts have given special attention to urban-rural contrasts in reporting on the 1970 Malaysian community group data. The census defines as urban (bandar) those populations living in metropolitan places (populations in excess of 75,000) and large towns (10,000 persons and over). Rural (luar bandar) populations are defined as those in small

TABLE 1. THE CHINESE COMMUNITIES OF PENINSULAR
MALAYSIA IN 1970*

Community (dialect) group	Population	Percentage of total Chinese population
Hokkien	1,068,803	34.2
Hakka (Khek)	690,821	22.1
Cantonese	617,588	19.8
Teochew	387,048	12.4
Hainanese	145,758	4.7
Kwongsai	77,577	2.5
Hokchiu	57,095	1.8
Henghua	16,924	0.5
Hokchia	9,039	0.3
Other Chinese	51,697	1.7
Total	3,122,350	100.0

*Based on Chander 1972: Table VIII, p. 28

towns (1,000 to 9,999 persons) and in all other rural settings. The term "urban connurbation area" is also used, denoting "the totality of the gazetted area of the town being discussed and the built-up areas lying outside its boundary" (Chander 1972:292). Ten urban connurbation areas are thus defined for Peninsular Malaysia, including Kuala Lumpur (708,191 persons), Malaysia's capital city, and Alor Star, Georgetown (on Penang Island), Ipoh, Johore Baru, Kota Baru, Kuala Trengganu, Kuantan, Melaka (Malacca), and Seremban. The principal towns of 3 of these connurbations (Kota Baru, Kuala Trengganu, Kuantan) fall short of the metropolitan definition, however; Peninsular Malaysia has a total of 8 "cities"—7 of the above and Klang in coastal Selangor.

On the basis of the rural-urban definition above, 47.4 percent of the Chinese were urban and 52.6 percent rural, while 14.9 percent of the Malays were urban and 85.1 percent rural in Peninsular Malaysia in 1970 (Table 2). Among the Chinese 29.1 percent were concentrated in the eight metropolitan places and another 18.3 percent were found in large towns. Small-town Chinese constituted another 23.4 percent, and the remaining 29.2 percent of the Chinese population was distributed in other rural places.

In the connurbation area of Kuala Lumpur 394,517 Chinese constituted almost 56 percent of the population in 1970. Similar percentages for other connurbation areas on the western side of the Peninsula are Alor Star (48 percent Chinese), Georgetown (70), Ipoh (69), Malacca (73), and Seremban (60). In the East Coast and southern Johore connurbation

areas the Chinese proportions of the populations are generally lower—
Johore Baru (39 percent), Kota Baru (23), Kuala Trengganu (15), and
Kuantan (50).

Chinese community (dialect) group composition varies greatly from
state to state. Table 3 summarizes data for each state for the 5 major
dialects: Hokkien, Cantonese, Hakka, Teochew, and Hainanese. Hokkien
speakers predominate in 8 states, Cantonese in 2 (Pahang and Perak),

TABLE 2. THE MAJOR COMMUNITIES AND DEGREES OF
URBANIZATION IN PENINSULAR MALAYSIA IN 1970*

Community	Urban areas (places with 10,000 persons or more)		Rural areas (places with less than 10,000 persons)		Total	
	Population	Percentage (for each community)	Population	Percentage (for each community)	Population	Percentage
Malay	699,372	14.9	3,986,466	85.1	4,685,838	53.2
Chinese	1,479,225	47.4	1,643,125	52.6	3,122,350	35.4
Indian	323,435	34.7	609,194	65.3	932,629˙	10.6
Others	28,401	40.8	41,130	59.2	69,531	0.8
Total	2,530,433	28.7	6,279,915	71.3	8,810,348	100.0

*Based on Chander 1972: Table XI, p. 30

TABLE 3. POPULATIONS OF MAJOR CHINESE COMMUNITY
(DIALECT) GROUPS BY STATE IN 1970*

State	Total Chinese population	Hokkien	Cantonese	Hakka	Teochew	Hainanese
Johore	502,978	217,310	43,477	99,830	78,150	30.790
Kedah	184,263	60,004	25,037	28,218	57,974	4,565
Kelantan	36,668	21,179	4,812	4,272	1,499	3 023
Malacca	160,084	68,005	14,410	40,163	13,501	15,900
Negri Sembilan	183,444	47,723	43,524	63,665	4,717	9,341
Pahang	157,666	34,064	39,575	37,881	6,125	9,187
(also 26,112 Kwongsai)**						
Penang	435,366	195,538	70,081	41,544	103,044	14,324
Perak	666,237	144,295	187,738	174,519	67,777	17,541
(also 27,540 Hokchiu—21,689 Kwongsai—5,186 Hokchia)**						
Perlis	19,571	6,402	2,219	6,062	3,133	732
Selangor	754,348	266,163	183,866	192,175	49,932	34,967
(also 4,192 Henghua)**						
Trengganu	21,725	8,120	2,849	2,492	1,196	5,388
Totals	3,122,350	1,068,803	617,588	690,821	387,048	145,758

*Source: Chander 1972, from tables between pages 48 and 83
**Additional figures for special concentrations of minor dialect groups

and Hakka in 1 (Negri Sembilan). In second order of predominance, Hakka speakers lead in 6 states, Teochew in 2 (Kedah and Penang), Cantonese in 1 (Kelantan), and Hainanese in 1 (Trengganu). The same table demonstrates the concentration of the Chinese population in the western states on the Peninsula; the east coast states of Kelantan and Trengganu have very small Chinese populations, and that of Pahang is also relatively small given the large size and total population of the state. Perlis, in the far north, is a very small state with a total population of only 120,991 in 1970.

Chinese Immigration and Settlement in the Southern Malay Peninsula

Before 1800 few Chinese were resident in the southern Malay Peninsula except in the seaport town of Malacca, although the history of Peninsular trading contact with China extended back many centuries. By the time of the Dutch conquest in 1641 Malacca had a population of 300 to 400 Chinese (Newell 1962:7 and Purcell 1967) and by 1750 the town's total population of 9,630 included 2,160 Chinese (Ooi 1963:107). Growth in the Peninsular Chinese population began to accelerate after 1800. By 1822, Singapore, founded in 1819, already had a population of 4,700, including 1,150 Chinese; by 1820 there were 8,300 Chinese in Penang; and Malacca's Chinese population had reached 4,100 by 1826 (Ooi 1963: 106–108). It is estimated that there were about 17,200 Chinese in all of the Straits Settlements by 1834 (Newell 1962:7) and in the Malay States at about the same time (1830) Ooi's estimate is 15,000–20,000 Chinese in mining, trading, and the cultivation of pepper and gambier in southern Johore.

In 1850 rich tin deposits were discovered in the Larut district of Perak. This discovery set off a mining rush that marked the beginning of massive immigration from China. Immigration was encouraged by the British, even to the extent of active recruitment of laborers for the mines. The immigrants came primarily from the southeast of China, from the provinces of Fukien, Kwangtung, Kwangsi, and the island of Hainan. Malaya was seen as a land of special opportunity in mining and trade; population pressures and·limited natural resources at home provided further stimuli to immigration (Ooi 1963:110). In commenting on the Chinese immigration phase as a whole, that is, especially the period from the 1850's until 1930, Ooi (1963:111–2112) states:

> The characteristic feature of Chinese migration to Malaya was that it was motivated entirely by economic reasons. The Chinese came to the country with but one desire—to make their fortunes before returning to their original homes. Few had any intention of settling permanently in the Peninsula. Movements of Chinese to and from south China were therefore extremely fluid. . . . The frequency and directions of these movements were highly geared to the existing state of the Malayan economy, periods of economic boom resulting in a net influx of labor and periods of depression causing a return flow of migrants to China.

Newell (1962:9) remarks that the immigrants came as individuals, rather than as whole village groups. They were free to settle where they wished, in towns or rural areas. Most tended to settle with others of the same dialect group, and very often with those from the same village in China. Male immigrants substantially exceeded females in numbers throughout the earlier immigration years.

In the 1880's tin mining expanded very rapidly to meet great demand and high prices. Thus in each of the years 1899 and 1900, 100,000 immigrants reached Malaya from China, and for the period 1881–1900 a total of nearly 2 million Chinese migrants came into the Federated Malay States (Selangor, Perak, Negri Sembilan, and Pahang) (Ooi 1963: 110). By 1901 there were more Chinese than Malays in Selangor and Perak. After 1900, rubber provided an additional economic opportunity for the migrants, so much so that by 1931 35 percent of the total population in rubber cultivation was Chinese. Chinese migration reached a new annual record of 278,000 in 1913, fell during the war years, and then climbed to an all-time peak of 435,708 in 1927 (Ooi 1963:112). In that same year, however, 303,497 Chinese left Malaya, so the net gain was only 132,000. Immigration restrictions were applied for the first time, affecting males only, in August 1930. Direct immigration into the Federated Malay States was stopped, and quotas were set for the Straits Settlements. Female immigration restrictions were added in 1939. Ooi (1963:113) cites estimates that at least 5 million Chinese entered Malaya during the nineteenth century and 12 million between 1900 and 1940. Of these 17 million at least 14½ million returned to China eventually. The net result in 1941 was a Chinese population of 2,418,615 constituting 44 percent of the total population of Malaya.

After the disruptions of World War II the postwar Chinese population of the Federation of Malaya stabilized, with relatively little movement to and from China. The Chinese population in Malaya in 1954 stood at 2,216,105 (Newell 1962:1). While immigration and emigration effectively ceased during the "emergency" years, Malaya's rural Chinese population was uprooted, relocated, and regrouped in more than 600 new settlements, primarily in 480 "new villages" (Sandhu 1973). The effects of these operations are still evident in the distribution of Chinese on the land in Peninsular Malaysia today (Nyce 1973).

Health Sectors and Health in the Chinese
Communities of Peninsular Malaysia

Descriptions of health conditions below the regional or national level generally depend upon subdivision of populations into geographical, political-administrative, or ethnic units. Thus the state of health of a nation's people may be described in terms of rates for diseases and disorders calculated upon the base populations of each of its states, districts, or other smaller components. Similar rates may be calculated for populations according to their geographical disposition, e.g. coastal in comparison to inland, lowland in comparison to montane. Ethnic (or linguistic,

or racial) subdivisions are also commonly employed in examining variation in health conditions within national populations.

The "political-administrative boundary" approach is convenient because
each political entity usually coincides with the data collecting entity for
the land and population under its jurisdiction. Population and health data
whose limits are defined by political boundaries are readily available
(although of uneven quality and scope) for many nations. Unfortunately
these data often obscure or cut across physical environmental and cultural
boundaries; the broad picture that emerges is distinctly unecological.

The geographical and ethnic group approaches to broad characteriza-
tions of health are useful but each method, employed alone, may obscure
or fail to reflect the man-culture-landscape interactions that underlie every
condition of human health. Thus a composite approach to the description
of health status appears necessary; such an approach must take into
account cultural and physical environmental settings, and will ignore
political boundaries, except in so far (1) as they coincide with the edges
of cultural and geographical domains, and (2) as they represent lines
between substantially different patterns of organized (private or public)
medical care. For some time I have been attracted to this concept of
the "cultural-ecological unit" (Dunn 1972:107) and recently I have
begun to use the expression "health sector" as an equivalent term to
represent the composite approach to health characterization mentioned
above. A health sector may be defined as a cultural-ecological unit whose
human population shares common broad patterns of disease and disorder
and thus a common range of health levels.

In theory there could be as many as 50 basic health sectors in Peninsular Malaysia (Table 4). As the table shows, however, many such sectors
do not exist; only some 30 sectors need be considered. By definition each
sector requires characterization with respect to health. Each ethnic grouping in a sector must also be described as to state of sociocultural stability
or change. For an ecologically coherent general description of health
in Peninsular Malaysia descriptions of health in these basic sectors would
suffice. Obviously the number of sectors can be increased by further
ethnic or geographic (i.e. settlement category) subdivision. For certain
purposes each Chinese dialect group might be considered separately in
relation to settlement, or estates might be further subdivided by type
(rubber, oilpalm, coconut, etc.) or by physical setting (coastal, inland,
etc.) in relation to one or more ethnic groups. It is important to appreciate, however, that there is much blending of ethnic (or dialect) groups
in certain settlement categories in certain areas of the country. For example, in the coastal coconut-growing lowlands of the west coast many
Chinese smallholders or traders live in single-family homes in close
proximity to smallholder Malays, essentially as co-residents of the same
ill-defined villages (*kampung2*).

Table 4 shows that the Chinese population is represented in substantial
numbers in all major settlement categories. In order to describe the
health of the Chinese it would therefore be necessary, at a minimum, to

TABLE 4. BASIC HEALTH SECTORS IN PENINSULAR MALAYSIA

Settlement categories	Major communities (ethnic groupings)				
	Chinese	Indians	Malays	Orang Asli (Aborigines)	Others (Europeans, Eurasians, etc.)
Metropolitan (75,000 persons or more)					
"Adapted" populations	+	+	+	—	+
"New" populations	+	+	+	—	+
Large towns (10,000–75,000)					
"Adapted"	+	+	+	—	—
"New"	+	+	+	—	—
Rural					
Small town (1,000–10,000)	+	+	+	—	—
Village (*kampung*)	+	—	+	+	—
Resettlement scheme	+	+	+	+	—
Estate	+	+	+	—	+
Mining settlement	+	—	—	—	—
Forest (including forest product camps)	+	—	+	+	—

Each health sector identified by a (+) has a *substantial* population (for that ethnic group) in the settlement category.

Each health sector identified by a (—) has only a *minimal* population, or sometimes *no* representation by that ethnic group in the settlement category.

describe the health conditions in 10 basic health sectors. At this time such an undertaking is not feasible; new survey data will be required for many health sectors and new analyses of existing data are also needed. The collecting and processing of health statistics is well advanced in Peninsular Malaysia, but the data are collected and organized in terms of political-administrative entities (states, districts, towns, etc.) and major ethnic (community) groups. Thus it is feasible to compare morbidity and mortality rates between major communities in the various divisions of the country, but it is not as yet possible to compare the health, for example, of Chinese living on resettlement schemes with that of Chinese miners; of Indian rubber estate workers with their counter-parts who have recently settled in metropolitan places; or of Malay villagers with Chinese small-town residents.

Comparative studies of health sectors should add a new dimension to understanding of the state of health, and should enable public health and other medical workers to define priorities even more closely than in the past.

The discussion above hints at the complexities and challenges that lie ahead in health research in Malaysia, with respect to the Chinese and all other communities. Only superficial, and possibly inaccurate state-ments can be made about the health of Chinese in most of the basic sectors at the present time. Since this paper is primarily intended to be a review of medical care as it affects the Chinese, the discussion of Chinese health is not carried beyond this point. However, attention is called to the opportunities that exist for analytical epidemiologic research in the complex and diverse cultural-ecological matrix that has been described. Many possibilities for differential epidemiologic study exist in Malaysia and only a few leads have been followed to date. Cancer research possibilities appear to be particularly promising, as sug-gested by data presented by Shanmugaratnam and Wee (1972) and by Ahluwalia and Duguid (1966), and several differential studies of naso-pharyngeal cancer are now in progress at centers in Kuala Lumpur and Singapore (R. W. Armstrong, personal communication, 1973). Similar opportunities are certainly present in several other fields such as cardiovascular disease research (Balasundaram 1970).

Medical Care in the Chinese Communities

In the foregoing sections we have seen the Peninsula States to be diverse culturally and ecologically, with this diversity extending to the Chinese communities whose numerous dialect groups and categories of settlement combine to form many Chinese health sectors. The status of health in these sectors is influenced by diseases peculiar to Malaysia's tropical setting, but the assemblages of disease and disorder are basically those of developed countries everywhere. This is especially true at the urban end of the rural-urban axis of settlement. Malaysia is a rapidly-developing country with some highly developed sectors, and others, less so, that are experiencing rapid change toward greater economic strength.

One manifestation of Malaysian diversity and development is a con-siderable range of options for medical care. Malaysian Chinese can and do seek medical advice from private or government-supported practi-tioners trained in the cosmopolitan Western system, or from practitioners and other sources of therapeutic support within the Chinese cultural tradi-tion, or from practitioners of the other schools and traditions—including Malay, Indian Ayurvedic or Unani, and Orang Asli—that the country affords.[2] The potential range of options is as great, of course, for other Malaysians, and for many the perceived range of choice must be as great as that indicated for the Chinese. This brings the writer to a series of questions for future research. What is the perceived spectrum of options for medical care in each of Malaysia's health sectors? What therapeutic alternatives do people actually consider when confronted with threats to health of various kinds? What actions do they finally take, and in what sequence if several types of practitioners are consulted? Very little information is available on the behavior of Malaysia's health care "consumers," and much is needed. To these questions can be added others, equally demanding of research, about the practitioners of traditional medicine and their behavior. Who enters such practice, and how, and with what motives and values? What kinds of relationships exist between practitioners of different schools and traditions? How do these relationships, or their lack, influence patient access to care? Little has been written to date about these matters in Malaysia; indeed the author knows of only one formal contribution in this field, a brief critique of "unlicensed" practitioners by Chen (1971).

In the following pages is offered a preliminary view of Chinese health behavior and medical care in Peninsular Malaysia. The discussion begins with cosmopolitan (Western) medicine, both private and public-supported; continues with traditional medicine other than Chinese; proceeds to personal health behavior, paramedical practitioners, and other paramedical supports within the Chinese tradition; and concludes with a study of Chinese traditional medicine.

Cosmopolitan (Western) Medicine

Peninsular Malaysia's citizens are the beneficiaries of a sturdy governmental system of public health and medical care. Current health expenditures account for 6.5 percent of total government expenditure and 1.9 percent of the gross national product (*Malay Mail* 1973). The system is strengthening each year as it is extended farther into the rural health sectors. Most urban residents are already within range of one or more government hospitals, and the people of the small towns and other rural places are increasingly served by Main Health Centres (44 in 1970 in Peninsular Malaysia), Health Sub Centres (180 in 1970), and Midwife Clinics (943 in 1970) (Noordin 1973). Newly-graduated doctors now face terms of compulsory government service and these newcomers, together with doctors recruited from abroad on contract, are making it possible to increase the staffing at the professional level in rural areas.

The ratio of registered physicians in 1971 reached 1 to 5106 people and this figure continues to improve each year. These physicians are drawn from all of the Peninsula's ethnic groups, but those of the Chinese and Indian groups are in the majority. Malaysia has one medical school (at the University of Malaya, Kuala Lumpur), is opening a second, and receives new graduates from medical schools abroad that accept considerable numbers of Malaysian secondary school graduates. The Faculty of Medicine in the University of Singapore has contributed many medical graduates to Malaysia, and is the former school of most of Malaysia's physicians who completed their training prior to the late 1960's. Physicians in Malaysia have their own vigorous organization, the Malayan Medical Association, which in turn supports a number of specialist groups such as the Public Health Society.

Physicians in private practice are still concentrated in the larger urban places, but intense competition in metropolitan practice is beginning to attract more private practitioners to work in the large towns. In a separate category are those physicians who work—on a full-time or parttime basis—for the rubber and oilpalm estates, and other firms that provide company-financed programs of medical care for their employees.

For Malaysian Chinese, cosmopolitan medicine thus offers the alternatives of government-subsidized care in hospitals or clinics; care by private physicians in group or solo practice; or private care through a company plan. Economic, linguistic, and other cultural considerations have a profound influence on choice among these options.

All informants agree that there has been a substantial shift in attitude toward cosmopolitan medicine in the Chinese community since about 1950. Prior to that time many Malaysian Chinese turned to this system of medicine, and especially to hospitalization, as a last resort. But in recent years more and more Chinese have reversed their choice, at least for organic diseases, and turn to Chinese medicine only if cosmopolitan care fails to provide relief. Thus today the Western-trained practitioner oftens sees the common infectious diseases and everyday complaints of young and middle-aged Chinese, but the stubborn problems of old age, the chronic disorders such as arthritis, and the incurable diseases continue to receive the Chinese physician's supportive care, in many instances.

Willingness to accept Western-style hospitalization has also increased in recent years. The Tung Shin Hospital, established in Kuala Lumpur in 1892 (as the P'ui Shin Tong Chinese Hospital), served for many years as the only hospital in the city providing traditional Chinese outpatient and in-patient care (Chai 1964:198; Field 1951). In recent years the hospital has offered both cosmopolitan and traditional Chinese care, with outpatient clinics for the two systems operating side by side, and ward care based upon a blend of the two systems (Tung Shin Hospital 1967). This hospital is now in the process of shifting its orientation even more strongly away from Chinese tradition. The traditional outpatient clinic will soon be shifted to an older separate building, slightly downhill and symbolically removed from the main reception block, and new wards soon to be opened or constructed will operate, it is said, with greater emphasis than in the past on cosmopolitan practice. Chinese practitioners will, however, continue to work at the hospital into the indefinite future and it is apparent that this recognition of tradition is very important in retaining community support (for the hospital depends upon private financial contributions from the Chinese community of Kuala Lumpur and environs).

The Tung Shin Hospital is located beside the large modern Chinese

Maternity Hospital (established in 1924). This hospital, operated strictly along Western lines, is symbolic of the Chinese preference, probably throughout the Peninsula, for Western obstetrical care. Similar Chinese maternity hospitals or homes are found in at least nine other Peninsular cities and large towns. Home delivery is apparently now rare, not only in the cities but also in rural areas. A recent study of a predominantly Chinese "new village" in Selangor showed that 81 of 84 children in the study households had been born in hospitals, 69 in the nearest district hospital (6 miles away) and 12 in hospitals in Kuala Lumpur (20 miles away); only 3 had been delivered at home (Soong 1973).

Little is known about the utilization of government or private Western medical facilities by rural Chinese. The "new village study" (Soong 1973) cited above focuses on immunization status and demonstrates that government facilities rather than general practitioners are preferred by these villagers for the purpose of receiving immunizations. An extensive study of Chinese new villages by Nyce (1973) has little to say about health and medical care, but the importance of spirit mediums, as persons to be consulted for cures, is brought out. Nyce (1973:94,134) reports the presence of at least 15 or 16 such mediums in 5 new villages not far from Kuala Lumpur. This, and other urban data discussed below, suggest that Jain's (1973:157–158) comments about the medical views of South Indian Tamils on a Malaysian rubber estate may apply with equal force to the rural Chinese:

> The cost of medical consultations and medicines is another drain on the laborers' earnings. This is somewhat paradoxical, considering that medical services are provided free to all estate workers and their dependents. These services are fairly comprehensive and include treatment at the estate dispensary, hospitalization . . . and reimbursement of transportation costs for patients authorized . . . to visit an even bigger hospital at the national capital. The paradox is resolved, however, when it is realized that estate workers have a deep-seated mistrust of Western medicine and an equally strong faith in the efficacy of the indigenous pharmacopoeia.

Traditional Medicine Other Than Chinese

Jain, the author of the quotation in the preceding section, continues with a brief description of some of the Tamil forms of personal health behavior and indigenous medical practice. It is evident from this discussion that a rich and strong tradition of South Indian medicine persists in the rural Malaysian Tamil community, but little is known of it and almost nothing has been written on the subject. In the cities, traditional Indian practitioners are far less conspicuous than their Chinese and Malay counterparts. The "yellow pages" of the January 1973 telephone directory for Peninsular Malaysia carry dozens of listings relating to Chinese medicine but only two under the heading "Homeopathic & Ayurvedic Physicians." Friends in the Kuala Lumpur South Indian community tell the writer that there are a number of Ayurvedic dispensaries and practitioners in the city, but that most are not doing very well in competition wih the various forms of cosmopolitan (and Chinese?) practice. Thus it appears that Ayurvedic practice may be less vigorous in the urban than in the rural areas of the Peninsula, but this again is an hypothesis awaiting investigation. In any event the writer has not talked with any Chinese informants in Kuala Lumpur who are familiar with Indian medical traditions, and none is aware of friends or relatives who have visited Indian practitioners. Indian fortune-tellers, however, are consulted by members of all ethnic groups, including the Chinese. These persons, like their Chinese counterparts, offer a sympathetic (some might say, psychiatric) ear and on occasion provide preventive or curative advice. Thus they are marginal but not necessarily unimportant members of the supportive primary health care "system" in Malaysia.

Indian Unani (Arabic-Persian) medicine undoubtedly has its advocates and adherents in Malaysia, at least in the Indian Muslim community, but this subject, too, requires future study. The Arabic-Persian tradition is, of course, also represented in Malaysia as one element of contemporary Malay medicine (Gimlette 1929:18). As mentioned earlier, Malay medicine has been extensively studied by a long succession of scholars and scientists. The practitioners—the *bomoh,* the *pawang,* and the *bidan*—continue to be important and influential figures in many Malay communities, and without doubt will long continue to provide preventive, supportive, and even definitive care in the Malay health sectors (Chen 1969; Colson 1971). The *bomoh* is seen as an important resource by many non-Malays as well. Informants of varied ethnic background have told the author of their first-hand—or, more often, second-hand—knowledge of the value of a consultation with a *bomoh* for certain conditions of ill-health, especially those thought to be manifestations of intervention by supernatural forces.

The *bomoh* practitioners or *halak* (*halaa'*) persons of the Malayan aborigines (*Orang Asli*) are seen by some traditional Chinese, Malays, and other non-Orang Asli as even more powerful allies in mediation with the supernatural world because of their knowledge of the forest and the secrets of their natural surroundings. Two of the parttime *bomoh2* in a Temuan village where the writer once lived offered their specialist skills to outsiders. One, a young man of considerable renown in northern Selangor, was frequently consulted in 1966—1968—and still is today—by Chinese, Malays, and others of the town and countryside on behalf of relatives suffering from epilepsy and other forms of mental disorder. The writer witnessed one of his extraordinary curing performances and learned from him of other successes, and failures. The other *bomoh,* who has since died, was primarily an herbalist. An expert botanist, he searched the forests for herbs and sold them, with specific therapeutic instructions, to a circle of rural residents of all ethnic backgrounds. He also marketed herbs in bulk, supplying medical halls through one or several Chinese traders.

Personal Health Behavior Within Chinese Tradition

T'ai Chi Chuan

Chinese philosophic tradition contains a strong preventive element, closely tied to the balancing dualism of *yin-yang*. The *T'ai Chi* or "Great Origin" of all things, which produced the two interacting principles of the *yin-yang*, is indeed incorporated in the name *T'ai Chi Chuan* ("Great Origin Fist") given to those calisthenics that are perhaps the most conspicuous expression of one's personal commitment, as a Chinese, to health maintenance through preventive behavior. Although these exercises are often associated with "self-defense" it is only the advanced student, in command of the classic 128 movements, who can make full use of the art for such purposes. For most Chinese the basic movements simply provide exercise, with emphasis on relaxation and control, in the interest of continued good health (Cheng 1973). *T'ai Chi Chuan* is widely practiced in Malaysia and Singapore, although more often by middle-aged and older men than by women or younger men. For women, especially, it tends to be identified with an economic status that allows for leisure-time, and thus for practice of the exercises. But on any rainless evening, just at dusk, one may see dozens of male *T'ai Chi* enthusiasts at their exercises on the lawns and playing fields of central Kuala Lumpur. *T'ai Chi* classes are popular, and a school, recently established in the city, now has some 300 students of all ages and both sexes. Instruction in Chinese medicine is considered a normal part of the training to become a *T'ai Chi* instructor, and many instructors are said to be skilled in bone-setting and the treatment of sprains and strains. One of the most famous *T'ai Chi* instructors in Kuala Lumpur, an elderly man who received his training in China many years ago, is indeed famous locally as a bone-setter. It is clear that it is difficult to draw a line between *T'ai Chi Chuan* and preventive or even curative medicine.

Cuisine

Cuisine is another important and obvious expression of the preventive element in Chinese philosophy, for the balanced and considerate use of foods is considered essential to maintenance of good health. Malaysian Chinese cuisine is rich and varied, the subject of great interest both within and without the Chinese community. At table with Chinese friends, in home or restaurant, one never quite forgets that the arts of cooking and dining are intimately tied to biological and social health. Personal food behavior is subject to important modifications at certain points in the life cycle, and in case of illness the Chinese physician gives his patient's food habits special attention and often recommends temporary or permanent modifications in diet. Every Chinese practitioner with whom the author has talked in Kuala Lumpur has given some time to the subject of food in the course of describing his approaches to therapy. Without doubt, most Malaysian Chinese see food behavior and health as very closely tied together. Manifestations of this attitude include ideas about "balance" in cuisine, concepts of "hot" and "cold" foods, wide recognition of the need to observe certain food taboos during confinement, and the widespread use of medicinal teas and herbal or other remedies that border on being "foods."

Medicinal teas

In old Kuala Lumpur, in the vicinity of Petaling Street, one can find more than 20 medicinal tea stalls, patronized with great regularity by the Chinese citizens of the neighborhood and by visitors to the thriving evening street markets of the area. Each stall—a wooden box on wheels with an upright advertising frame—supports fine brass brewing vessels, cups and glasses, and the other paraphernalia required for preparing herbal teas. The stalls are located in traditional streetside spots and are usually handed-on from parents to offspring. At one such stall the young man in charge told us of his 8 years in service on the same site since inheriting the stall from his father. He works from 11 in the morning until 11 at night, selling four varieties of tea—sugarcane and *lallang* root extract as a "cooling" tea (10 Malaysian cents); "cooling" chrysanthemum tea, especially good for eye conditions (20 cents); *wong loh khat,* dark bitter medicinal tea, very popular in Kuala Lumpur as a preventative (30 cents); and Korean *ginseng* flower tea, especially for sore throats (50 cents). Hundreds of passers-by purchase these and similar teas every day, not only at this site, but in many such localities up and down the length of Peninsular Malaysia. The customers are predominantly but not exclusively Chinese. The popularity of these teas is still another measure of adherence to Chinese health tradition.

Confinement

Confinement behavior in the Chinese community provides one of the finest illustrations of the continuity of tradition in Malaysia. This is a little-investigated field that merits attention, not only in Malaysia, but on a comparative basis in Chinese communities in other parts of the world. The details of observance, their variety and specificity, studied comparatively, could be a valuable measure of adherence to tradition in matters of personal and family health. Described are Cantonese confinement customs as they obtain today in the states of Selangor and Johore. Informants repeatedly emphasized that confinement practices differ among the dialect groups, but the author did not question outside the Cantonese community.

During pregnancy there are few food taboos to be observed, even in the most traditional households. Mutton is often forbidden, however, because of a common belief that its consumption may cause the child to be epileptic. This is related to the similarity of the words for "lamb" and "epilepsy" in Cantonese. "Cooling" foods are generally avoided, although not forbidden. Alcohol consumption is permitted but only in small quantities. Special herbal teas are taken, as tonics in early pregnancy and to "strengthen the womb" in the eighth month. There is a general belief that overeating should be avoided to prevent the development of an overly heavy fetus. No feasts or special foods are associated with pregnancy in Malaysian Cantonese custom.

Delivery is normally accomplished in a hospital or maternity home, as above noted, this generalization applying even in the most traditional families. During labor the prospective mother is encouraged to chew dried *ginseng* for strength. This appears to be a common practice, regardless of where the delivery takes place. After a normal delivery the mother and child usually remain 4 or 5 days in hospital and then return home, to seclusion if the family is traditional. This seclusion may last only a few days if the family is poor and the mother must return to work, but in normal circumstances the postpartum period of seclusion lasts 1 month, that is, 28 days according to the Chinese lunar calendar. Today, a name for the newborn is generally selected before birth so that the name can be provided for hospital and other records shortly after delivery. In the past the first proper name that the baby would be given would be determined during the postpartum confinement month, upon consultation with an astrologer. A practice still widely observed is to keep the child's time of birth secret, to prevent the child from being exposed to danger.

The period of postpartum confinement is a time of pollution, for the new mother, her child, and those who assist in her care. If members of the family participate in her care they cannot pray at the home shrine or at the temple until they have cleansed themselves ritually at the end of the period of seclusion. If the family can afford her, a specialist servant *(p'ui yuet)* is employed for the first postpartum month. These servants are in considerable demand; they cook and care for the mother and child, thus freeing the family from polluting influences. The servant knows how to prepare and serve the traditional foods, and how to protect the mother and child from untoward influences. The mother and child must be kept warm, away from draughts, secluded in the house and away from people. All bathing and drinking water should be warm, fans are forbidden, and warm clothing is required.

Throughout the seclusion period there is a taboo on "cooling" foods such as green vegetables, fruits, and fish; and on meat other than chicken and pork. (A young, well educated woman of the author's acquaintance teaches home economics at the secondary school level; she is well-versed in the principles of good nutrition, i.e. in Western terms. While prepared—during a recent confinement—to accept all of the restrictions that her mother-in-law imposed upon her, she nevertheless quietly supplemented her diet with quantities of vitamin C tablets because of fears that her own health and that of her breastfed baby would otherwise suffer from a lack of fruits and vegetables.)

While many foods are taboo, others are specially indicated during the seclusion period. Instead of the normal light breakfast and two full meals per day, the mother is encouraged to take four full meals, with stress on "warming" foods. Rice, pork, and chicken are acceptable foods.

Alcohol consumption is strongly encouraged, especially brandy or Bene-
dictine (for those who can afford it), or at least rice wine. The 12th
postpartum day is marked by a special meal which is prepared in the
home and carried around to friends and relatives in the neighborhood.
This event provides public recognition of the birth. The special foods
for this feast include pig's feet cooked with fresh ginger and dark vinegar,
and a rich chicken wine soup prepared with sliced ginger, peanuts, and
dark fungus. The same special meal is prepared again on the "Day of
the Full Moon Ceremony," the end of the seclusion month, announced
by sending red-dyed hard-boiled eggs and pickled ginger to the homes of
relatives and friends. But on this occasion the feast is consumed in the
home, after the mother and child have been bathed, freeing themselves
of the "milk scent," and after the mother has prayed. Family members
who have provided care during seclusion must bathe and pray in the
same fashion. On the Full Moon day close friends and relatives visit
the home, bringing *angpow* (red packet) gifts of money, or pieces of
jewelry for the infant. Depending upon the views of the family the baby
may or may not be protected at this stage, and for months or even years to
come, by wearing an amulet to ward off evil forces.

The practices outlined above are interwoven with ideas about protection of the mother, the child, and the household from misfortune, and
especially from disease. Many of the customs may indeed be protective,
especially against such hazards as staphylococcal infection of the newborn
and maternal mastitis. According to informants this Cantonese pattern
of behavior is still widespread in Malaysia and unlikely to fade away.
The guardians of these traditions are the mothers and grandmothers;
their daughters, however non-traditional their views, will generally accede
to their elder's wishes at the time of their confinement, and so the tradition is maintained.

Self-medication

The above section on medicinal teas lists a few varieties available at
one of the stalls in Kuala Lumpur. These fall into two categories: curative teas (such as *ginseng* flower tea when used for sore throat) and
preventative teas (such as *wong loh khat*). The Chinese medical halls
(herbal medicine shops) of Malaysia's towns and cities make available
a great array of other preparations, especially tonics and ointments, that
may be purchased for prevention or cure, either upon the advice of a
Chinese physician or upon one's own initiative (or that of a relative).
In discussions with the proprietors of several medical halls the author
learned that self-medication is widely practiced in the Chinese community
but chiefly through the use of patent preparations and widely-advertised
tonics (including certain popular alcoholic beverages). Traditional herbs,
or herbal mixtures, are much less often purchased for personal use
without the guidance of an herbalist-medical hall proprietor or a Chinese
physician. To this there are exceptions, however, such as the widespread
use by Malaysian Chinese women of herbal tonic teas, for example

tang kuei (Angelica sinensis), for "cleansing the blood" after the end of the menstrual period.

Charms and talismans

Still another element of personal health behavior is that directed toward one's relationship with supernatural forces. Of the types of behavior so far considered, that in this category would seem least likely to survive among those whose orientation is strongly modernist. The author's informants are agreed, however, that many "superstitious" people still resort to charms and talismans, and consult temple spirit mediums or sidewalk fortune tellers for medical advice. Even the *Tung Seng* Chinese almanac, widely purchased each year and consulted by many Malaysian Chinese families, provides a section on charms and spells. Many hawkers of talismans, especially itinerant Nepalese, do a thriving streetside business in the cities and larger towns of the Peninsula. Topley (1953) has described in detail the paper charms and paper sheets employed as adjuncts to Chinese worship in Singapore some 20 years ago. Their use continues today in Kuala Lumpur and undoubtedly elsewhere in Malaysia and Singapore. They may be burned, fastened to walls or door frames, or used as amulets to protect against evil spirits and influences. They may also be taken as medicines, either by compressing them into pellets for swallowing or by burning them and collecting the ashes for consumption with water or tea.

Paramedical Practitioners and Other Supports Within Chinese Tradition

In this brief section note is taken of several types of "paramedical" support that should not be overlooked in any holistic consideration of Chinese medical care in Peninsular Malaysia.

Several kinds of paramedical workers have already been mentioned, medicinal tea vendors, for example, and fortune tellers. Many of the latter, described as "streetside psychiatrists" by one informant, are good listeners who provide sympathetic advice to those who consult them. The "fortune" that the bird, cards, sticks, or palm-reading produces may, in many instances, be less significant than the "therapeutic conversation."

The presence of temple mediums in Chinese rural villages—former new villages—has also been noted. Nyce comments (1973:134):

> "Certain families are known to patronize mediums. Perhaps the most common reason for consulting a medium is to seek a cure for illness. . . . The medium, after dialogue with the gods, which may or may not be accomplished through a trance, may prescribe a particular herb, instruct what else is to be done, or may even advise hospitalization."

Such mediums are associated with urban temples as well, in Kuala Lumpur and throughout the Peninsula. Spirit mediums have been studied rather extensively in Singapore (e.g. Elliott 1955; Topley 1956) but have received less attention in Malaysia (although see Stirling 1924).

A useful summary of spirit mediumship in Malaysia can be found in Chen (1971), and a discussion of its psychotherapeutic aspects has recently been published by Teoh (1973).

Another community resource worthy of note is the residential religious institution, a category which Topley (1956) prefers not to include in her classification of Chinese "temples." Some of these institutions play important sociomedical roles as lodging places for the old and dying. Topley, in another paper (1954), has described the functioning of one such set of institutions: the Chinese women's vegetarian houses in Singapore. Comparable residential arrangements for the very old can be found in Kuala Lumpur in what are familiarly referred to as "temples" on the outskirts near the city's largest Chinese burial ground. Other lodging places in Kuala Lumpur for the very elderly and chronically infirm are run on non-religious lines. The Tung Shin Hospital also provides ward space for very elderly persons who do not necessarily require clinical care.

Chinese Traditional Medicine in Peninsular Malaysia

The tradition of Chinese medicine is strong and growing stronger every year, notwithstanding the strength and growth of cosmopolitan medicine in Malaysia. The Chinese community supports traditional medicine and turns to it for many health problems. Even the least traditional of Malaysian Chinese seem to turn back to Chinese medicine for selected medical complaints, especially after failing to gain relief from other sources. Furthermore, non-Chinese frequently consult Chinese physicians and medical-hall herbalists. International interest in medical developments in China—especially in acupuncture—has stimulated younger, modernist Malaysians to learn more about these practices and associated traditions. Increasing numbers of foreign visitors to Malaysia have also been seeking out Chinese physicians for treatment by or instruction in acupuncture technique.

Interest within the Chinese community is further sustained by *The China Press* (a Chinese-language newspaper published in Kuala Lumpur) which devotes a half-page every Thursday to Chinese medicine. The issue of November 15, 1973 carried number 1245 in a series started in 1948 and edited for many years by Mr. Ngeow Sze Chan, one of Malaysia's leading Chinese physicians. The contributions are written locally or edited from material published elsewhere, including both modern and classical articles from China. Number 1245 carried four articles under the following titles: "Correction of false theory on typhoid and dysentery," "Talking about physiotherapy," "Memoir of my village clinical study" (in China), and "General outline of damp sickness" (that is, rheumatism, etc.). A study of this immense collection of published materials, written and assembled over a span of 25 years, might prove very rewarding. Cuttings from the newspaper are collected and bound at quarterly intervals for distribution to the members of the Chinese Physicians' Association of Central Malaya.

The beginnings of Chinese medicine in Malaysia are commented on by Dr. Gwee Ah Leng, a Western-trained physician of Singapore with a keen interest in Chinese medical theory and practice:

> Malaysian Chinese came to Malaya at a period when Chinese medicine was at its height, and its concepts were being accepted officially and privately as the basis for health and illness. The absence of a comparable system of medicine at that time in Malaya permitted Chinese medicine to flourish, and become firmly entrenched, so that the Malaysian health concept even to the present day has a very strong Chinese medical flavor (Gwee 1971:102).

In the early days of settlement in the Peninsula all fully-trained Chinese physicians obtained their education in China, and this continued to be the case until after World War II. Other practitioners, who had received more limited training as apprentices, also began to work in the Peninsula at an early stage, and some continue even today to establish themselves, usually after apprenticeships, as self-proclaimed *Sinseh* practitioners. After 1945, some of those Chinese physicians who had received their training in China, concerned about maintaining good standards of practice, established a school for Chinese physicians in Singapore. The first group of students began studies in 1948 and graduated in 1952 after completing a 4-year parttime course. Some of these graduates are today among the leading Chinese physicians of Singapore and Malaysia. The Singapore school continues to offer a 4-year course, now nearly full-time (requiring afternoon and evening study). A new group of 20 students begins the course of study every 2 years.

World War II and the postwar period brought to a halt the easy movement back and forth between the Peninsula and China that had prevailed in earlier decades. A sense of isolation, and an appreciation of the need to rely on local resources, grew up in Chinese medical circles in Malaya and Singapore in postwar years. This was probably a major factor behind the educational and associational movements that emerged in the years after 1945. Possibly this sense of isolation accounts for differences between the Peninsula and Hongkong in this respect. Marjorie Topley (personal communication, July 1971) has noted the limited tendency toward creation of traditional Chinese medical associations in Hongkong.

In Malaya the first step toward nationwide association took place on December 19, 1946 when the Malayan Chinese Medical Association (MCMA) was established. By the end of the year 87 members were listed, with their registration confirmed by the Kuomintang in China. In 1948 another association, the Chinese Physicians' Association (CPA) of Central Malaya, was set up without ties to China. On January 1, 1954 the MCMA merged into the CPA of Central Malaya. In the spring of 1955, a broader organization—the Pan Malayan Chinese Physicians' Association—was founded, also without any ties to China. This Pan Malayan organization represented the CPA of Central Malaya, and Chinese physicians' associations in other Malayan towns and Singapore.

More recently the Pan Malayan CPA became the Federation of Chinese Physicians & Medicine-Dealers Associations of Malaysia-Singapore, but in the fall of 1973 a cleavage occurred as the CPA of Singapore left the Federation. At this writing the Federation of Malaysian associations brings together the CPA of Central Malaya and CPAs of Sabah, Sarawak, and several Malaysian towns including Penang, Ipoh, Seremban, Johore Baru, and Kuantan—as well as a group of medicine-dealers' associations. Mr. Ngeow Sze Chan, previously mentioned as editor of *The China Press* medical series, has been behind many of the developments described above. A leading and very active Chinese physician, educated in the prewar period in China, he is currently Chairman of the Federation, Chairman of the CPA of Central Malaya, and Principal of the Chinese Medical Training Institute of Malaya.

In November 1973 the membership of the CPA of Central Malaya (that is, Kuala Lumpur and environs) stood at 157. Mr. Ngeow estimates that the total number of Chinese physicians in Peninsular Malaysia today is about 1,000. Most are speakers of Cantonese, Hakka, or Hokkien. Of these about 500 are members of CPAs and thus are recognized by their colleagues as fully qualified. Of these physicians about 200 were educated at the Chinese Medical Training Institute in Kuala Lumpur; an unknown number at similar institutes in Penang, Ipoh, and Batu Pahat (a school in Johore, now defunct); and most of the remainder at the institute in Singapore. Of those who came to prewar Malaya after completing their training in China, only a dwindling few continue in practice. Most of the 500 non-CPA physicians in Peninsular Malaysia are men who have entered practice on their own, usually after completing apprenticeships. Many are specialists in such fields as bone-setting, treatment of nasal disorders, and treatment of piles. About 100 of these are in practice in Kuala Lumpur. The CPA physicians tend to regard these practitioners with some concern lest their actions impair the public image of the profession as a whole. Mr. Ngeow's estimate for Singapore is a total of about 500 Chinese physicians and other less fully qualified practitioners.

The Chinese Medical Training Institute of Malaya began accepting students in August 1955 and was officially opened October 1, 1955. The first class met in a school building near the Tung Shin Hospital. In the spring of 1959 the institute moved into its present three storey building where classes are held on the floors above a free medical clinic. Volunteer instructors, other physicians, and students of the institute work together in the clinic, which is open to the public from mid-morning until mid-afternoon, and in the evening, every day except Sunday. Since 1971 the Institute has also offered postgraduate instruction for advanced clinical investigation. Averaging about 20 graduates every 2 years since 1954, the alumni so far number about 200. There were 26 graduates in the 1970 class, one of the largest groups to finish the course.

The institute course extends over a 4-year period, with 3 terms per year. Instruction is carried on every evening except Sunday for 3 to 4 hours. Tuition is 15 Malaysian dollars per month, and admission depends upon attainment of at least the Form 5 level School Certificate, and proficiency in *gwo-yu* (Mandarin). The students seem to be drawn primarily from the Hakka, Hokkien, and Cantonese dialect groups. The most recently admitted class, now in its second year, began with about 50 students and has trimmed down to about 30 who are expected to complete the course. (It is estimated that there are about 80 students in Malaysia's 3 institutes at this writing.) [3] Many of the dropouts are women who leave because of marriage; a few of the continuing students are female but most of the graduates will continue to be male, as in the past.

Instruction stresses Chinese medical theory, diagnosis (with special attention to pulses), and herbal, acupuncture, and moxibustion therapy. Traditional massage and bone-setting are not included in the curriculum. Texts, anatomical models, acupuncture supplies, and periodicals come from China, either directly or through Hongkong. Instruction is also offered in Western medical theory and therapeutic principles, and diseases are considered from both perspectives. Thus the graduates have the potential training for cooperative practice with their Western-trained counterparts. At the Tung Shin Hospital this cooperative or blended approach to medical care has been in effect for some years, but there are no other institutions in Kuala Lumpur where Chinese and cosmopolitan practice normally intersect. At the end of each year of work the students take a series of examinations, and upon graduation they receive a certificate that is recognized by the various Chinese Physicians' Associations, but not by the government.

Many Chinese physicians who are members of the CPA of Central Malaya are in favor of government registration, but only for those who have completed training in one of the institutes. Early in 1973 the Ministry of Health gave some consideration to the possibility of such registration but, for the present at least, no action is likely, in part because of difficulties in deciding who should or should not be registered, and in part because of opposition to the idea from cosmopolitan-trained physicians. However, as in many other countries, there is an increasing awareness in Malaysia of the importance of non-Western practitioners and other indigenous paramedical workers as contributors to the national medical effort. Such a view was expressed several years ago by the Editor of the *Medical Journal of Malaya,* under the title "Medical manpower in a rapidly expanding population": Chinese herbalists, *sinsehs* (Chinese physicians), and others "who practice traditional and indigenous forms of medicine should be taken into consideration when assessing the medical manpower of the country since they represent the unmet demands for qualified medical personnel" (Sandosham 1968:150).

The new graduates of the institute in Kuala Lumpur face considerable competition, like their Western-trained counterparts, if they choose to stay in the city. It is said that comfortable practices can readily be established in Malaysia's towns, but most graduates prefer to stay in the largest cities. Some support themselves in other jobs and practice parttime or as volunteers at the free clinic attached to the institute. Many other graduates take positions as resident physicians in association with medical halls (herbal medicine shops). Typically, the physician holds office hours throughout the day when the hall is open. He provides prescriptions which the patient can fill immediately in the shop, and he, or an assistant, may also employ acupuncture-moxibustion therapy. Often the physician also provides psychotherapeutic support and advice on diet and exercise. Quite often he will recommend that a patient see a Western physician or go to the government hospital. A few successful physicians own their own medical halls, but most are dependent upon their modest fees, which are standardized by the CPA. Most of the writer's informants in Kuala Lumpur agree that about 25 to 30 percent of their patients are not Chinese; this is also the approximate percentage of non-Chinese customers in the medical halls. The percentage of customers other than Chinese is probably even higher in most small-town medical halls.

A few Chinese physicians in Kuala Lumpur practice in Western-style offices or office suites, as individuals or in small groups. Like medical hall proprietors they must purchase business licenses but are not subject to other government regulation. These physicians tend to place greater emphasis on acupuncture-moxibustion than on herbal remedies, and some are nearly full-time acupuncture specialists of considerable renown. They keep abreast of current developments in acupuncture therapy in China and elsewhere, and use this form of treatment in a truly innovative fashion, often with electrical stimulating equipment and complex manipulations of needles, voltage, frequency, and stimulation time. Among the most recent institute graduates are at least a few young physicians with strong interests in research, especially in acupuncture therapy. One spoke with the author of his future hopes for a Chinese medicine research institution in Malaysia. These physicians prefer to prescribe packaged and standardized herbal medicines, imported from China, rather than the dried herb preparations that are compounded in the local medical halls. Especially they emphasize the predictability of results that standardization of dosage provides; of course most medical halls also sell these imported preparations.

It has been difficult to collect data on the medical halls. Certainly they can be found in every Malaysian town and in great numbers in the cities. According to best estimates there may be 200 such shops in Kuala Lumpur alone, and more than 1,000 in Peninsular Malaysia. An inspection of the "yellow pages" in the January 1973 Peninsular Malaysian telephone directory revealed the following: 33 "pharmacies" (6 in Kuala Lumpur)—these are the only legal outlets for Western prescription drugs; and 261 listings under "herbs" or "medical halls" (53 in Kuala Lumpur)—outlets for medicinal herbs and patent medicines as well. Almost all of the names in the listings under herbs and medical halls are Chinese, certainly including surnames representative of all the major dialect groups. These listings reveal a geographical distribution of shops which correlates well with the distribution of the Chinese population in the Peninsula. The traditional herbal medicine shop carries a formidable inventory of crude herbs and other preparations. An inventory taken in Chinese medical halls in Singapore in the 1920's totaled 456 drugs— 415 of plant origin, 29 from animal sources, and 12 minerals (Hooper 1929). Many shops today carry similar arrays of drugs, supplemented by scores of patent medicines.

To return to the beginning of this brief survey, the author is convinced of the continuing strength of Malaysian Chinese traditional medicine. The findings of Gwee and coworkers (1969) for Singapore surely apply as well to Kuala Lumpur, and to the Peninsular States in general. Gwee found, in a 1958 survey of Chinese hospital patients in one medical unit for acute conditions, that at least 90 percent admitted to having received Chinese medicine prior to admission, or were still receiving such medicine. Other studies by Gwee nd colleagues in 1966–1967, reported in the same paper, also demonstrate the continued adherence of Singapore Chinese to their medical tradition. No similar publications or other documentation seem to exist for Kuala Lumpur or other Malaysian cities, but the strength of this medical system is amply reflected in the vigor of the Chinese physicians' associations and training institutes, the abundance of prospering medical halls, and the comments of many informants—practitioners, patients, lay observers, and students.

Summary and Concluding Comment

In this paper is attempted an overview of medical care in the Chinese communities of Peninsular Malaysia. The Chinese are first examined in terms of their representation in the national population, their ethnicity (dialect groups), and their settlement preferences. The idea of the health sector is discussed, and the basic Chinese health sectors are noted. Medical care is then described, beginning with Chinese utilization of the cosmopolitan or Western medical system and the other non-Chinese traditional systems of the Peninsula. Personal health behavior, paramedical practitioners, and institutional supports that conform to Chinese tradition are examined next, and the description concludes with a review of *contemporary* Chinese *traditional* medical practice in the Peninsula States.

These words—contemporary and traditional—are deliberately employed together to emphasize that Malaysian Chinese medicine today, although firmly rooted in tradition, is also a modern, innovative, changing system. The youngest Malaysian practitioners, and some of their elders, are alert to new developments within their therapeutic domains, show a strong interest in research and in maintaining high educational standards, and are trying very hard to determine how their practice fits within the broader system of Malaysian national health and medical care. They are not alone in this search, for some of the most thoughtful practitioners and proponents of Malay medicine (and, undoubtedly, Ayurvedic medicine) are asking the same questions. On the other hand

—in the cosmopolitan tradition—there is a growing awareness of the significance of traditional medicine as a medical resource, but much more exchange of information and two-way communication is needed, as in the United States and so many other countries with diverse medical traditions. In the face of rapid population growth and limited resources for expansion of cosmopolitan care, it is obvious that traditional medicine is not going to diminish or disappear from Malaysia in the decades ahead. On the other hand, in the present state of knowledge, it is impossible to make any predictions about possible blending or merging of some of Malaysia's diverse forms of medical care. This is an important research question for the future—as a part of a much-needed development of Malaysian research in comparative medical systems.

Acknowledgments

The author is indebted to many persons in the Chinese community of Kuala Lumpur who generously gave time for interviews. To all of those who are not mentioned by name sincere gratitude is acknowledged. Particularly thanked is Mr. Ngeow Sze Chan, Principal of the Chinese Medical Training Institute in Kuala Lumpur, for his courteous support and aid. Above all, thanks to the author's good friend, Mr. Yap Loy Fong of the Institute for Medical Research, for his invaluable assistance in arranging and conducting interviews, and for his advice and guidance in so many other ways.

NOTES

1. A recent special issue of the *Scientific American* devoted to "the role of medicine in human life" (with special reference to the United States) has nothing whatever to say about alternative or traditional modes of medical care, even in the otherwise excellent introductory article by White (1973).

2. An additional option for medical care open to Malaysian Chinese or, of course, to other Malaysians is the trip "in search of a cure," perhaps to China or Hongkong. This option does not require further discussion here.

3. A new class of 50 students, selected from about 80 applicants, began studies at the institute in Kuala Lumpur on January 7, 1974.

REFERENCES

AHLUWALIA, H. S. and J. B. DUGUID
1966   Malignant tumors in Malaya. British Journal of Cancer 20: 12–15.

BALASUNDARAM, R.
1970   Cardiovascular disease in a West Malaysian town. A survey in general practice. Transactions Royal Society Tropical Medicine & Hygiene 64:607–614.

CHAI, H. C.
1964   The Development of British Malaya 1896–1909. London, New York, and Kuala Lumpur: Oxford University Press. 364 pages.

CHANDLER, R. ed.
1972   1970 Population and Housing Census of Malaysia. Community Groups. Department of Statistics, Malaysia; Kuala Lumpur. 292 pages.

CHEN, P. C. Y.
1969   Spirits and medicine-men among rural Malays. Far East Medical Journal 5:84–87.

1971   Unlicensed medical practice in West Malaysia. Tropical and Geographical Medicine 23:173-183.

CHENG, M. C.
1973   T'ai Chi Chuan. A Simplified Method of Calisthenics for Health and Self Defense. Malaysian Edition. Ipoh, Malaysia: Strand Book Co. 170 pages.

COLSON, A. C.
1971   The Prevention of Illness in a Malay Village: an Analysis of Concepts and Behavior. Developing Nations Monograph Series II, No. 1, Overseas Research Center, Wake Forest University, Winston-Salem, North Carolina. 156 pages.

DUNN, F. L.
1972   Intestinal parasitism in Malayan aborigines (Orang Asli). Bulletin World Health Organization 46:99–113.

ELLIOTT, A. J. A.
1955   Chinese Spirit-Medium Cults in Singapore. London School of Economics Monographs on Social Anthropology No. 14. London: The Athlone Press, University of London.

FIELD, J. W.
  1951 The historical, racial and cultural background of Western medicine. *In* The Institute for Medical Research 1900–1950. Studies from the Institute for Medical Research, Federation of Malaya, Jubilee Volume No. 25 Chapter I, pp. 1–36. Kuala Lumpur: The Government Press.

GIMLETTE, J. D.
  1929 Malay Poisons and Charm Cures. Third Edition. J. & A. Churchill, London. 301 pages. Reprinted as Oxford in Asia paperback, 1971. Kuala Lumpur and Singapore: Oxford University Press, 156 pages.

GWEE, A. L.
  1971 Traditional Chinese methods of mental treatment. *In* Psychological Problems and Treatment in Malaysia, N. W. Wagner and E. S. Tan (editors) pp. 102–114. Kuala Lumpur: University of Malaya Press, 156 pages.

GWEE, A. L., Y. K. LEE, and N. B. THAM
  1969 A study of Chinese medical practice in Singapore. Singapore Medical Journal 10:2–7.

HOOPER, D.
  1929 On Chinese medicine: drugs of Chinese pharmacies in Malaya. The Gardens' Bulletin, Straits Settlements 6:1–163.

JAIN, R. K.
  1973 South Indians on the Plantation Frontier in Malaya. University of Malaya Press, Kuala Lumpur and Singapore; and Yale University Press, New Haven and London. 460 pages.

MALAY MAIL, THE
  1973 "Good news! You will live longer." Anonymous newspaper article. Issue of 8 December 1973, page 24.

NEWELL, W. H.
  1962 Treacherous River. A study of Rural Chinese in North Malaya. Kuala Lumpur: University of Malaya Press, 233 pages.

NOORDIN, R. A.
  1973 Health and social programmes for the pre-school child—1. Ministry of Health. Bulletin, Public Health Society, Malayan Medical Association 7:35–39.

NYCE, R.
  1973 Chinese New Villages in Malaya. A Community Study. Singapore and Kuala Lumpur: Malaysian Sociological Research Institute, 278 pages.

OOI, J. B.
  1963 Land, People and Economy in Malaya. London: Longmans, Green and Co., 426 pages.

PURCELL, V.
  1967   The Chinese in Malaya. London, Hongkong, and Kuala Lumpur: Oxford University Press, 327 pages. (Originally published in 1948.)

SANDHU, K. S.
  1973   Introduction. Emergency resettlement in Malaysia pp. 24–65. *In* Nyce, R. Chinese New Villages in Malaya. A Community Study. Singapore and Kuala Lumpur: Malaysian Sociological Research Institute, 278 pages.

SANDOSHAM, A. A.
  1968   Medical manpower in a rapidly expanding population. Medical Journal of Malaya 23:146–151.

SHANMUGARATNAM, K. and A. WEE
  1972   Ethnic/dialect group variations in cancer incidence in a Chinese population pp. 16–17. *In* Abstracts of Papers, B. Applications, Abstract 8. Conference on Host-Environment Interactions in Etiology of Cancer in Man—Implementation in Research, Primosten, Yugoslavia, August 27–September 2, 1972.

SKEAT, W. W.
  1900   Malay Magic. An Introduction to the Folklore and Popular Religion of the Malay Peninsula. London: Macmillan & Co. (Second impression, 1965, Frank Cass & Co., London) 685 pages.

SOONG, F. S.
  1973   The immunization status of some pre-school children in a new village in West Malaysia. Bulletin, Public Health Society, Malayan Medical Association 7:50–53.

STIRLING, W. G.
  1924   Chinese exorcists. Journal of the Malayan Branch Royal Asiatic Society 2:41–47.

TEOH, J. I.
  1973   Chinese spirit-mediumship: its sociocultural interpretation and psychotherapeutic aspects. Singapore Med. Journal 14:55–61.

TOPLEY, M.
  1953   Paper charms, and paper sheets as adjuncts to Chinese worship. Journal of the Malayan Branch Royal Asiatic Society 26:63–80.

TOPLEY, M.
  1954   Chinese women's vegetarian houses in Singapore. Journal of the Malayan Branch Royal Asiatic Society 27:51–67.

TOPLEY, M.
  1956   Chinese religion and religious institutions in Singapore. Journal of the Malayan Branch Royal Asiatic Society 29:70–118.

TUNG SHIN HOSPITAL
  1967   Rules of the Selangor Tung Shin Hospital, Kuala Lumpur. 25
         August 1967. Booklet in English and Chinese. Kuala Lumpur:
         The China Press.

WHITE, K. L.
  1973   Life and death and medicine. Scientific American 229(3):
         23–33.

CHAPTER 8

COMMENTS ON CONTEMPORARY SOCIOCULTURAL STUDIES OF MEDICINE IN CHINESE SOCIETIES

BERNARD GALLIN

The six chapters[1] presented in this section of the book raise questions: Why are social scientists involved in a conference on the comparative study of traditional and modern medicine in Chinese societies? What are the reasons for and the value of their study of the phenomena of health, illness and medical practice in China? The reason for the participation of some derives from an interest in the ways in which the culturally-derived concepts of a society influence health, illness and medical delivery systems. The reason for the involvement of others lies in a concern with the ways in which cultural and social factors influence people's perception of and response to medical care. The ultimate value of these social scientists' study of these phenomena, however, is that it provides insights into the dynamics of culture process and culture change in China.

As Fabrega and Silver have noted: "The perception of illness, in effect, is one more example of the way behavior is structured and organized by underlying culture rules. And an analysis of medical treatment may allow access to beliefs regarding religious and malevolent agencies, giving the anthropologists some idea of the ultimate values that the culture holds sacred" (1973: 4). In addition, they say that ". . . changing strategies when dealing with disease often initiate and always reflect other complex changes that can be observed in a social-cultural group, giving the anthropologists a rich area for development and testing of theory" (1973: 4).

It is unfortunate that until recently little attention has been given to culturally-derived concepts and perceptions of health and illness in China. Social scientists concerned with the interrelationships between culture, society, health and illness, seldom have focused their research on China. Those scholars who have worked in China usually have superimposed separate and distinct Western categories such as philosophy, religion, politics, social structure, or economics on the Chinese reality; rarely have they allowed the Chinese interactional view of the world to come to the surface. These six chapters, however, all authored by social scientists specializing in the study of Chinese society, represent a different approach; they look at health and illness in China in terms of a larger cultural picture. They make it abundantly clear that an understanding of medical phenomena in China is possible only if it is based on a thorough knowledge of the Chinese cultural and historical context.

Several themes concerning the relationship between health, illness and culture in Chinese society emerge out of these chapters. (I apologize in advance if I seem to neglect some of the chapters; all of them have influenced and stimulated my thinking.) One theme runs through all of them; perceptions of health and illness in China are influenced by—in a sense are intertwined with—its values and world views, religio-philosophical beliefs, and even its political thought and system. For example, Anderson in his paper describes the way in which the Chinese dietary system, and consequently nutrition and health, are influenced by the folk concept of hot and cold; a concept closely related to certain philosophical and religious aspects of Chinese life. As Anderson notes, ". . . dietary beliefs center around maintaining harmony, conceptualized as part of the need to maintain a general harmony of *yang* and *yin* in the system, and balance . . ."[2]

Political philosophy and the concept of "moral uprightness" also are related to health and illness in China. For example, it long has been believed in China that moral breakdown in a ruler or in any person of high standing eventually will cause a breakdown in the entire sociopolitical system. Such a breakdown can be remedied only by the righting of the moral problem of the ruler, or by changing the ruler: a change which is legitimized through the concept of the "Mandate of Heaven." The relationship of the concept of moral uprightness and moral breakdown to the general health and welfare of the population is neatly paralleled in the conceptualization of illness and its causes in China.

In my own research we found that the explanation more frequently given for many illnesses brought to ritualistic curers and to secular traditional Chinese medical practitioners was some kind of moral breakdown in social behavior. Commonly the many traditional curers, after some probing and perhaps prior inquiry, quickly elicit from a patient, or the latter's representative, indications of anxiety which have been generated by nonfulfillment of responsibility toward elders—either living or dead. Similarly, Ahern and Gould-Martin also point out that the etiology of illness frequently is attributed to some kind of moral turpitude such as unfilial behavior or other breakdown in interpersonal relations. And Margery Topley notes in her paper that, in the event of illness, " . . . prevention is first moral reform and then protection by liturgies and charms. Cure is by secular means, medicine, but only after moral reform."

An understanding of the above relationships allows us to appreciate the dichotomy which exists in the Chinese perception of types of illnesses: as Gould-Martin writes, illness "from outside the body" and "from within the body." Illness "from outside the body" may be attributed to the activities, interference, or possession by negative-type spirits responding to social or familial moral breakdown. Ahern and Gould-Martin describe how the patient or victim suffers from a "fright" *(ching),* manifested in a physiological or psychological "breakdown." Such an illness usually can be diagnosed only by supernatural means, by a diviner of some kind; its cure requires sacred or ritualistic medical treatment as well as rectification of the moral breakdown.

Illness "from within the body," however, is the result of a physiolog-ically-based problem; it is not considered to be related to supernatural causes. This type of illness responds to secular medical treatment, e.g., as administered by a Chinese herbalist, bone-setter, acupuncturist, or a Western medical practitioner. These practitioners deal directly with the physiological symptoms through the application of biomedical techniques.

Here, then, we have the basis for the use, even in modern Chinese societies, of different kinds of medical systems, often simultaneously. As Topley notes, one should ". . . not regard secular and non-secular medi-cine as being in opposition, but as complementary or possibly supple-mentary techniques." Frequently in Chinese societies' there is initial dependence on Western or Chinese secular medicine in order to deal with the symptoms of an illness: then, either simultaneously or at a later time, sacred medicine may be utilized to determine or explain the cause of the illness. The patient and/or his family, in order to prevent the recurrence of the illness, attempt to deal with its causal factors by rectifying the breaches in filial piety, ancestor worship, mistreatment of ancestors, and so on, which have been brought to light by the non-secular practitioner.

The practice of non-secular professionals, however, may be com-promised by political authorities. For example, in Taiwan during the Japanese occupation when public health facilities were improved and Western medicine made more available, shamanistic healing rituals were "outlawed" or, at least, restricted by police surveillance. Nevertheless, shamans apparently continued to be called upon to perform in secret. However, in the absence of arbitrary political interference, as Topley notes, ". . . both secular and non-secular professionals might coexist. This is the situation we have in Hongkong." It is also the situation in Taiwan in recent years as we have seen in a number of papers. In places such as modern Western-oriented Taiwan—under both the Japanese and the Nationalist Chinese—and in colonial dominated Hongkong, regardless of the supposed coexistence of secular and non-secular professionals, there has been a decidedly official government preference given to the secular over the ritualistic, and to the modern Western over the Chinese traditional curing methods and practitioners.

Such a preference is clearly related to the high status and prestige accorded Western-style physicians who, in both Taiwan and Hongkong, usually are drawn from among the better educated and well-to-do classes. As a consequence of their stature, many of these people are elected or appointed to important government positions in which they can exert influence to strengthen their own interests. For example, such modern Western-style medical people have been highly instrumental in the or-ganization and operation of government health services and medical agencies, and, of course, often in the licensing of medical practitioners in Taiwan and Hongkong . The political influence of Western-style physicians has therefore been highly significant in promoting the influence of Western medicine—often to the detriment of traditional Chinese secular and ritualistic curing. This can be seen in Hongkong- particularly in the work of Margery Topley, and also in Taiwan as more generally observed by numerous researchers and in the daily press.

Under the present Nationalist government, both rural and urban Taiwanese, especially the lesser educated population, continue to call upon shamans for ritualistic healing. The greater availability of Western medicine and the influences of modernization still have not undermined the need for and the use of Chinese sacred medicine, in conjunction with Chinese or Western secular medicine; this is not unexpected, however, given the religio-philosophical belief system of the Chinese and the often limited efficacy of Western and Chinese secular medicine.

In addition, the Chinese sacred medical system has certain positive attributes which contribute to its continued use. The traditional sacred system is functionally relevant; and because it is an integral part of the total Chinese culture system, it meets the psychosocial needs of much of the population. By searching out evidence of moral breakdown as the cause of illness, the sacred medical system instills and reinforces moral behavior. It does not simply offer treatment of the symptoms and the illness itself, but instead, attempts to prescribe for and treat their basic causes in order to return the patient and his family to a state of harmony and peace (*p'ing-an*).

The system also satisfies other psychosocial needs through the curing rites performed by its practitioners. The ritual which frequently accompanies the diagnosis of illness serves as a kind of group therapy session in which concerned participants discuss problems and their sources. At the same time, this ritual, in its resemblance to a social event, provides a certain amount of levity, or release of tension.

The curing rituals of sacred medicine also function to displace responsibility from the patient's family or from the patient himself to the practitioner, the *tang-ki*. The explanation of illness and the prescriptions which these practitioners offer are known to some degree by everyone, but they are solutions which most would be loath to prescribe on their own. Since the *tang-ki*, as indicated by Gould-Martin, are likely to know and reflect local folk customs, they are better able than Western-style doctors to serve as a "receptacle" for the responsibility.

Still another function of sacred medicine (and, to a lesser degree, traditional Chinese secular medicine) is that it focuses on the patient rather than on the disease. As Anderson and several other writers have pointed out, the cure involves the participation and cooperation of the patient, his whole family, and, sometimes, his whole community. The patient, placed in the center of all the activities of his family and community, thus is provided with significant moral comfort and support.

On a more practical level, sacred medicine also deals with social, familistic, or psychological problems in situations where professionals often are unavailable. Tseng points this out in his paper, although he seems to consider such non-professional services to be effective only in the area of less serious types of psychological problems. Tseng is probably quite correct when he suggests that such traditional services do not provide very much help for the more serious psychoses or deeper psychological problems. But when dealing with serious psychoses, it is worth asking: How high a rate of cure has psychiatry had in the West?

Having said this, it seems appropriate to present some thoughts which these papers have raised in my mind. Most of them, particularly those of the anthropologists, present an extremely positive view of Chinese traditional sacred and secular medical systems and a more negative view of Western medical systems, especially as they exist in Chinese societies. It is curious, and at the same time interesting, to note that only Tseng and Lee are not so completely positive about the Chinese medical systems and so completely negative about the Western medical system. (I leave the interpretation of this datum up to each individual reader.) Tseng, for example, expresses what is taken to be some unhappiness with the Chinese system when he writes in his paper, "The effectiveness of traditional medicine may be over-described beyond its own actual pharmaco-medical capacity." In addition, both he and Lee are critical of Chinese practitioners: Tseng because he believes that the non-transmission of secret prescriptions by herb doctors is an obstacle to the continued development of this form of medicine; and Lee because he believes that, socially and technically, Chinese practitioners, as opposed to the Western doctors in Hongkong, are secretive, "non-cohesive" and non-cooperative.

Why then have most Western observers, including this writer (Gallin 1966: 231–269), generally been so positive about Chinese sacred and secular medical systems? Why have we found no apparent negative attributes within these systems? It seems worthwhile to speculate on some answers; they could help us to arrive at a more balanced and, therefore, more credible picture of Chinese traditional medical systems.

For some Western anthropologists, including myself, the answer to these questions may reside in what I conceive of as a "reverse" or "inverted ethnocentrism": an extreme cultural relativism expressed through an overly rational functional approach. It seems to me that when we adopt such an integrative approach to a cultural system, we tend to see anything reinforcing that system as essentially good. Our situation may be likened to that of Robert Redfield, who posited a totally positive view of peasant culture as he described Yucatan. Redfield's admiration for the peasants, and the non-industrial lifestyle they represented, caused him to look for those factors which demonstrated that their life was well integrated and beautiful. Oscar Lewis later disputed this view of peasantry. He saw the peasants' poverty and suffering, and sought those factors which would help him to understand their causes and consequences. Each, of course, found what he was looking for, and the extreme differences in their findings may be attributed, at least in part, to the differences in their approaches and views of life.

Similarly, anthropologists and other social scientists, as a result of their selective interests, may only see and report on the positive side of traditional healing systems within the communities they study. Their findings, however, may tell only a part of the story. It is true that many villagers, including the more sophisticated and better educated local elite, do usually utilize and participate in the rituals of traditional secular and sacred Chinese medicine. These phenomena are part of the established social patterns of behavior within their communities. Utilization of the traditional systems, however, does not necessarily imply belief in these forms of medicine. Many people "go through the motions"—especially when it comes to the shamanistic healing rituals of the *tang-ki*—to satisfy social expectations and pressures. They realize that if a patient should die without having had the possible benefit of the healing rituals, his family would be blamed and subjected to extreme criticism. As a consequence then, even the well-to-do and relatively better educated residents of the rural villages frequently participate in such healing rituals. Their participation may be for the benefit of their own family members or as part of a community display of concern for the illness of some fellow villagers. Young people in high school or in higher education may actually openly scoff at the various kinds of ritual activities, especially those for curing that take place in the village. However, should they remain in the village and take on family and other community responsibilities, then social expectations and pressures usually ensure their participation in such ritualistic activities. The only ones who maintain their incredulous attitude toward such village ritualistic behavior—attitudes which frequently become an important source of division in the community—are those who soon leave the rural area for the city where they may become free from pressures for their ritual participation. (However, the large number of shamans engaged in ritualistic curing in the large cities of Taiwan causes one to question how totally free such modernized, educated, rural migrants to the cities are from the social pressures and pangs of conscience which help to assure the continuance of such activities among their rural relatives.)

But, just as the above forces help to provide continuity in the use of ritualistic curing, "it is probably these [same] two factors of social pressure and fear of leaving any method untried, which opened the way for the very notable acceptance of Western medicine in Taiwan. While the skeptic is thus forced by them to call upon the shaman, the traditionalists are likewise forced to call upon Western medicine when traditional methods have failed" (Gallin, 1966:267). The anthropologist, therefore, has an obligation to delve into significant attitudes and analyze the ways in which social forces within the local area may influence the overt behavior he observes.

Our view of the local medical scene in a village or a community also may be influenced by our frequent emphasis on the "dramatic." Frequently we are preoccupied with the performance of shamans during curing rites. As a result, we may under-report the more ordinary and less dramatic activities of Chinese herbalists, bone-setters, midwives, or Western medical practitioners, presenting only a partial picture of Chinese medical systems.

Extending this discussion further, I would like to ask: Might not some occidental social scientists harbor a basic negativism toward Western medicine which influences their viewpoint? Several authors have clearly indicated their displeasure with Western medicine's traditional concern with the disease and not the patient. Most consider the patient-oriented approach of Chinese medical systems to be their strong point, and the disease-oriented approach of the Western medical system its weak point. I might ask, however, how many deaths or disabilities have resulted from an over-reliance on the subjective approach of traditional sacred medicine?

Regardless of the answer, I hasten to add that the Western social scientist is not alone in holding biases. I find it interesting that Lee only mentions Chinese secular medicine and Western medicine in his paper; it is as if Chinese sacred medicine did not exist in Hongkong or had no bearing on medical beliefs, needs, and behavior. Of course, sacred medicine was not the defined topic of Lee's paper and I cannot fault him for his omission. Nevertheless, I think it is unfortunate that many Chinese social scientists, usually people from the middle or upper classes, generally tend to disregard or ignore the existence of sacred medicine.

I certainly found this to be the case in Taiwan. In 1965, during my second field trip there, I live in Taipei in a compound owned by the National Taiwan University. Next to the compound was a small village in which shamans (tang-ki) held ritualistic healing sessions almost every night. When I told some Chinese anthropologists and sociologists about these activities they refused to believe me, remarking that nothing of that sort was to be found in "sophisticated" Taipei. I finally was able to convince them only by leading them to some of the many places where they could observe shamans perform.

The point to be made, then, is that if we are to arrive at a balanced picture of Chinese medical systems we all need to be aware of our own biases. In addition, we can and should strive for this balance in other ways. First, we need to document more adequately the frequency of cases when we study illness and the use of medical systems; too much of our reporting has depended on impressions and, unfortunately, our attitudes frequently are reported as facts. Second, we, that is Western and Chinese social scientists, must engage in more cooperative research so that we might counteract each other's biases. Third, we must conduct more complete studies of process type, providing detailed analyses of illness histories. Such studies should include information on the "before, during, and after" of illnesses as well as complete observations and in-depth interviews by researchers well-versed in both Chinese culture and society and health and illness.

Finally, we must be more careful not to attribute the same knowledge, perceptions, and behavior to all members of Chinese society. For too long, we took for granted the universality of the knowledge, and even the behavioral manifestations, of the tenets of the great Confucian tradition among the Chinese population. Just as we are now aware of the diverse influences of regionalism, class, education, and religio-philosophical sophistication on knowledge and behavior, so too must we be cognizant of the ways in which these factors influence individuals' conceptions and behavior regarding health, illness and medical systems.

In conclusion I would like to note that most of the authors of these papers share the common belief that in Chinese societies the explanation of the cause of an illness is just as necessary as the curing of its symptom. So long as traditional Chinese values persist it is likely that the efficacy of secular Western and Chinese medicine will be fully realized only if they are utilized in combination with traditional sacred Chinese medicine. Curing requires a concern for both the physiological and socio-psychological aspects of illness. So long as secular medical systems do not demonstrate both of these concerns, then we can expect to find the continued utilization of the sacred medical system along with them. In addition, so long as secular, "scientific" biomedicine remains fallible, even those illnesses perceived to be caused from "within the body" will continue to be treated by traditional Chinese sacred medicine. Given the fact that the Western medical system is not integrated into the Chinese psychocultural system, it does not seem likely that it will be able to stand on its own and satisfy Chinese perceptions of health needs.

NOTES

1. Gallin's discussion in *Medicine in Chinese Cultures* (Kleinman et al, eds. Bethesda, Md.: Fogarty International Center, N.I.H., 1975; pp. 273-280) is based on 6 chapters in that book, which appear as chapters (2), (3), (4), (6), (15), (16) in the present volume. His discussion does not include chapters (5) and (7) in this section, because the former was written after the conference at which Gallin acted as a discussant, and because the latter was formerly in another section of the conference and of *Medicine in Chinese Cultures* (Editors' note).

2. All quotations are taken from the original versions of six papers presented at the conference.

REFERENCES

FABREGA, H. and D. SILVER
   1973   Illness and Shamanistic Curing in Zinacantan. Stanford: Stanford University Press.
GALLIN, B.
   1966   Hsin Hsing, Taiwan: A Chinese Village in Change. Berkeley: University of California Press.

Part B
Other Asian Societies

CHAPTER 9

DO CULTURAL DIFFERENCES MAKE ANY DIFFERENCE? CHOICE POINTS IN MEDICAL SYSTEMS AVAILABLE IN NORTHWESTERN THAILAND

PETER KUNSTADTER

This chapter considers choices in medical care, using data from northwestern Thailand. Other chapters have studied medical systems largely as if they are the result of independent cultural traditions. They have implied the "traditional," "popular," "folk" or "classical" medical system was integrated into the society and culture within which it exists, and have looked at "Western," "modern" or "cosmopolitan" medicine as intrusive, and thus poorly integrated. We may ask what happens when there are customarily available to the same people two or more alternative systems of explanations and behavior with regard to health, illness and the treatment of illness. The author believes this is not an unusual situation, since alternative systems are often available, not just as an artifact of contact between "Western" and traditional societies.[1] Indeed this may be a general situation, inherent in all medical systems, since none is completely deterministic and all must deal with unanticipated or undesired outcomes. Further, the writer would argue that it may be psychologically and perhaps socially conservative (i.e., 'tending to induce stability in the system) to have alternatives, given the uncertainties involved in any medical situation with uncertain knowledge and imperfect control over natural events. This assertion seems contrary to the predictions resulting from the "cognitive dissonance" argument that conceptual inconsistency or ambiguity produces social and psychological ambiguity. At least it raises the question of the definition of cognitive dissonance (or consonance) and, implicitly, the definition of the "rationality" of man. It also suggests it may *always* be appropriate to look for the alternative systems of explanation and action as a normal (not deviant or intrusive) part of any social subsystem.

The multi-ethnic society, with a variety of traditional beliefs and practices, offers an opportunity to examine the activities of people for whom many alternative medical systems are customarily available, where viewing these alternatives as "intrusive" is of no particular utility in understanding the processes of choice. We may consider the cultural, technical, and social aspects of the medical systems, that is, the systems of belief and evaluation concerning health and illness, the medicines and other items of technology used to influence health, and the regularities of organized social behavior associated with illness and the promotion of health. As used in this discussion the term "medical system" thus includes medical practitioners using various therapeutic devices, interacting with patients (or populations) to treat or prevent illness, and also the definitions and means of recognition of health and illness (the ways of deciding whether a particular condition belongs in the category which requires healing or even preventive action, if available); diagnosis (identification of the illness, classifying its appearance by history, circumstance or symptoms, often involving attribution of cause of classification into a category of conditions for which appropriate actions are known); treatment (application of actions understood and intended to modify the causes or effects of the illness); and evaluation of the recognition-diagnosis-treatment in view of the outcome of the case.[2]

The thoughts and actions implied in this paradigm are, of course, embedded in a social system of larger scope. For some purposes the logic of any given system may be treated in isolation, but because our interest is in choices among alternatives, we must also consider cultural and social settings in which health activities take place.

Choice is possible at many points along the sequence of events we have outlined. Some of the choices may be idiosyncratic, resulting from individual differences in the actors; some are probably social-situational, relating to differences in the positions of the individual vis-à-vis relevant resources such as geographical or social distance to a health facility, or the economic requirements of the facility; and some of the factors of choice relate to the recognized availability of alternatives. It is the two latter categories we will emphasize in a consideration of the multi-ethnic society. This will allow us to consider the question of cultural differences and cultural conflicts in medical systems: how do cultural differences make any difference at the various choice points in the system outlined above?

Our tasks in this paper will include outlining the social setting and medical systems in northwestern Thailand along the dimensions indicated, giving some abbreviated examples of how people work within the systems including an indication of points at which choices are blocked, and attempting to interpret our observations as they may relate to the questions of choice within and between systems, and eclecticism versus cultural conflict.

Ethnic Characteristics in Northern Thailand [3]

Northern Thailand is an area of a few broad and many narrow valleys, relatively densely settled, interspersed with more sparsely peopled rolling mountains reaching a height of over 2,500 meters. The Northern Thai majority people live mainly in the valleys in small rural communities and in a few large towns. Their predominant activity is wet rice cultivation, and their dominant religion is Buddhism, represented in every village by a temple usually with several resident monks. Chinese and "Indian" (usually Chittagonian Muslim) merchants, Central Thai white collar workers and officials, and a few Christian missionaries generally live in the towns. The hills are occupied by a variety of minority people, including Lua' and Karen who are mainly animistic subsistence farmers of hill rice, and who often supplement their meagre income with wage work for lowland employers. A substantial number of Karen and Lua' people live in the lowlands where their economic activities resemble those of the Northern Thais in similar communities, and where many of them consider themselves to be Buddhists (as well as animists). Some Northern Thais have moved into the hills in search of small patches of marginal agricultural land, or to gather forest products. Also in the hills are a number of groups such as Hmong (Meo), Yao, Akha and Lahu, hill farmers raising cash crops such as opium, for ultimate sale in lowland markets. Most of what follows refers to Lua', Karen, Northern Thai and Westerners in Mae Sariang District of Mae Hongson Province, not far from the Burma border.

Ethnic Groups, Cultural Traditions and Social Interactions

By ethnic group is meant a population self-consciously associated with a pattern of beliefs and customary actions, the members of which usually identify themselves as such, and who are usually identified by others as members of that group. For the purposes of this paper are included some religious groupings under the category "ethnic," since, for example, being or becoming Christian involves accepting specific and consciously-recognized beliefs as distinct from being an animist or a Buddhist, just as being or becoming Karen, Lua' or Northern Thai involves accepting specifically and consciously recognized beliefs of these groups, as distinct from one another. As will be shown, ethnic self-identity is clearly related to acceptance of some medical beliefs and practices, and some patterns of association with different parts of the multi-ethnic medical system.

The definition implies that the populations and boundaries of the groups depend on the particular "pattern of beliefs and customary actions" and on who is perceiving and acting on the basis of these patterns. Thus, for some purposes it is appropriate to make a distinction between all Lua' and everyone else, or between Lua' animists and Lua' Christians, or between all Christians and all non-Christians. Some roles, which in some senses determine individual behavior, are associated with ethnic "status," but it should become clear in what follows that ethnic status is mutable, and that depending on the context, one or another ethnic status may be assumed by or assigned to any one individual.

The common presumption that ethnic groups are clearly bounded populations sharing amongst themselves a common and unique set of understandings of cultural traditions, and confining their social interactions to people within that group with whom their culture is uniquely shared, is probably not quite true anywhere. It is certainly an unacceptable distortion of the facts in Southeast Asia, where the demographic boundaries of groups are permeable, where the existence and content of several cultural traditions is known and positively or negatively valued by members of other groups, where social contacts are not expected to be confined to a single group, and where membership in another group may be the subject of a realistic aspiration. Medical systems are one focus for interaction between individuals from supposedly distinct groups, and may be a reason for maintaining or changing ethnic affiliation.

The diversity of cultures in northern Thailand is large, and a great variety of medical care systems is available to such minority groups as Lua' and Karen who have been in contact with each other and with Northern Thais and other groups for hundreds of years. In general the cultural traditions, or elements thereof, which have been available here have been freely offered, and have not been seen by their bearers as mutually exclusive or necessarily in conflict. Although it is possible to determine boundaries between the groups bearing these traditions, a Lua' may become Karen or Thai, and movement in the opposite direction, though less frequent, is possible and has also occurred.

Religious eclecticism is well known in Southeast Asia. Thais, for example, recognize that they respect simultaneously Buddhism as prescribed by Pali texts, as well as practicing (or having practiced for them) Brahmanistic and animistic rites appropriate to certain times, places or occasions. The major exceptions to this eclecticism are in Christianity and Islam, which have tended to be exclusivistic religions, drawing the hard line that an individual cannot subscribe simultaneously to more than one "all-encompassing" tradition.

Medical practices and theories have been attached more or less clearly to the different ethnic and religious traditions, and to the people identified most clearly with them, though the boundaries between medical systems are even fuzzier than between religious traditions or social groups. The same herbal remedies, for example, may be claimed as "traditional" by adherents to different cultural traditions. General concepts of supernatural cause, diagnosis, treatment and prevention of disease are considered by Lua', Karen, and Northern Thai people, who speak languages of completely different families, to be more or less equivalent and for some purposes interchangeable. One may conclude from this that the efficacy of the medical activity in question is not believed by the actors to be dependent on the ethnic group of the doctor or patient, but is believed to be dependent on the nature of the illness, the qualifications (training, experience, previous success) of the practitioner, and the strength of his medicines, surgery, sacrifices, prescriptions or incantations. In general these activities are not viewed as potentially conflicting: use of one system does not preclude use of other systems of diagnosis or cure, nor does it prevent simultaneous belief in other theories of disease, or even consultation with qualified members of other ethnic groups.

The exception may be the modern (Western) medical system, which has been associated in part with Western Christian missionaries, who sometimes have tended to draw a hard line between their medicine (and its underlying theories) and other ("unscientific") medical systems. Pharmacists and peddlers, of course, have offered Western drugs without requiring a "cultural loyalty oath." Western medicine is a complex phenomenon including an exclusivistic and naturalistic theory of the "cause" of disease, but it has been obvious to all that the very effective Western medical techniques do not require adherence to any particular theory beyond the practical one that they work. As with other medical techniques, Western medicine has been a focus for contact between members of different ethnic groups. In Thailand, in contrast, for example, to India (Brass 1968; Leslie 1967) this contact has not been a point of major political conflict between organized groups, perhaps because the traditional practice of medicine in Thailand has never been the exclusive prerogative of any group. (See also Chapter 11.)

Definition and Recognition of Illness and Health

Illness is recognized among the people of northern Thailand in terms of symptoms such as pain, fever, chills, coldness of hands or feet, weakness, loss of appetite, some unusual sensitivity to odors, diarrhea, constipation, injuries, failure to heal, psychological disturbances, general physical appearance (thinness), skin color (paleness), body form (swelling etc.), in other words, abnormality. Common conditions, such as coughs, "cradle cap," seen on almost every small child, or smarting eyes, which everyone has from time to time due to smoky house-interiors, are considered of no importance, apparently because they are so common. Serious illness involves interference with normal physical or psychological function, or expectations of function given a person's age. Thus an infant's failure to thrive and develop "normally" would be considered to be a sign of illness, even though no specific emphasis is put on age of first walking or talking; weakness and progressive thinness is expected with old age, or perhaps is interpreted as a sign of old age, and is not, in itself, considered to be illness.

Beyond such general concepts, recognition of illness must anticipate a discussion of diagnosis and treatment. Recognition is, in fact, a preliminary stage of diagnosis in which the appearance or behavior is classified into one of several categories which are more or less clearly distinguished from each other in terms of the relationship of signs and symptoms to presumed cause and appropriate treatment, as well as the predicted outcome of the illness. The differences between the classification of illness seem most clear when comparing various traditional categories (which seem to be widely shared amongst the various ethnic groups) and modern "Western" medical categorization, which does not classify some symptoms into similar kinds of categories as do the several local traditional systems, and which may recognize illness in symptoms which are overlooked by the local systems.

An Outline of Theories of Disease

A number of theories of disease are extant within the knowledge of most people in the multi-ethnic system. The practice of diagnosis and treatment appropriate to these theories is more or less widely distributed, depending on the availability of the required knowledge. The theories of disease "nature" or "cause" include: spirits of many varieties, soul loss, incantations or sorcery, "sin" or lack of merit, "little bugs" or germs, and natural or accidental injuries or conditions that "just happen." [4]

Initial categorization of illness

Once a person believes himself to be ill, or is seen by others as ill, the patient or the observers generally place the illness in one of a number of categories. They do so by using certain ethnically determined assumptions, and several kinds of information, including symptoms, past history of the patient, recent history of the patient, and general recognition of the local epidemiological scene (with respect to diseases like measles, smallpox or malaria).

The most difficult task of diagnosis is involved in conditions for which there is believed to be no necessary connection between specific symptoms and cause. Two major categories, diseases caused by spirits and diseases caused by incantations may be found with almost any variety of symptoms. In both, not only is the cause obscure, but also there tends to be little relationship between diagnosis and symptomatic treatment, since the attributed cause is outside the patient's body, and the patient's condition may be thought of as only incidental to the cause. For other categories of illness, the cause may be much more obvious: snake bites are caused by snakes and burns are caused by fires. Remedies are directed at relief of the symptoms, but an ambiguity may arise if the apparent illness persists (e.g., due to infection) beyond a normal healing period, or if there is no apparent external cause (e.g., for a condition like boils). Differential diagnosis between and within categories in which there is no necessary relation between cause and symptom is difficult, and may be done simply by trial and error (or, more accurately, trial and success). The interpretation of symptoms may depend on a combination of observations: roughly the same symptoms reported by two women may be interpreted differently, depending on whether one of them has recently given birth and thereby is liable to have the common postpartum illness which is understood to be subject to herbal and behavioral remedies, or has not delivered recently and thus is liable to have a spirit-caused illness which is understood to respond to proper identification and propitiation of the spirits.

Spirits (*phi*)

A widely known and apparently accepted folk tale is that in the past, when spirits were handed out, the Lua', in order to carry them home, put them in a tightly woven, closely covered basket, thereby managing to prevent all of them from escaping. The Karen put them in a basket without a lid, and many of them bounced out along the trail and were lost, while the Thai just threw them in a loosely woven basket, and arrived in their village with only a few. Thus as compared with other groups in this multi-ethnic society, all people generally concede the Lua' have more spirits in their surroundings, have more obligations to them, and suffer more from the demands of the spirits than do the Karen or

Thai. This is probably one reason (or rationalization) for the pattern of consultation for medical assistance: Lua' will seek aid from any source, including Karen and Northern Thai specialists, but Northern Thai will rarely need aid from Lua' and Karen spirit specialists, because Thai believe they have relatively few spirits bothering them. In what follows, then, the writer indicates what applies mostly to Lua' villagers, and what is understood and accepted as well by Karen and Northern Thai rural villagers.

In general, spirits are not considered to be malevolent, but they are believed to cause illness in order to call human attention to their desire to be fed an animal sacrifice. If the correct spirit can be determined, and the correct offering is made, the victim will recover. Meanwhile the patient is also given supportive therapy for relief of symptoms, including much moral support from relatives and friends.

There are many kinds of spirits which follow this general pattern, including primarily spirits which are believed to inhabit the forests. Thais, living in the irrigated lowlands, escape most of these spirits. Ancestral spirits, usually believed by Lua' to dwell in or near the cemetery (though they may be fed at home or in the fields), are usually considered to be the source from which many blessings flow, but they also occasionally cause illness in one of their descendants in order to be fed. Karens subscribe to this belief, but it is unimportant to Northern Thais. People who die away from home or die a violent death are generally believed to be transformed into powerful and often malevolent spirits which may strike anyone who happens to be near the place the death occurred. This belief is generally recognized by Karen, Lua', and Northern Thai villagers. A particularly virulent type of spirit (phi ka') is believed by Karen, Lua' and Northern Thai [5] to be created as a result of violations of incest or exogamy taboos, and this spirit may devour the liver or other organs of anyone in the village (not the taboo-violating couple). In such a case, unlike other spirit-caused illnesses, the solution is not to attempt to appease the spirit, but rather to drive the spirit out of the affected person and force the offending couple (and with them, the dangerous spirit) out of the village. Villagers do not always know that such spirits have been created in their midst. Some Lua' and some Karen villages have the reputation of harboring many such spirits and may be shunned by outsiders for this reason.

Ubiquitous spirits (phi nyat) are believed to be able to cause widespread illness, which is not subject to any but symptomatic treatment. Diagnosis of this category of illness is based on the nature of the disease, especially how common it is. Epidemic or widespread "common" diseases, including measles, chicken pox, smallpox, and the common cold, are believed to be caused by this spirit. They are believed to be subject only to symptomatic treatment if the preventive action of annual feeding of village guardian spirits and, when necessary, closing the village to all persons who wish to come in or through, is unsuccessful. This concept seems widely held by the various ethnic groups.

Lua' believe another class of spirit-caused illness is recognized by symptoms of aberrant psychological behavior and the individual's past history of episodes of this type. This type of illness is believed to be caused by heaven-dwelling spirits and can be treated only by members of a hereditary priest lineage. This class of spirits is not recognized by Karens, or necessarily in all Lua' villages, though the class of spirits is reported to be recognized in some Northern Thai villages.

For most spirit-caused illnesses, however, there is no necessary relationship between symptom and cause. Fever, headache, persistent infection, diarrhea, and so forth may be caused by any one of a number of forest-dwelling spirits, and most diagnostic efforts are directed at determining which one of these spirits wants what kind of an animal sacrifice. Meanwhile, symptomatic relief is offered in the form of herbs, massage, cool baths to reduce fevers, etc. This view of cause is held in common by Lua' and Karen, but seems unimportant to Northern Thai who rarely or never make animal sacrifices for individual curing rites.

Diagnosis of spirit-caused illness

Several methods of diagnosis are known to the Lua', including taking a small handful of uncooked rice from the patient's household and counting out the number of grains into which the diagnostician has whispered his proposed diagnosis. The initial verification of the diagnosis is determined by whether the number of grains is even (correct) or odd (incorrect), and whether or not the procedure can be repeated without receiving an odd number of rice grains. Other techniques include staring into a cup of rice wine, and more direct communication with spirits by means of a trance. Karens often diagnose by thrusting slivers in the vein holes of a pair of chicken femurs and observing the angles they make with the shaft of the bone.

The quality of the diagnostician is determined by the frequency of his successes, and diagnosticians with good reputations draw cases from surrounding communities many miles away. Practically every adult male Lua' knows how to count rice grains, but staring into wine and direct communication with spirits by means of trance are practiced by only a few specialists.

Diagnosis is usually tentative at first, and will generally be reinforced, at least in the case of serious or prolonged illness, with an intermediate step: summoning the spirit by name and offering a pledge as a token of the animal to be sacrificed to the spirit which has been named in the tentative diagnosis. If the patient shows signs of improvement, this suggests the diagnosis and proposed treatment (sacrifice) were correct, and the animal sacrifice will be carried out. If the patient shows no improvement after the pledge, or after the sacrifice, this suggests the diagnosis was in error, and the diagnosis and pledging processes will be repeated. These processes are diagrammed in Figure 1.

The diagram is simplified in that it does not distinguish, for example, between different classes of specialists associated with diagnosing and treating, nor does it indicate that patients, diagnosticians and curers need not be from the same ethnic group. It does indicate, however, that in moving through this portion of the system, an individual may return to begin at an earlier choice-point, if he has been unsuccessful at a later stage.

The diagnoses resulting from this system are subject to empirical confirmation (and thus the theory is subject to support) or disconfirmation, depending on the condition of the patient following the pledge or prescribed sacrifice to the named spirit. One might ask why the unsuccessful diagnoses do not lead to the abandonment (instability) of the theory. The answer seems to be in part that the system enjoys many more successes than failures. Most people do not die of most illnesses.

Beyond this, there is, of course, uncertainty in the diagnostic outcome of a specific combination of spirit and animal sacrifice, which makes disconfirmed diagnoses (unsuccessful pledges or treatments) understandable as mistakes of the diagnostician, not a basic error in the system. The number of spirits which can cause illness is believed to be very large, and the number and type of animal sacrifices which they might want further increases the total number of possible permutations. Disconfirmation of the diagnosis thus may be interpreted as a mistake in communication with the spirits (leading to the wrong spirit + sacrificial animal combination). Thus, if the patient dies, the survivors need not feel guilty, since everything that could be done was done, but the spirit proved uncommunicative. There is no interest in a *post mortem* attempt to reach the spirit, since nothing further can be done for the patient.

Given the assumptions under which it operates (spirits cause human illness, spirits respond to being fed animal sacrifices), the system seems to be "rational," in the sense that it is internally consistent, and is subject to almost continual empirical testing by leading to predictions, the outcomes of which are observed. This is not to say that the system is "scientific," inasmuch as there is no traditional method for examining and testing the underlying assumptions, logically, observationally or probabilistically, through the design of crucial experiments.

Incantations (*katha*)

As already indicated there is thought to be no necessary connection between symptoms and diagnosis of a disease caused by incantations or *katha,* thus it is not immediately obvious that a particular illness is caused by someone casting a spell *(tu katha)* in order to do deliberate harm, rather than by spirits wishing to be fed. The preliminary clue to the diagnosis may be that circumstances of the patient suggest he may have angered someone who put a curse on him, or paid someone else to do so, as a consequence, for example, of a dispute over land rights. The reason for the curse may or may not be known or understood by the victim or the diagnostician.

Correct diagnosis and treatment of this type of illness can only be made by someone who is also adept at *katha,* preferably someone whose

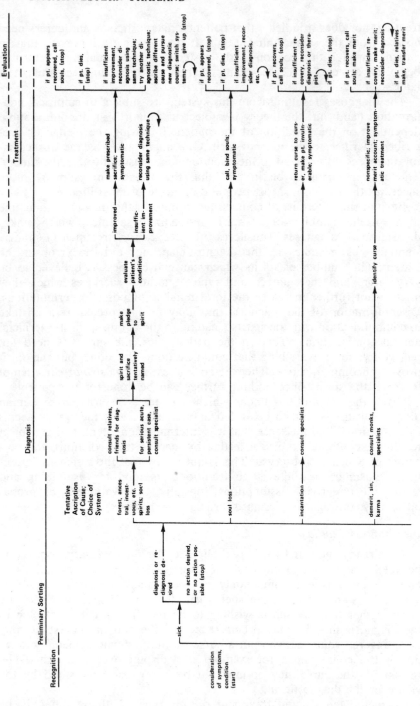

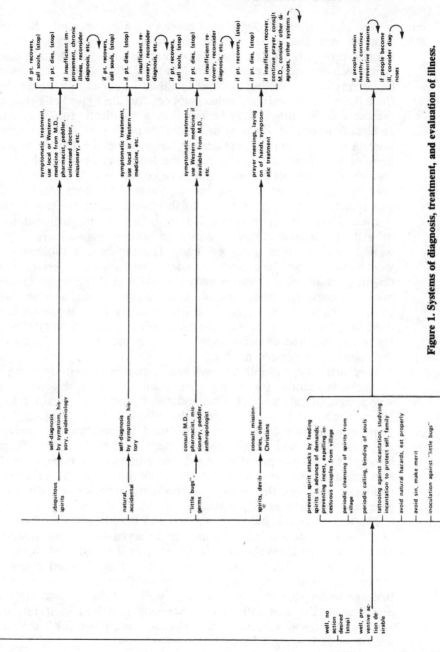

Figure 1. Systems of diagnosis, treatment, and evaluation of illness.

powers *(khang)* are stronger than those of the curser, and who can thus turn the incantation back on its originator. The verification of correct diagnosis, once the illness has been tentatively assigned to this category, is the recovery of the patient, but failure of the patient to recover may be interpreted as resulting from the fact that the curser's *katha* are stronger than those of the curer. Further support for the hypothesis that this is the cause of the illness may be found in a recollection of quarrels, but, as already indicated, this sort of "proof" is not essential, nor is there any attempt to prove that the presumedly angered person has made incantations or hired someone to do so. In the few cases of which the writer is aware, the parties to disputes who have considered that *katha* may have been directed at them believe that the cursers are from another village, and sometimes (though not necessarily) from another ethnic group.

Incantations, often accompanied by tattooing, are believed to ward off evil, and are commonly used as a preventive against knife or gunshot wounds, animal bites, etc., or curses. The tattoos are thought by their wearers to be more decorative reminders that *katha* have been performed on their behalf rather than protective devices in themselves. The tattoos may contain words or letters, often in scripts or languages the wearers cannot read, which may refer to words or letters in the incantation. When used for protection or curing, the incantation is said to be "blown" *(pao katha)*, as the practitioner whispers or blows the words of the chant into the rolled up fingers of his fist.

Special training, usually study under a master, sometimes using books of *katha* (common, for example, in Burma, from where many of the *katha* used in this part of Thailand have come), is required to learn incantations of various sorts, including those used for cursing, for preventing or turning curses, and those used by specialists to cure or to tame elephants and break them to harness. Belief in the efficacy of incantations is widespread among the several ethnic groups. Even Christian elephant owners openly accept incantations as the only effective technique and seek the services of specialists who know incantations to give them power over elephants.

Katha powers are jealously guarded and may have to be "fed," much in the way spirits are fed; they are not believed to be inexhaustible, but may be used up if invoked too frequently, or if transferred, by teaching, to someone else. Many men will admit to having studied a few minor incantations, but often claim to have given them up. Because *katha* are believed to be able to cause harm, as well as being potentially helpful, and because the incantations are ordinarily practiced in secret, specialists are both respected and feared, and the more powerful *katha* varieties are not eagerly sought by all.

Soul loss

People, and some animals (buffalos, elephants) are believed by Lua', Karen and Northern Thai to have a number of souls *(khuan)*. The number of souls varies according to the ethnic group, but the general belief is shared that souls influence health. Some souls are believed to be associated with particular parts of the body, but the association is not completely clear. Separation of one or more souls from the body is believed to weaken the individual, resulting in chronic weakness, failure of children to thrive, or inability to ward off illness. Symptoms of "soul loss" may be similar to those which are usually considered to be caused by spirits, except that soul loss would not be suspected as the cause of a sudden acute attack of illness. Soul loss may be a diagnosis which results from an attempt to determine which spirit is causing an illness, particularly a chronic illness, or from failure to make a prompt recovery from an acute attack, a bad cold, and so forth.

All three groups believe that pollution of men (and elephants) may result from being physically beneath women, or by coming in contact with women's skirts. Such a condition is felt to weaken the man (or elephant) and the treatment is identical to that for soul loss. The author is not sure whether this form of pollution is believed to produce soul loss, or merely to produce weakness and thus vulnerability to soul loss.

Souls are summoned and fed at times when people are felt to be in a weakened or vulnerable condition, either as curative or, more generally, as preventive or supportive therapy. Times or conditions of weakness or vulnerability include infancy and youth, recovery from illness regardless of the believed cause of the illness, moving from accustomed place of residence or revision of living arrangements as with marriage, travel away from the home village, completion of the year's work in the fields and thus abandonment of customary place of work, etc. On such occasions, the souls are called to the body of their owner, induced to enter food which the patient then eats, and bound into the patient by tying cotton string around his or her wrists. A similar ceremony may also be held in behalf of an old relative, symbolically demonstrating wishes for health and long life. Souls are not believed to cause illness directly, but separation of souls from the body may exacerbate illness or delay recovery.

Many people share the knowledge of techniques for summoning souls, and most household heads can and do perform the appropriate ceremony for their household members.

Sin, lack of merit

The concepts of "merit" *(bun)* and "demerit" or "sin" *(bap)* are generally believed both by actors and observers of Thai society to be central to Thai Buddhist practice and belief. These concepts are generally understood and can be fairly directly transplanted into Lua' and Karen language, belief and actions. Both merit and demerit can be accumulated, and in the Thai belief, transmitted to other people and transmitted from past to future incarnations. The balance between merit and demerit, as well as their absolute quantity, is believed to influence one's fate or reincarnation, and is believed by many people to be effective in this life as well as in the next. Thus "be good, get good" is a prescription for prevention of illness and misfortune, as well as for a better life, perhaps now and perhaps in the future.

Belief in the efficacy of merit, accumulated by adherence to Buddhist precepts, is widespread among Lua' and Karen people, even though belief in reincarnation may not be entirely clear, especially among the Lua'. Adherence to Buddhist proscriptions against the taking of life and the ingestion of intoxicants could not be absolute in combination with non-Thai animist traditions which require animal sacrifices and use rice liquor as an essential social and ceremonial lubricant. Nonetheless, the "important" parts of the prescriptions to do good can be followed (by being generous), while the greatest sins (killing people, stealing) can be avoided, thus making it possible to achieve a favorable balance even in the absence of the Buddhist clergy in many non-Thai villages. Merit is made and shared as a deliberate preventive measure, with the aid of Buddhist monks, in both Northern Thai and non-Thai communities. Making merit is much more common among Northern Thais than among the non-Thais, and may be the prescribed method for them to deal with offenses to spirits, hoping that the prayers of the monks will redress any offenses to spirits.

The interpretive value of these concepts for their adherents is high, though their predictive value for any individual is low. One's condition depends both on present and past amounts and balances of merit and demerit, and any actions now may not necessarily overturn the total balance. Overly large amounts of demerit are not believed to be reflected in any particular symptoms, and accumulation of merit is more likely to be used as a preventive rather than a curative action. Buddhist monks may be consulted by both Thais and non-Thais for traditional cures of specific health problems.

The Christian concept of sin which is held by Lua', Karen, and Northern Thai Christians seems to this observer to be roughly the same as the Buddhist concept of sin. For the Christian, the result of sin may not appear until after death (going to heaven or hell), and is not associated with a doctrine of reincarnation in one or another ranked form (worm, pig, woman, man, king, etc.) in another worldly life. It is not clear to the writer whether sin is believed by Christians in northern Thailand to be a direct cause of illness, or whether avoidance of sin is believed to prevent illness, much in the way accumulation of merit is used by Buddhists.

"Conditions, symptoms"

The condition which is known as *"lom"* in Thai, meaning air or wind, is widely accepted as a diagnostic category, though the causative origins of this sort of illness are not clearly known (at least to this author). One commonly accepted diagnosis among the several ethnic groups, *lom phit dyan,* is associated with postpartum, or sometimes menstrual irregularities. Its symptoms are weakness, perhaps nausea, and sometimes hypersensitivity to odors. The usual preventive action include wrist binding (prevention of soul loss), and food and activity taboos on a woman who has given birth, which restrict the kinds of foods she can eat and require her to be heated by lying near the fire for a certain number of days, the number is sometimes regulated by phases of the moon (*dyan*). Diagnosis of this illness is by symptom and history. Treatment, if the condition appears more serious than "normal," is by ingestion of "hot medicine" *(ja hawn)*, composed of a large number of herbs and spices, which is believed to "clean out" the stomach (or uterus), thereby preparing it for future pregnancies. Persistent cases may be treated by traditional specialists (herbalists), or may be considered to be caused by spirits or incantations, and thus subject to further diagnostic differentation and appropriate treatment.

Lom awk hu, literally "wind coming out of the ears," is a symptom, a sense of pressure in the ears, such as occurs with a head cold or ear infection, or when changing altitude walking up or down a hill. It is considered abnormal, but as such the symptom is not considered serious, and no cause (other than the circumstance) is attributed to it, nor is there any attempt at further diagnosis or treatment.

The diagnostic category *lom* ("wind," without any qualifier) is apparently associated with symptoms of faintness, loss of consciousness, and occasionally seizures (perhaps epileptic) or, as observed in a Lua' village, talking meaninglessly or incoherently, and uncontrolled trembling of the limbs. This extreme condition, labeled *lom,* is interpreted as a situation in which the patient is in direct uncontrolled contact with the land of the spirits. Contact with the spirits may be consciously desired, as a diagnostic device sought by spirit medium specialists, or by nonspecialists in direct contact with ancestral spirits during ceremonies. In these cases, speaking in ways which are not representative of the normal speech of the speaker is not labeled *lom,* nor interpreted as a symptom of illness. Most cases of *lom* are not so serious, and do not involve apparent loss of conscious control of speech.

Neither *lom phit dyan,* nor *lom* (unqualified) are recognized by Western-trained physicians as "reasonable" categories or syndromes, although there is virtually universal acceptance of these as important categories among the non-medically-qualified multi-ethnic population. Because this category seems primarily to be a symptom (in the local understanding) this may be a major area of potential conflict or misunderstanding between Western medical practitioners and Northern Thai, Lua' or Karen patients. To complain of *lom* is simply not meaningful to the Western-trained practitioner, and further symptomology or history (which is perhaps embarrassingly obvious to the patient or patient's relatives) must be sought.

Many expressions in the Lua', Karen and Northern Thai languages refer to the heart, in apparent reference to a person's psychological, moral, or even social position. Such expressions may be literally translated as "hot heart" (nervous), "cool heart" (relaxed, cool headed), "long heart" (generous), "old heart" (respected elder), "fallen heart" (surprised), "to enter the heart" (to understand), "hurt, broken heart" (disappointed, saddened), "healthy, happy heart" (healthy, happy, contented), "shaking heart" (palpitations, nervousness), etc. With the exception of the last one, such expressions seem most properly interpreted as metaphors similar to usages in English, rather than being anatomical or physiological descriptions. This inference is drawn from the fact that no direct attempt is made in any of the traditional medical systems to determine the physical condition of the heart, nor to influence directly its size, shape or condition, with the possible exception of "shaking heart" which is sometimes considered to be a symptom of illness. There seems to be no conception of using "hot" or "cold" medicine to influence the temperature of the heart (and thus influence the emotions of the individual) suggesting that this form of linguistic interpretation should not be pushed too far.

"Little bugs"

There is general recognition among many members of the multi-ethnic society that "little bugs" (maeng) can cause illness. This appears to be a local interpretation of the germ theory of disease. There is no elaborate association of particular symptoms or syndromes with particular varieties of "little bugs," nor does anyone claim to have seen them. Western (modern) medicine is believed to be effective against these bugs, although the mechanism involved is not clearly understood by the patients. The causation of symptoms by "little bugs" apparently does not rule out, for Lua' and Karen non-Christians, the alternative theories of disease cause. The spirit, soul loss, or incantation cause, if not identified and treated, may cause further outbreak of illness either in the present patient or some other patient, even if the symptoms of this particular illness are successfully removed. At a minimum, a patient with a disease successfully treated with medicine against little bugs should also be given the wrist-binding treatment for soul loss, to be sure that he is not left with residual weakness.

Natural causes

There is a clear understanding that "natural" causes may operate to cause illness, or at least injury. People have frequent experience with snake bites, burns, broken limbs, and similar, and the direct cause is clearly understood. Such illnesses are subject to symptomatic treatment, sometimes by modern medical practitioners or pharmacists, but often by specialists with knowledge of herbs, splinting, etc., many of which appear to an outside observer to be quite effective, as are some of the herbal and other remedies aimed at relief of symptoms believed caused by spirits, incantations, and so forth. Likewise addictions (to opium, alcohol) are traditionally thought of as natural, the result of exposure and "sticking" to the substances. A variety of cures may be sought, including proprietary drugs and Buddhist or Christian religious guidance.

Simple, direct treatment of apparently naturally-caused illness may leave unresolved the question of why a particular individual received a particular injury at a particular time. Thus a further cause (spirits, incantation, etc.) is sometimes sought, and, minimally (if recovery is prompt and "normal"), the patient's soul will be summoned and his wrists will be bound when it appears he is well on his way to recovery.

Spirits, devils

Animists who convert to Christianity do not thereby give up the theory that spirits cause illness, but they do abandon the idea that spirits can and should be propitiated, substituting the idea of appeal through prayer to a more powerful spirit. Vague symptoms which would have been ascribed to spirits by animists may be ascribed to devils and combated, without elaborate diagnosis, by prayer.

Evaluation

Evaluation by the system's participants of the diagnosis, treatment and underlying theory evidently proceeds on two levels, one referring to the particular case, and the other to the general theory. In general a successful cure supports the theoretical system and its application. Failure in a particular case is not considered to invalidate the general theory, though failure may lead an individual to try another subsystem. This is implied in the general acceptance of multiple theories of causation. This means there is *always* some place to go. People may be driven from one to another subsystem because of scarcity of resources, but this does not require that they change their entire belief systems. In fact, it is only the practitioners in the Western system who require "proof" of the effectiveness of a particular technique and categorically reject "supernatural" causes. As far as the customers are concerned, proof of the theory or the technique in a statistical or logical sense is never really available. Aside from anecdotal information on efficacy, accepting chemotherapy or modern surgery must be just as much an act of faith as is accepting the theory that spirits cause disease and that identifying and feeding the proper spirit with the proper sacrificial meal will cure a particular ailment. The test of the correctness of the "theory" must be whether it is perceived to work, at least some of the time. Under these conditions there is no adequate disproof of a theory if it does work some of the time, and it is perhaps best to consider that it is practice and practitioner not theory which is evaluated.

The description of theories, diagnostic principles, categorization of conditions and patterns of treatment suggests a fair degree of uncertainty is operating in the overall system of response to illness. We turn now to the question of how people choose within an overall system which has a variety of explanations, or levels of explanation, for many illnesses and a variety of possible responses once an explanation has been tentatively accepted.

A Paradigm of Medical Choices in a Multi-Ethnic Setting

In the previous descriptions it is apparent that there are several alternative choices of action or interpretation at most points in the process from recognition of illness through diagnosis, treatment and evaluation. A flow chart of the situation suggests an incompletely-deterministic branching stochastic process, with many possible loops, rather than a unilinear unidirectional deterministic flow (compare Figures 1 and 2). The writer believes this is true of all medical systems, though the details are bound to vary.

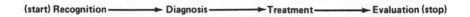

(start) Recognition ⟶ Diagnosis ⟶ Treatment ⟶ Evaluation (stop)

Figure 2. Unilinear-unidirectional deterministic model.

Number of Available Choices and Probabilities of Their Use

The nature of the systems in northern Thailand is such that starting at the point of recognition, the path by which a patient may travel to successive points is not determined, though by virtue of individual or group characteristics some subsets of paths may be more probable than others. Rules may be outlined describing the order in which some choices are made (recognition usually comes before diagnosis), but at many choice points the patient may "return to start" or "return to diagnosis," etc. for another set of choices, which, when rice grains are used for diagnosis, may be more or less randomly assigned. Within the overall system, including more or less discrete subsystems, it is possible to describe rules or probabilities that certain kinds of choices may be made by certain individuals (Christians are restricted from choosing spirit techniques in all but a very small number of cases—see Figure 3B).

The writing of a complete set of rules for the overall multi-ethnic system is beyond the scope of this paper, but we may consider the subsystems, in terms of the composition of the groups which enter them, as being ordered in terms of numbers of alternatives, from Lua' (the most complex and varied number of alternatives) through Karen and Northern Thai, to Western (missionary), the subsystem whose adherents have the fewest choices (or which has the lowest probabilities of making any but a restricted number of choices). We must review the social setting in which the potential interactions take place. It should be recognized that there is a rough parallel between this pattern of available choices and the prestige ranking of the subgroupings: hill minorities have the lowest prestige, Westerners have the highest. Of course prestige is *not* unilinearly ranked for all purposes and in all social contexts. This is so in part because even though Westerners are generally considered materially most powerful and rich, they are not necessarily considered culturally or morally superior. Also, it seems conceptually impossible for any non-Westerner to "become Western," or for any Westerner to "become Thai" (or Lua' or Karen) to the same extent that a Lua' may "become Karen" or "become Thai." In part the prestige rankings represent aspirations for social mobility which can realistically be accomplished. The prestige rankings also are not unilinear because, although both Karen and Lua' villagers readily admit their economic and political inferiority to the dominant Thai society, they both claim cultural and moral superiority to some important aspects of Northern Thai culture and behavior (especially marriage patterns), and they also both claim cultural superiority to each other. In spite of this, Lua' and Karen consider themselves, especially vis-à-vis Northern Thai, to be "like brothers and sisters," and Karen myths speak of similar relationships with Westerners.

Animist-Buddhist Lua' individuals may and do enter any part of the multi-ethnic health system as customers. Missionaries, and their strict followers, partake in a much more restricted segment of the total system (including Western medicine practiced by missionary doctors, Western drugs purchased from pharmacists, traditional Western home remedies, Christian prayer).

The boundaries of the social groups themselves are not complete barriers, and individuals may and do move from one to another, as shown in Figure 4.

Social Influences on Choice: Systems Boundaries

We may ask if position in, or movement from one to another part of, the social space represented in Figure 4 affects movement through the medical system, or restricts choices within it. Clearly a difference or change in ethnic group does influence and often inhibits choices, sometimes deliberately so. A person who starts as an animist-Buddhist Lua' and becomes a Protestant or Catholic cannot return to animist Lua' diagnostic and treatment systems for spirit-caused, incantation-caused, or soul-loss illness without leaving the Christian group and sub-culture, and resuming Lua' animist identity and group membership. Occasionally this has been done and has been accompanied by a re-acceptance of traditional techniques. More often the Lua' has become Christian to escape the burdens of supporting spirits through the traditional techniques, and also, explicitly in some cases, to get aid from the missionaries in receiving Western medicine.

We have suggested there is a general parallel between prestige ranking of the ethnic groups within the multi-ethnic social system and use of the various medical subsystems by members of the different ethnic groups. In general, it appears that in seeking medical help one looks to an equal or higher social level in a way that parallels both the prestige ranking and the general pattern of attempts at social mobility. It is relatively rare for a Northern Thai to become Lua' or Karen, and it is unlikely that a Northern Thai would seek a Lua' or Karen medical specialist— he would probably feel loss of status in doing so. Lua' individuals and families do occasionally become Northern Thai and do occasionally seek medical assistance from Northern Thai healers, both traditional her-

Young adult Lua' male

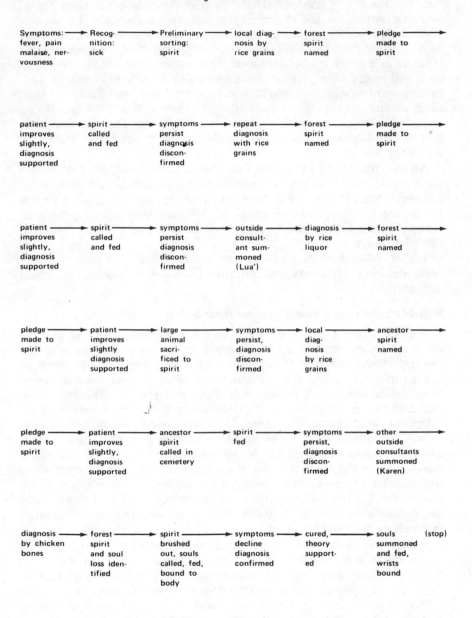

Symptoms: → Recog- → Preliminary → local diag- → forest → pledge →
fever, pain   nition: sorting: nosis by   spirit   made to
malaise, ner-   sick   spirit   rice grains   named   spirit
vousness

patient → spirit → symptoms → repeat → forest → pledge →
improves   called   persist   diagnosis   spirit   made to
slightly,   and fed   diagnosis   with rice   named   spirit
diagnosis   discon-   grains
supported   firmed

patient → spirit → symptoms → outside → diagnosis → forest →
improves   called   persist   consult-   by rice   spirit
slightly,   and fed   diagnosis   ant sum-   liquor   named
diagnosis   discon-   moned
supported   firmed   (Lua')

pledge → patient → large → symptoms → local → ancestor →
made to   improves   animal   persist,   diag-   spirit
spirit   slightly   sacri-   diagnosis   nosis   named
           diagnosis   ficed to   discon-   by rice
           supported   spirit   firmed   grains

pledge → patient → ancestor → spirit → symptoms → other →
made to   improves   spirit   fed   persist,   outside
spirit   slightly,   called in   diagnosis   consultants
           diagnosis   cemetery   discon-   summoned
           supported   firmed   (Karen)

diagnosis → forest → spirit → symptoms → cured, → souls   (stop)
by chicken   spirit   brushed   decline   theory   summoned
bones   and soul   out, souls   diagnosis   support-   and fed,
             loss iden- called, fed, confirmed   ed   wrists
             tified   bound to   bound
                         body

Note persistent actions during illness, especially at times of crisis: relatives, neighbors and friends gather around patient, massage wrists and legs, display emotional involvement with patient; patient's family continues to participate in community rituals.

Figure 3. Examples of cases. (A) (above) Young adult Lua' male; (B) (facing page) young adult married Lua' female.

Patient: young adult married Lua' female

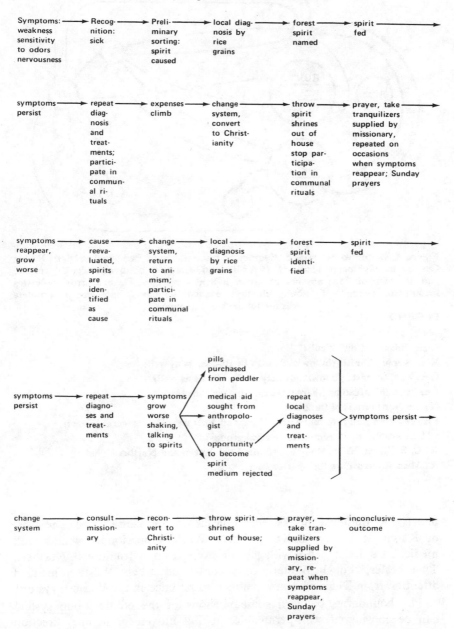

Note persistent actions during illness, especially at times of crisis: relatives, neighbors and friends gather around patient, massage wrists and legs, display emotional involvement with patient; patient's family participates in community rituals only during periods of animism.

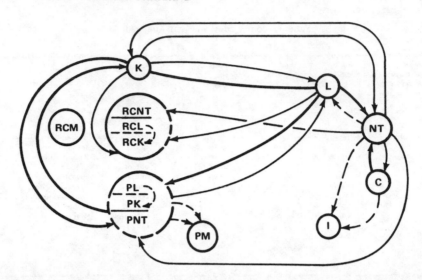

Figure 4. Simplified Schematic Diagram of Interchange of Personnel between Ethnic Groups in Northwest Thailand. (Breadth and direction of arrows signify volume and direction of flow; absence of arrow indicates no flow. Dashed arrow indicates incomplete change of ethnic identity; dashed boundary indicates incomplete distinction between groups.)

LEGEND:

C = Chinese "Confucianist"
K = Karen animists (in lowlands may be Buddhists as well)
L = Lua' animists (in lowlands may be Buddhists as well)
I = "Indian" Muslims (there are also Chinese Muslims)
NT = Northern Thai Buddhists
PK, PL, PNT = Protestant Karen, Lua' and Northern Thai (several groups)
PM = Protestant Missionaries (several groups)
RCL, RCK, RCNT = Roman Catholic Lua', Karen and Northern Thai
RCM = Roman Catholic missionaries

balists and Buddhist monks. Missionaries do not aspire to become Lua' or Karen. It is very unlikely that a Western missionary would seek medical aid from a hill villager, or even from a traditional Northern Thai healer, though Western missionaries do accept Western medical attention from Thais who are qualified to practice in the Western system.

The boundaries between some portions of the ethnic group system can be considered semi-permeable, in that movement in one direction is much more common than movement in the other. Position in the ethnic structure restricts availability of alternative choices socially in terms of patterned interactions between groups (as outlined above) and culturally (in terms of belief systems shared or not shared with other individuals). In this context the conceptual conflict between theories is clear: Christians may believe in souls, but not in soul-loss as a cause or concomitant of illness, nor in wrist-binding as a therapeutic activity. They are allowed to believe in devils, but are not allowed to believe that forest spirits can be propitiated by direct animal sacrifices; thus traditional techniques depending on communication with these spirits are no longer relevant, nor is consultation with native specialists, except for symptomatic relief by use of herbs, or other physical or material techniques. Lua' and Karen who convert to Christianity believe in part they are doing so in order to reduce their burdens of obligations to potentially hungry spirits. Their change in belief is symbolized by literally throwing the spirit dwellings out of their house at the time of conversion.

It seems clear from the way in which these people act that *they* recognize fairly explicitly the difference between operating at the conceptual realm (including beliefs in spirits and souls) and operating at the physical or material realm (Seijas 1973). Their ideas of "cause" may involve both realms, and clearly their ideas about treatment and prevention involve both. They have techniques for dealing with both realms, and their physical or material techniques are often quite effective. They know when they are dealing with one or the other realm, as well as recognizing the culturally or socially determined boundaries between different subsystems dealing with these realms. Physical effectiveness in dealing with symptoms is quickly appreciated, but is not necessarily a reason for accepting the underlying theory which may be in the mind of the therapist, nor is it necessarily a reason for rejecting traditional beliefs that spirits cause disease, even if the idea that germs cause disease is accepted.

The existence of fairly firm lines between subsystems of the spiritual realm is not confined to the distinction between Christianity and animism. Lua' people may "convert" to become Karen, or to become Northern Thai, by moving into appropriate communities, with the intention of thereby removing themselves from obligations to Lua' spirits. Karen beliefs include acceptance of a tattooing ritual (*cekosi*), perhaps originally Buddhist-Brahmanist, for doing away with the extremely demanding obligations to ancestral spirits, by making a token offering of a pledge which can never be redeemed (roasted, sterilized seeds are offered with a promise to make further offerings only after they have germinated and flowered). After this ceremony has been performed on behalf of a household, they say that the household members and their descendants are no longer subject to demands from the ancestor spirits, that is, that their ancestral spirits can no longer cause them illness in order to call attention to their needs. (This pattern of belief is regarded as hypocritical by those Karen who continue to serve their ancestral spirits.)

The multi-ethnic social system is populated by groups of people who hold different, partially overlapping, partially exclusive, theories or assumptions regarding the nature and recognition of illness and the appropriate techniques for diagnosing, treating and evaluating the treatment of illness. Restrictions on movements between different parts of the system lie at different points on the paths from recognition through treatment and evaluation of treatment. Mutual acceptance of underlying assumptions is not necessarily required for participation in interaction across some of the boundaries between the groups, and in fact might inhibit such interaction. One obvious example is that a Lua' patient need not know modern physiology, nor accept the germ theory of disease, in order to accept treatment from a Western practitioner who bases his "rational" therapy on that theory. Nor does the Western therapist necessarily have to know or accept the patient's theory of the illness cause, so long as there can be some communication regarding the symptoms and desired outcome of the relationship between the parties.

Lack of mutual acceptance of theories underlying the actions does not necessarily inhibit some potential interactions. Missionaries do not accept completely Lua' theories of disease diagnosis and cure. There is agreement on the theory that diseases can be caused by spirit forces, but missionary methods (exorcism, expulsion) are incompatible with traditional diagnostic and curing techniques (appeasement after establishing communication). Thus, though it is possible for a Lua' to accept simultaneously Lua' theories of disease cause, diagnosis and therapy while participating in Karen animist or Northern Thai folk-Buddhist curing rituals, when he becomes a Lua' Christian, he must reject (and usually *wants* to reject) a series of traditional Lua' diagnostic preventive and curing techniques along with their expensive sacrifices. Becoming Northern Thai does not require this sort of rejection, though it may make some of the specific disease causes irrelevant or remote, because becoming Thai requires movement away from the hills where many of the spirits causing disease for Lua' mountain dwellers are believed to live.

Social Influences on Choice: Within and Between-Group Variation

Aside from the existence of such boundaries imposed by the nature of the medical subsystems themselves, the members of the multi-ethnic society appear to behave as members of their respective groups in responding to the health services which are available to them from other ethnic groups. By this is meant that their behavior in health contexts is similar to their behavior in other inter-ethnic contexts. Examples of this generalization may be seen in patterns of use of a Western medicine mission clinic, where the following observations were made: Age distribution of patients in the clinic, when classified by ethnic group, reflects a basic difference in travel patterns between Lua' and Karen. Despite an overall similarity in age structure, there are fewer Lua' children than Karen children seen in the clinic. This is an example of the general behavior pattern in which Karens frequently travel as complete family groups (including infants and young children) when going to visit or to market, while Lua' families frequently send only the adult or young members to visit or to market (Kunstadter, Chiewsilp and Yuill 1968).

Ethnic differences in use of the clinic for birth control reflects not just the "need" (as defined by Western-trained personnel, including missionaries), but rather the reproductive controls of the ethnic groups prior to the availability of medical birth control techniques (Northern Thais in the community have had lower fertility, and are now the most liable to seek birth control information and services). The sex ratio of Lua' and Karen patients (more males than females) probably reflects the dominance of males in inter-ethnic or commercial activities of Lua' and Karen villagers, while the prominent place of women in Northern Thai commercial and inter-ethnic activities is reflected in the fact that there are slightly more female than male Northern Thai patients. These relationships are probably "real," not the spurious effect of differential proximity of the different ethnic groups to the clinic, which is located in the midst of a predominantly Karen community, but within easy walking distance of Northern Thai and predominantly Lua' communities in the same town.

Summary and Conclusions

The data reviewed in this paper regarding medical systems in their social settings may be summarized as follows:

In a situation where multiple subsystems are available, cultural differences regarding theories of illness may make a difference in the perception of illness and use of techniques for diagnosing and treating illness. Sometimes these differences may be deliberately manipulated in order to produce a desired effect, i.e., an individual may change his culture or a portion of it in order to avoid using a portion of his culture. The drawing of lines between subsystems is not unique to Western theories of illness, though Western theories tend to be more exclusivistic and universalistic than traditional ones in northwestern Thailand.

Use of medical systems across boundaries of ethnic groups and their cultural subsystems may be a principal focus for inter-ethnic relationships in a multi-ethnic society. Differential use reflects *general* patterns of social relations within the user group, and between user and outside groups, regardless of the specific content of the interactions.

Individuals make changes in regard to the practice of a particular traditional (non-scientific?) subsystem, not because of conclusive scientific proof of theoretical correctness but rather for more "practical" or empirical reasons, including immediate availability, convenience, low cost, high perceived effectiveness, satisfaction of the need to feel something is being done, appropriateness for the immediate social situation, and perhaps social prestige (including affiliation with a group perceived to be powerful, successful and benevolent). Perception of effectiveness, in the absence of statistical tests, is unlikely to be anything but anecdotal. Given the uncertain outcome of illnesses (from which most people are going to recover most of the time), "proof" of the superiority of any system is unlikely to be completely scientific, though it may be "rational" on the basis of available evidence and the acceptance of recognized authority.

Multiplicity of choices is probably beneficial to the perpetuation of any one of the subsystems to the extent to which it allows any possible outcome of a series of uncertain events to be interpreted, understood and accepted, without calling for revision in the system if things do not work out the way they are "supposed to." Multiplicity of interpretive systems increases ambiguity beyond the level achieved even in a system as ambiguous as the diagnosis of spirit-caused illness. Complete consistency with a single theoretical system is not required to make people happy. Ambiguity may be preferable in the face of an uncertain and uncontrollable world. This may be both an explanation of why diverse systems persist and a reason why they should be allowed to persist, even in a society supposedly as scientific (and exclusivistic) as our own. This is not a plea for the Age of Aquarius, but rather a suggestion that diversity may give strength.

Comparative Studies of Medical Systems in Various Societies: So What?

This chapter began with the question: Under what circumstances do cultural differences make a difference? This question may be important, first, because an answer may lead to improved understanding of human behavior under the common situation of confrontation of two or more different cultural traditions, and second, because if we are concerned with medical systems for the propagation of human welfare, cultural differences may inhibit the transfer of life-saving knowledge and practices. Are there general theoretical lessons to be learned from the analysis of choice points in the medical care systems of northwestern Thailand and in the other papers presented at this conference?

There are frequent references in other chapters of this book as well as in the literature to the humoral, *yin-yang,* cold-hot, or "Hippocratic" classifications of illness and treatment. The general theory associates an illness with a class (hot or cold, etc.), which in turn is conceptually associated with a parallel classification of medication or other treatment. Anthropologists have often asserted that there are conflicts between these traditional classifications and their associated theories of disease cause and cure, on the one hand, and modern Western, or cosmopolitan, medical practice on the other. The usual form of the argument is that, when Western practice applies treatment which is perceived or classified as inappropriate in the local system for the category in which the disease is locally placed, treatment will be rejected because of the "cultural conflict" or "cognitive dissonance" generated in the patient.

A more general statement of the theory is that people are "rational" in attempting to make their behavior conform to a single consistent set of general cultural rules (or "cognitive maps," or ethno-theories of how the world is or should be structured) which determine how individuals will behave in any real situation. Derived from this theory is the hypothesis that an item will be accepted or rejected depending on its agreement (congruence, consonance) or disagreement (incongruity, dissonance) with the traditionally established classifications and their associated behaviors. Is the theory sound, and does the material presented in this chapter and elsewhere in this volume help us in evaluating the theory or hypotheses derived from it?

The writer believes the theory is seductive but not basically sound, or, at best, it is incomplete. This is said in part because the writer does not believe people ordinarily intellectualize their behavior in the sense of making everything consistent, neither is it believed they could do so even if they wanted to. This is not to say that people are not "rational," in the sense of trying to make their actions appropriate to their goals and modifying their actions in the light of experience, but rather to suggest their rationality (or their rationalizations) applies in limited contexts at any one time, that they have multiple goals and values and that their values and goals are often mutually contradictory. The ordinary human game, the writer believes, is *not* the intellectual one of conforming to a single set of rules, applicable in all situations, to reach a single goal. Rather, it involves multiple rules applicable in some but not all situations, and requires balancing between several simultaneously desired goals or values. If we no longer believe in "economic man" or "political man," why should we believe in "rational-consistent man" behaving only with respect to a single set of principles?

One bit of evidence supporting this argument is the existence of multiple theories of illness and treatment which ordinarily have not been made to conform in a single consistent system of theory and behavior. The situation in northwestern Thailand may represent a higher than usual number of available subsystems, but in having alternatives it is not unique among Asian or Western societies. This suggests that people need not put any novel event automatically into one or another mutually exclusive category. Evidently, for some items or events the hot-cold, etc. classifications are considered by users of that system to be irrelevant.

Another bit of evidence is the common report (Anderson, Chapter 4) that the classifications may not be applied similarly by members of different subcultures within the same (Chinese) culture, or, for some events or items, there may be differences in application of the classification system by individuals within the same subculture or ethnic group.

Beyond these arguments, which are essentially ahistorical, one may ask the question of how cultures may change in the face of a "strain for consistency." The concept might be useful for understanding persistence, but seems of no help in explaining invention or cultural change.

These arguments suggest that if the "strain for consistency" has utility, the context of consistency must be considered. Is there any reason why there must be only one kind of consistency? It is suggested that the evidence which is occasionally presented to support the cognitive dissonance hypothesis be re-examined in two ways: (1) Is lack of consistency used as a handy *ex post facto* rationalization for rejecting an item already rejected on other grounds? and (2) if so, what other explanations are there for the initial rejection? The writer feels there are many other possible factors, including such things as economics (too expensive), geographical distance (too far), social distance (too high or too low in the social ranking system, or too unfamiliar, or involving people with whom there are no other social connections), fads (why else would acupuncture become so popular in the West, roughly simultaneous with President Nixon's visit to Peking? Surely this has nothing to do with classificatory consonance in our medical culture), or perceived success or lack of success (many people die in hospitals, etc.). All such reasons are in some sense "rational" and all in some sense can be seen to conform to some cognitive map (perhaps constructed after the event). They cannot all be referred to a single goal or value.

The author suggests that greater emphasis be placed in future studies in looking at the section of the process labeled "preliminary sorting" (Figure 1), which may be a point at which the selection is made of systems with which to maintain consistency. It is also suggested that a more detailed look be made at the conditions associated with a return to an earlier point in the paradigm (once diagnosis or treatment have been performed), and at the question of evaluation as it extends to earlier as well as later events in the paradigm.

Perhaps making these arguments specific will encourage research designed to test relevant hypotheses beyond the level of seeking mere plausibility.

Throughout this chapter assertions have been made concerning practices, beliefs and interpretations. In general these are based on direct observation of the practices and responses to the writer's direct requests for explanation of these practices. The writer has tried to indicate by qualifying statements ("it appears," etc.) where belief is inferred rather than having being directly communicated.

As regards interpretation or explanation, some of this derives from direct observation and response to questioning (e.g., explanation of reasons for religious conversion), but in some places the inferences are the writer's, unverified by direct questioning (e.g., the assertions that there really is a "system" and that ambiguity tends to maintain conceptual systems associated with uncertain events). No doubt the writer has imposed his own concepts of orderliness (although pointing out ambiguities which are believed an essential feature of the system). It is wondered if the author's informants would agree with this interpretation, and how the author would interpret their response, regardless of what it was. Is the ordered ambiguity "really" out there, or is its functional beauty only in the mind of the beholder?

Ideally these different levels of observation and interpretation should be clearly separated and used as the basis for future research, but that is beyond the scope of this already long chapter.

NOTES

1. It is perhaps characteristic only of the orthodox medical professionals of modern Western middle-class society to deny the existence of medical systems other than the (for them) approved, legitimate professional system. Despite their doctors' belief in the superiority of "official" professional medicine, Western middle-class people use massive amounts of non-professional and unorthodox treatment systems (e.g., patent and proprietary drugs). They also evidently rely on a variety of explanatory theories or hypotheses which are only incompletely, or not at all, integrated into orthodox professional medical practice (e.g., diet, exercise, stress, recreation, prayer, exorcism, moral support, etc.). Some of these are the basis for more or less organized alternative medical systems which, though usually denounced by the professional establishment, persist in Western societies (chiropractic, Christian Science, diet fads, faith healing, etc.).

2. The "medical system" thus defined may be considered to be related to the "health system" which includes the ecological conditions influencing the distribution of health and illness in the population. The health system also includes characteristics of the natural environment (including disease organisms, reservoirs, and vectors), the economic system which determines the distribution of goods and services and thus may influence the distribution of malnutrition or access to medical care, and the social system which influences contacts between people and thus possibly affects the transmission of disease organisms, whether or not it is intended or understood to function in this way. For a recent comprehensive review of the field of medical anthropology see Lieban (1974), cf. the distinction between "sociology of medicine" and "sociology in medicine" (Lieban 1974:1033ff., citing Kendall (1963) and Straus (1957)).

3. General ethnographic background on Lua', Karen and Northern Thai in Mae Sariang District, northwestern Thailand, may be found in Kunstadter (1965, 1966, 1967, 1969A, 1969B, 1970, 1972). For additional information on medical systems and customs elsewhere in Thailand see Anuman Rajathon (1961), Blanchard et al (1958), Cunningham (1970), Cunningham, Doege and Bangxang (1970), and Hanks (1963); for an outline of the formal structure of health systems in Thailand see Research Analysis Corporation (1968); for a description of a health system in another upland minority group see Durrenberger (1972); and for a description of the role of Buddhist monks in curing, see Tambiah (1970).

4. Other causes are reported for other parts of northern Thailand. Examples include one specialist in Chiang Mai who treats imbalances of the elemental components of wind, water, earth and fire (*thaat lom, thaat nam, thaat din, thaat fai*). Excessive weakness or strength (*thaat awn, thaat kae*) of these components may appear in various

symptoms, may be diagnosed by physical examination and treated with herbal remedies. Compounding the prescriptions may involve a theory of hot and cold and seasonal variations as well as practical knowledge of the effects of herbs. Women mediums *(chao nai),* who specialize in diagnoses of illnesses through trance or spirit possession, are found in many Northern Thai communities. Chinese drug stores, found in all sizeable towns, sell Chinese herbal, mineral and animal medicines usually along with an array of "patent" and "ethical" products. Ideas of causality associated with these modes of curing apparently are not familiar to the rural people in Mae Sariang District, and are not included in this description of their alternative systems. Some of these people may use these specialists (especially Chinese pharmacists) for diagnosis and prescription of cure.

5. In other parts of Thailand *phi ka'* is thought to be a spirit genetically inherited in certain family lines. The spirit is also believed to enter and devour the organs of its victims, its presence may be confirmed by a spirit doctor who can cause the spirit to answer questions through the vicitm. Preventive action is to avoid offending the people who are reported possessors of this spirit, but no attempt is made to expell them from their village.

REFERENCES

ANUMAN RAJATHON *Phraya*
1961   Life and Ritual in Old Siam: Three Studies of Thai Life and Customs. Translated and edited by W. J. Gedney. New Haven: Human Relations Area Files Press.

BLANCHARD, W., H. C. AHALT, A. BELL, M. GRESHAM, B. HOFFMAN, J. MCEWEN, and J. SCHARR
1958   Thailand, Its People, Its Society, Its Culture. New Haven: Human Relations Area Files Press.

BRASS, P. R.
1968   The politics of Ayurvedic education: A case study of revivalism and modernization in India. *In* Education and Politics in India: Studies in Organization, Society, and Policy. Susanne H. Rudolph and Lloyd I. Rudolph, eds. Chapter 14, pp. 342–371. Cambridge: Harvard University Press.

CUNNINGHAM, C. E.
1970   Thai "injection doctors": Antibiotic mediators. Social Science and Medicine 4:1–24.

CUNNINGHAM, C. E., T. C. DOEGE, and H. NA BANGXANG, eds.
1970   Studies of Health Problems and Health Behavior in Saraphi District, North Thailand. Chiang Mai, Thailand: Faculty of Medicine, Chiang Mai University.

DURRENBERGER, E. P.
1972   The ethnography of Lisu curing. Ph.D. dissertation, Department of Anthropology, University of Illinois, Champaign-Urbana, abstract published in Dissertation Abstracts International 32(10):5585–B, April 1972.

HANKS, J. R.
1963   Maternity and its rituals in Bang-Chan. Cornell Thailand Project, Interim Report Series, No. 6. Data Paper No. 51. Ithaca, N.Y.: Southeast Asia Program, Department of Asian Studies, Cornell University.

KENDALL, P. L.
1963   Medical sociology in the United States. Social Science Information 2:1–15.

KUNSTADTER, P.
1965   The Lua' (Lawa) of Northern Thailand: Aspects of social structure, agriculture and religion. Princeton University, Center of International Studies Research Monograph 21. November 1965.

KUNSTADTER, P.
1966   Residential and social organization of the Lawa of Northern
       Thailand. Southwestern Journal of Anthropology 22(1):61–
       84. Reprinted *in* Introductory Readings on Sociological Con-
       cepts, Methods and Data, M. Abrahamson, ed. New York:
       Van Nostrand Reinhold Company, pp. 74–84, 1969.

KUNSTADTER, P.
1967   The Lua' and Skaw Karen of Maehongson Province, North-
       western Thailand. *In* Southeast Asian Tribes, Minorities, and
       Nations, P. Kunstadter, ed. Princeton: Princeton University
       Press, pp. 639–673.

KUNSTADTER, P., D. CHIEWSILP and T. M. YUILL
1968   Social integration and ecological isolation: a report of a medi-
       cal survey of a Lua' village in Maehongson Province, north-
       western Thailand. Bangkok: SEATO Medical Research Lab-
       oratory, mimeo. 67 pp.

KUNSTADTER, P.
1969A Hill and valley populations in northwestern Thailand. *In* P.
       Hinton, ed., Tribesman and Peasants in North Thailand.
       Chiang Mai: Tribal Research Centre, pp. 69–85.

KUNSTADTER, P.
1969B Socio-cultural change among upland peoples of Thailand: Lua'
       and Karen—two modes of adaptation. Proceedings of the
       VIIIth International Congress of Anthropological and Eth-
       nological Sciences, 1968, Tokyo and Kyoto, vol. II, Ethnology,
       Tokyo: Science Council of Japan. pp. 232–235.

KUNSTADTER, P.
1970   Medical care systems available to upland minority peoples.
       Paper prepared for Symposium on the Culture of Health and
       Illness in North Thailand, C. E. Cunningham, Chairman,
       American Anthropological Association, 69th Annual Meeting,
       San Diego, November 1970, mimeo. Abstract published in
       Abstracts of the meeting.

KUNSTADTER, P.
1972   Spirits of change capture the Karens. National Geographic
       Magazine, February: 267–284.

LESLIE, C.
1967   Professional and popular health cultures in South Asia:
       Needed research in medical sociology and anthropology. *In*
       Understanding Science and Technology in India and Pakistan,
       W. Morehouse, ed., Occasional Publications No. 8, Foreign
       Area Materials Center, University of the State of New York.

LIEBAN, R. W.
1974 Medical anthropology. *In* Handbook of Social and Cultural Anthropology, John J. Honigmann, ed. New York: Rand McNally College Publishing Company, Ch. 24, pp. 1031–1072.

RESEARCH ANALYSIS CORPORATION, FIELD OFFICE—THAILAND
1968 Health Improvement Organizations and Programs, prepared by Research Analysis Corporation, Field Office—Thailand, for the Joint Thai-US Military Research and Development Center, sponsored by Office of the Secretary of Defense, Advanced Research Projects Agency, Counterinsurgency Organizations and Programs in Northeast Thailand (U), Volume 6. OSD/ARPA Research and Development Center, APO San Francisco 96346, Military Research and Development Center, Bangkok, Thailand.

RILEY, J. N. and SANTHAT SERMSRI
1974 The variegated Thai medical system as a context for birth control services. Bangkok: Institute for Population and Social Research, Mahidol University, Working Paper No. 6, mimeo. 71pp.

SEIJAS, H.
1973 An approach to the study of the medical aspects of culture. Current Anthropology 14: 544–545.

STRAUS, R.
1957 The nature and status of medical sociology. American Sociological Review 22:200–204.

TAMBIAH, S. J.
1970 Buddhism and the Spirit Cults in Northeast Thailand. Cambridge Studies in Social Anthropology 2. London and New York: Cambridge University Press.

CHAPTER 10

SUPERNATURALLY CAUSED ILLNESS IN TRADITIONAL BURMESE MEDICINE

MELFORD E. SPIRO

Introduction

Although traditional Burmese medicine recognizes both "natural" and "supernatural" causes of disease, the present paper is restricted to those of the latter type which, according to village estimates at least, accounts for about 25 percent of the total. This restriction is dictated by two considerations. First, in his own work in Burma the author was especially concerned with religion, and data on medicine were collected insofar as they were related to religious investigations.[1] Hence, the author's personal knowledge of naturally caused illness and its treatment is limited. Second, social science research in Burma has been confined to a small number of scholars, and these few have had little interest in medicine. As a result, the information available on the non-supernatural aspects of traditional Burmese medicine is scanty. For both reasons this paper is confined to supernaturally caused illness.[2]

Following a general sketch of what the Burmese villagers consider to be supernaturally caused illness, we shall turn to a more detailed examination of one of its sub-types—mental illness. In all cases the data to be presented here are based on the author's work in Upper Burma in the early 1960's and, more particularly, in villages within a 10-mile radius of the former capital of Mandalay. In short, this paper deals with supernaturally caused illness at the village level.

Disease Theory

Traditional Burmese medicine recognizes a variety of supernatural agents of disease (and death), the most prominent being witches, ghosts, and a type of evil spirits, known as *nat*. Beginning with the first, we may distinguish two types of witches—master witches (*aulan hsaya*) and ordinary witches (*soun*). The former are not only the more powerful, but they are male, while the latter are female; the former are hired by a client, the latter practice from personal spite; the former utilize ghosts, *nat,* and other evil spirits to achieve their nefarious ends, the latter achieve theirs by innate power or by the use of spells, rites, and material substances.

Based on acquired knowledge, the master witch causes illness by obtaining coercive power over various spirits who do his bidding. Power over a *nat,* for example, is obtained by making an offering consisting of opposite, sacred and profane, elements. The profane elements may consist of the beak of a crow, the penis of a dog, a woman's skirt (the latter being polluting), and earth from a cemetery, a latrine, and a *nat* shrine. The sacred elements may consist of a streamer adorning a Buddha image and earth taken from a monastic ordination hall. The master witch sets fire to this concoction, places it at the shrine of a powerful *nat* (the Mahagiri *nat*) who is repelled by fire, and thereby gains control over him.

Witches are much more prevalent than master witches; indeed, according to folk belief, there is a witch in one out of every seven houses who, as already indicated, is almost always female. Witches generally cause someone to become ill because he or she has offended them in some manner. The most typical witch-caused illnesses are eye, intestinal, and mental illnesses. Although there is a variety of techniques by which witches may achieve their end, the most prevalent technique is to introduce some foreign object, such as human hair, which they had previously cursed, into their victim's food, and thereby "poison" him.

There are at least three types of ghosts in Burmese belief; the type that is relevant for our purposes comprise the disembodied "souls" of persons who, as karmic punishment for sins committed in their previous lives, are reborn as ghosts (*tasei, thaye*). Typically invisible, they are described as monstrous in size, black, having huge ears, long tongues, tusk-like teeth, and repulsive in all ways. Usually living near cemeteries, where they feed on corpses, they enter a village when they are hungry or are in an especially malevolent state, in order to eat a villager or to cause him to become ill. In addition to individual illnesses, epidemics of plague and cholera are also caused by ghosts (and *nat*).

Nat refers to a class of supernatural beings who are more powerful than man and who can affect him for good or evil. Our concern here is with only one type, the so-called "Thirty-Seven *Nat*." These are malevolent spirits who had been human beings in their former lives and had come to sudden and violent deaths. Although they can cause various types of illnesses, they most prominently cause mental illness. Essentially irascible and quick to take offense, it is best to have nothing to do with them. Since, however, they cannot be evaded, discretion dictates that they be propitiated by means of food offerings. If they are not propitiated, or if they are offended in other ways, they may cause harm, including (among other things) illness and death.

Based on surveys in the villages of Upper Burma in which the author worked, we can make the following generalizations concerning the types of diseases that are supernaturally caused. The most frequent supernaturally caused children's diseases ("disease" refers to those conditions which the villagers identify as disease) include prolonged crying, abdominal pains, diarrhea, dysentery, fever, and body sores. For adults the list includes sore eyes, choking feelings, appetite loss, abdominal pains, diarrhea, dysentery, fright, and mental illness (including wandering about in a daze, falling unconscious, violent attacks, uncontrolled obscenity, fits, and trance states). The patients ("victims" is a better word from the Burmese point of view) vary with respect to age and sex. Supernaturally caused illnesses are generally restricted to those under 5 and over 14 years of age, and are rarely found during the so-called latency period of personality development. Again, in almost all cases, ghost-caused diseases (except for epidemics) are confined to children, *nat*- and witch-caused diseases to adults. Finally, adult females are more susceptible to supernaturally caused diseases than adult males.

Supernaturally caused illnesses occur in one of four ways: object intrusion, spirit intrusion, soul interference, and attack from a distance. Object intrusion, as has already been indicated, is the typical method of witch-caused illness. In "soul interference"—another method of witch-caused illness—the witch steals the patient's soul (or "butterfly spirit" as it is called in Burma). A brief absence of the soul results in illness, a prolonged absence results in death. In attack from a distance, illness results from the magical manipulation of the patient's exuviae. There are, finally, two types of spirit intrusion. In one type the soul of the *nat* unites with that of the patient; in the other the *nat* or witch himself/ herself enters the patient (in spirit form). If, to use our jargon, both types may be referred to as "possession," the former type occurs without trance, the latter occurs with trance. More is written about this below.

Preventive Medicine

For witches (including master-witches), preventive medicine consists in placing food for them to eat outside the home, the wearing of amulets, and the living of a proper Buddhist life. If, despite these precautions, a person is bewitched, and if, despite medical treatment, he should die, more rigorous techniques are used to prevent the witch from causing further illness or death. For example, a master-witch may be employed to harm the putative witch or to kill her. Either goal, needless to say, is achieved by ritual techniques.

The wearing of amulets is a widespread means of preventive medicine, not only with respect to witches but with respect to ghosts and *nat* as well. The type of amulet most frequently used is a small, cylindrical, metallic foil, over which an incantation or spell has been pronounced. The amulet is attached to a piece of string, and worn about the neck or wrist. *Aficionados* of the occult use even more powerful amulets, such as cabalistic symbols inscribed on paper or metal, and which sometimes are inserted into the flesh, or small alchemic balls, usually of mercury or iron, which are carried on the person. These amulets, it should be noted, not only offer protection against supernaturally caused illnesses, but also 'against other forms of supernatural and natural calamities.

To prevent plague or cholera epidemics, public ceremonies are conducted at seasonal changes. Fires are lit in various quarters of the village or town, accompanied by the beating, with fists and mallets, of gongs, tin roofs, wooden doors, pots and pans, and anything else that comes to hand. The combination of the brightness of the fire and the loud and cacophonous sounds is believed to frighten away the ghosts. To make sure that they stay away, a group of Buddhist monks walk in procession through the various quarters chanting Buddhist spells.

The most effective prevention of *nat*-caused illness, as has already been mentioned, is their regular propitiation, including prayer and offerings. Depending on the *nat*, propitiation may take place in the home, in the fields, or at a *nat* shrine. In addition there are elaborate public festivals for the Thirty-Seven *Nat*, at which time their propitiation also includes singing and trance dancing to the accompaniment of orchestral music.

Medical Practitioners

When illness strikes, the Burmese can choose among a wide variety of medical specialists, including modern physicians, herbal doctors, astrologers, shamans, exorcists, and many others. Even when they know that they are suffering from a naturally caused illness, however, Burmese peasants only infrequently consult modern physicians, if only because the latter are almost exclusively found in towns and cities. Instead, they consult, at least in the first instance, a traditional herbal doctor (*hsei hsaya*), of whom typically there is at least one in every village. The latter not only dispense the herbs and roots that are part of their extensive pharmacopoeia, but their treatment also usually includes some magical rite, in the belief that the latter practices enhance the therapeutic efficacy of the physical medicine. Should these doctors diagnose the illness as supernaturally caused, charms, spells, and amulets—as well as herbs—comprise the major components of their *materia medica*.

If the patient or his relatives believe that the illness is supernaturally caused, then, in the case of physical illness, they will usually consult either a herbal doctor—most of whom, as has been indicated, specialize in both naturally and supernaturally caused illnesses—or a shaman (whom we shall describe below). If, despite the efforts of the one or the other, the illness persists, or if antecedently it is assumed that the illness is supernaturally caused, they will consult an exorcist. Often, the herbal doctor is also an exorcist (in which case the patient need make no choice concerning the appropriate specialist) and it is the latter who, depending on his diagnosis, must choose which of his two therapeutic roles he should enact.

Since the shaman and exorcist are the two most important specialists for supernaturally caused illnesses, it is important briefly to describe these practitioners. With very few exceptions, shamans (some writers prefer to designate them as spirit mediums) are females. Indeed, one becomes a shaman *(nat kadaw)* by becoming the wife of a *nat*. With very few exceptions, shamans are parttime practitioners, and even then their major activity is not concerned with medicine, but with *nat* propitiation. Since, however, *nat* cause illness, a shaman is frequently consulted when it is believed that illness may have been caused by a *nat*. She determines which *nat* may have caused the illness, and how he might be pacified so that the patient may recover. Shamanism is an ecstatic role in that recruitment to the role, as well as its practice, is based on *nat* possession. A woman becomes a shaman only by marrying, in a formal wedding ceremony, the *nat* by whom she was possessed. Similarly, the shaman performs her role in a state of possession, in which state her *nat* husband reveals the identity of the *nat* who has brought illness to her client and how he is to be pacified.

Like shamanism, exorcism is a parttime specialty, but unlike shamans, exorcists *(ahtelan hsaya)* are exclusively males. There are important differences between these two roles, including their medical dimensions. Shamans are inferior to, and must therefore propitiate, the disease-causing supernaturals. Exorcists, because their practice is based on Buddhist-derived power, are superior to these supernaturals whom they control rather than propitiate. Moreover, unlike shamanism, exorcism is not an ecstatic role. The exorcist treats possession, but he does not become possessed himself, neither as a recruitment requirement nor as part of his practice. To become an exorcist one must be initiated into a quasi-Buddhist sect *(gaing),* as a member of which one learns to enlist various types of Buddhist forces and power, and to remain a member of which one must adhere to the moral precepts of Buddhism and practice Buddhist meditation. Most exorcists also practice herbal medicine, but the reverse does not hold true.

Diagnosis

Usually, as already mentioned, a herbal doctor (who might also be an exorcist) is consulted when a person feels ill. His first task, of course, is to make a differential diagnosis which means, given the Burmese world view, that he must determine whether the patient's illness is naturally or supernaturally caused. Often, this diagnosis is simple to make, and does not require the skills of a specialist.

Just as Westerners can usually identify the symptoms of some, at least, of the well-known diseases, so the Burmese can differentiate the symptoms of many supernaturally caused diseases. It is only when the symptoms do not permit of a ready diagnosis that a diagnostic specialist is required. If the illness is diagnosed as supernaturally caused, the specialist has other differential diagnoses to make, for in order to choose the proper treatment he must identify the type of supernatural agent responsible for the illness and, in addition, the particular member of the type. Finally (and this too is part of the diagnosis), in order to choose the appropriate treatment, he may also need to uncover the supernatural's motive for causing the illness.

As indicated above, the diagnosis of naturally- versus supernaturally-caused illness is often easy to make. If the symptoms are not self-evident, however, the doctor—at least the ones found in the villages with which the author is acquainted—may resort to a hand-trembling test. If, when the patient holds out his palm, his hand does not tremble, the disease is naturally caused; if it trembles, it is probably supernaturally caused and, depending upon the manner of trembling, the doctor determines whether it is witch- or *nat*-caused. These determinations, however, are taken as hypotheses to be further tested. It is only when these further tests—which need not be described here—confirm his earlier tentative diagnosis that the doctor moves to the next step, the specifying of the particular *nat* or witch.

Specifying witches is relatively simple. Since, so it is believed, witchcraft is almost always performed against a fellow villager or those in adjacent villages, the patient's relatives (and often the doctor himself) can usually recall some incident by which the patient offended a sweetheart, a mother-in-law, a neighbor, and so on, and that person is then assumed to be the putative witch. If the doctor is an exorcist, he can then confirm the hypothesis by inducing the alleged witch to possess the patient and, using the patient as his medium, interrogating the witch directly.

If a *nat,* rather than a witch, is believed to have caused the illness, the means for determining its identity depends on whether the specialist is a shaman or an exorcist. The shaman identifies the *nat* by one of two means. Sometimes she does so by judicious questioning of the patient or his relatives. Has the coconut offering to the house *nat* been changed at appropriate intervals? Has the annual tribute been offered to the hereditary *nat?* Did the patient perhaps urinate under a tree which is inhabited by a tree *nat*? And so on. Sometimes, however, the shaman may identify the *nat* by becoming possessed (in a state of trance) by her *nat* husband, who then communicates this information to her. The exorcist, like the shaman, may also employ possession in order to identify the *nat,* but instead of becoming possessed himself, he induces the putatively responsible *nat* to possess the patient, and he then proceeds to query the *nat* directly.

Treatment

Depending on the nature of the illness and on the type of medical practitioner, a variety of therapeutic techniques is available for the treatment of supernaturally caused illnesses. Basically, however, there are five techniques, of which the first three to be described are used for physical illness, the latter two for mental illness. These techniques—including propitiation, magic, a combination of propitiation and magic, exorcism without a séance, and exorcism with a séance—are briefly described.

If, in the case of a *nat*-caused illness, propitiation seems to be the indicated treatment, the specialist may instruct the patient to make an offering to the offended *nat,* on the assumption that, appeased by the offering, the *nat* will desist from his attack. In the case of ghost-caused illness or witchcraft, the specialist may prescribe the swallowing of water over which he has intoned an incantation, usually consisting of passages from Buddhist scripture. The efficacy of this "medicine," as it is called, derives from the magical potency of the incantation; hence, it is not to be confused with physical medicine, the curative power of which is in its natural properties. If the illness is deemed to require a more powerful treatment, but not as powerful as an exorcism ceremony, the treatment may consist of a combination of propitiation and magic. As in the case of magic alone, the incantation is always associated with Buddhist sacra and, hence, taps Buddhist sources of power.

As noted, these three techniques are only employed for supernaturally-caused *physical* illness. Supernaturally caused *mental* illness, however, is almost invariably treated by means of exorcism, either with or without a séance. Both types of exorcism, beginning with the first, require more extensive description.

Having diagnosed the illness as having been caused by witchcraft, for example, the exorcist administers a purgative to the patient in order that the witch's "poison" be ejected. This is usually insufficient, however, since the witch normally continues to control the patient's behavior, a control that can be handled only by exorcising the witch. This is accomplished in two ways: first, by having the patient worship the Buddha and vow to faithfully observe the Five Precepts the rest of his life; second, by the exorcist invoking the Buddhist gods *(deva)* and requesting them to protect the patient from the witch (and from any further affliction by any other supernatural being).

If this simple type of exorcism is ineffective, it is necessary to conduct an exorcism séance. In this ceremony, the *nat* or witch is induced (or compelled) by the exorcist to possess the patient so that, with the patient as his medium, the exorcist may engage him in conversation, discover the reasons for his anger, and finally subdue him. There are three invariable elements in such a séance. First, there are rituals which protect the patient from the malevolent action of the supernatural and which exorcise him by enlisting the assistance of the gods. Second, there is possession of the patient by the supernatural, in the course of which the exorcist converses with him and, by a combination of pleas, promises, and threats, induces or compels him to desist from his attack. Third, there are medicines, whose properties are magical rather than pharmaceutical, administered to the patient.

It is apparent, then, that the exorcism séance differs from other forms of therapy in two important respects: the invoking of the offending supernatural, and the active involvement of the patient. From the Burmese point of view, the efficacy of the séance rests on the same principle as the efficacy of other forms of therapy. In all of them, cures are achieved through the power of Buddhist supernaturals and the power residing in Buddhist symbols and Buddhist sacra, the assumption being that the forces of Good (the Buddhist forces) are more powerful than the forces of Evil (the anti-Buddhist forces).

Possession and Dissociation in Mental Illness

Following this brief sketch of Burmese traditional medicine as it relates to supernaturally-caused illness, including mental illness, we now take a closer and more detailed look at its theory and at treatment of the latter type of illness. Although physical illness is attributed by traditional Burmese medicine to both natural and supernatural causes, mental illness is attributed exclusively to supernatural causes. The patient, so it is believed, has come under the influence or control of a maleficent supernatural being—spirit, witch, ghost. Although the last statement seems fairly straightforward, it is in the author's mind more than a little ambiguous, if not in the minds of the Burmese.

In the scientific study of religion, the expression, "control, or influence by a supernatural" usually refers to a state of possession, *i.e.,* a state in which it is believed that some supernatural has literally entered the body of a person. Often, but not always, possession is accompanied by some form of psychological dissociation—such as trance, fugue states, unconsciousness, etc. It must be noted, however, that these three variables—supernatural influence, possession, and dissociation—are not only analytically independent, but also may be empirically independent of each other. The ambiguity in the author's understanding of the Burmese materials stems from difficulty in sorting these variables.

The Burmese term, *pude,* which is typically glossed as "possession," presents us with our first ambiguity. Thus, if "possession" is taken literally to mean body intrusion, the notion of witch possession *(soun pude)* is difficult to understand, unless it is taken to mean that the patient is possessed by the spirit of the witch or by the witch in some non-material guise. With respect to *nat* this problem does not of course arise, but even in their case body intrusion can be of two kinds. Thus, when, as is sometimes believed to happen, a *nat* falls in love with a person, it is assumed that the soul of the former has entered into and united with the soul of the latter. This union may be temporary or permanent, the latter occurring when, as in the case of a shaman, the human and *nat* are married, and their souls are "tied" in a formal wedding ceremony. Here, then, we see an instance of permanent possession unaccompanied by dissociation. On the other hand, when a *nat* wishes to harm someone, and causes him to become mentally ill, the *nat* himself, and not merely his "soul" enters the person's body. This kind of possession also occurs when an exorcist induces a *nat* to enter a patient during a séance, or when a shaman invites her *nat* husband to enter her so that she might practice divination. In all of these cases of temporary possession, dissociation not only accompanies possession, but the very fact of dissociation is taken to be the sign of possession.

In short, from the Burmese point of view, dissociation (in the sense both of loss of consciousness and of trance) may or may not accompany possession. Their relationship, however, is not haphazard, there being at least four experiences in which the two are invariably associated.

These include (a) the séance, in which the exorcist induces the supernatural to possess the patient; (b) divination, in which the shaman induces
her *nat* husband to enter herself; (c) shamanistic dancing at *nat* ceremonies, in which both shaman and *nat* seek each other; (d) mental illness,
in which the supernatural forces himself upon the patient. In the first
three experiences, the dissociational state is a trance state; in the fourth
it may consist either of trance or of unconsciousness.

Just as possession may occur without dissociation, so, it must also be
observed, dissociation may occur without possession, for although dissociational states are always supernaturally caused, they may be caused
by a supernatural attack as well as by supernatural possession.

It should be noted, finally, that mental illness can be caused merely
by personal encounters with supernaturals, encounters which involve
neither possession nor attack, and in which there is no dissociation.
Although from our point of view these encounters (depending on the
circumstances) must be either hallucinatory or illusory, they are not
dissociative in that the actor is both conscious of the experience while
having it, and capable of recalling and reporting the experience after
having had it. Thus, the author has recorded numerous instances in
which persons have "seen" or "spoken with" some supernatural, much
as they might see or speak with a human being. Sometimes the experiences are reported as having been pleasurable, sometimes as frightening,
but whether the one or the other, they often (though not always) lead
to mental illness. (Notice that it is not the encounter itself that is taken
to be abnormal—from the Burmese point of view such encounters consist of veridical perceptions—but only its bizarre behavioral consequences.)

A few examples of these various forms of mental illness might be
helpful. A 17-year-old, unmarried girl was viewed as mentally ill by
her parents when she exhibited the following symptoms: severe stomach
pains, sudden and unpredictable bursts of crying, disappearance from
her home and the inability, when she returned, to remember where she
had been. Again, two young men simultaneously and indiscriminately
attacked, and attempted to kill, everyone they met. In another case of
folie à deux, two young women roamed through villages with fancy
dress and painted faces in complete silence, neither speaking nor responding to anyone. Again, a young man, at intervals of 3 to 4 months,
exhibited the following behavior: he wandered through the fields in a
trancelike state, he went into a catatonic stupor, he engaged in violent
aggression against everyone in his sight. In a final example, a young
married man encountered a beautiful girl with whom he attempted to
make love, and who abruptly disappeared only to reappear at the top
of an adjacent hill, from where she told him that she was its guardian
spirit. From his, and the villagers', point of view, the encounter with the
spirit was a normal and veridical experience, but the consequences of
the experience—acute abdominal cramps, extreme fright, obsessive sexual desire for the spirit, inability to eat and sleep, the squandering of his

assets on drink—were taken as unambiguous symptoms of mental illness.

It might be noted, adverting to the last example, that there are at least two other types of encounter with supernaturals which we might interpret as abnormal, but which the Burmese take to be normal. Thus, shamans may consciously experience possession by their *nat* husbands, in which they have the conscious sensation of sexual union with them. Again, in Buddhist meditation, the meditator may experience ecstatic states in which, among other things, he has visions of Buddhist supernaturals. Both types of encounter, the shaman's with her *nat* and the meditator's with a god, are viewed by the Burmese as veridical perceptions.

It should now be abundantly clear that certain types of Burmese behavior, which modern psychiatry would take to be symptomatic of psychopathology, are viewed as normal by Burmese traditional medicine, and that other types are considered by both to be pathological (although they differ about their etiology). The author adds that he knows of no cases of Burmese behavior which Burmese medicine views as pathological but which modern psychiatry would view as normal.

That traditional Burmese medicine and modern psychiatry may sometimes differ in their interpretations of psychopathology is hardly surprising given the differences in their theories of mental illness (which in large part derive from their different *Weltanschauungen*). If, then, we were to contrast these two ways of looking at mental illness, we might do so in terms of four dimensions. First, traditional Burmese medicine attributes the cause of mental illness to supernatural action, rather than to mental conflict. Second, it views any experience with supernatural beings as being motivated in the first instance by them, rather than by the patient. As a result—and this is the third point— although it assumes that experiences with supernaturals may lead to pathological consequences, it does not view the experiences themselves as pathological. Finally, although it views the patient's bizarre behavior which follows a supernatural experience as pathological, it explains the behavior itself as instigated by the supernatural, rather than by the patient. In short, whereas modern psychiatry views the mind of the patient as being an active agent in his illness, Burmese medicine views the patient as a passive agent, a victim of forces outside himself. Hence, whereas in modern psychiatry therapy consists of changing certain psychopathological processes within the individual, in Burmese medicine it consists of changing certain pathogenic forces which are external to him.

Treatment of Mental Illness

Given the traditional Burmese interpretation of mental illness, we might wish to assume that its treatment is efficacious—and it often is efficacious—because a supernatural is exorcized, thereby accepting the notion that the illness is indeed caused by supernatural attack or possession. Alternatively, we might wish to identify those elements in the

exorcism ceremony which, albeit unintentionally, conform to acknowledged principles of psychotherapy, thereby adopting the view that the
phenomenological experience of a supernatural attack or possession in
itself conforms to, and can be explained by means of, known principles
of psychological projection, hysterical seizures, and trance states. On
the basis of the latter assumption, and without attempting to examine
the grounds for holding it, let us briefly examine the possible psychotherapeutic elements in the exorcism séance, of which we might mention
four.

First, there is the element of group support. Since the patient's
abnormal behavior, no matter how antisocial, is attributed to supernatural causes, he is absolved of all blame and, instead, is offered every
form of sympathy and emotional support. Moreover, by consensually
validating the supernatural interpretation of his behavior, the group also
offers him cultural support, for patient and group share the same cognitive assumptions regarding his emotional and mental state and both
share in a common faith in the cultural resources by which his suffering
can be alleviated. In addition, the group offers important instrumental
support; they finance the expensive exorcism, fetch the ritual objects
which are required in the ceremony, and offer him other forms of assistance. The patient knows, in short, that he has not been abandoned,
that he is not alone in his time of stress. Finally, the group offers social
support during the exorcism itself. The exorcism ceremony is always a
public ceremony, and the patient is surrounded by friends and relatives
who constantly offer advice, make comments, volunteer sympathy, etc.
In an important sense, patient, exorcist, and group comprise one inter-
locking system.

A second therapeutic element is the active participation of the patient
in the treatment. He perceives the rites that are conducted by the
exorcist; some of them (with the guidance of the exorcist) he performs
himself; most important, while possessed by the supernatural, in a state
of trance induced by the exorcist, he speaks the thoughts of the supernatural. The first two aspects of his participation may be said to offer
the patient faith and courage by exposing his conscious mind to the
potent sacred symbols in whose efficacy he himself believes. In essence,
an exorcist ceremony is a circumscribed and ritualized enactment of a
contest between the forces of Evil (the anti-Buddhist supernatural
forces) and the forces of Good (the Buddhist forces), and although the
contest is often a difficult and frightening struggle, its eventual outcome
is never in doubt. The patient, like everyone else, knows that the power
of Buddhism is incomparably greater than any other power. To believe
that such power is on his side in the contest must surely serve to reduce
the patient's feelings of depression and despair concerning his fate, and
thereby energize his will. The third aspect of the patient's participation—
and the most important—may be seen as confronting him with his
unconscious mind, for although it is believed that while in trance his
words are those of the supernatural, we can safely assume that they are

rather the words of his own unconscious. In short, the exorcistic trance permits some of the ego-alien wishes of his unconscious mind (which the writer assumes are at the root of his conflict) to be expressly articulated.

A third psychotherapeutic element in the exorcism is the personality and role of the exorcist. Buddhist power can defeat anti-Buddhist power only if the two meet in confrontation, and this can happen only if the exorcist is sufficiently powerful to compel the anti-Buddhist supernaturals to participate in the ceremony (by possessing the patient), and sufficiently pious to induce the Buddhist supernaturals to do battle against them. In short, for the ceremony to work, the patient must have absolute confidence in both the power and the piety of the exorcist. This confidence is inspired in the first place by the very willingness of the exorcist to expose himself to the great dangers entailed in invoking the presence of the evil supernaturals. (His willingness to assume this risk has, of course, yet another therapeutic element: it informs the patient of the exorcist's love and concern for him.)

Given his confidence in the exorcist and in the rites which he performs, the latter's therapeutic influence on the patient may be found in his behavior and personality. Since the exorcist establishes a supportive and nurturant tone—he rarely condemns or censures, but rather expresses his compassion and concern—the patient is free to express, while in trance, his shameful and forbidden ego-alien impulses. Thus, when the exorcist converses with the putative supernatural who has possessed, and therefore speaks through the patient, he is uniformly kind and understanding. He speaks of his "love" for the supernatural, refers to him as his "brother" or "sister," tells him that he will share his Buddhist merit with him (so that he can ultimately be reborn as a human being), and so on. But though gentle and kind, the exorcist is also firm, for if the supernatural proves to be intractable in his refusal to give up his hold on the patient, the exorcist warns him of the punitive consequences of his obstinacy. The successful exorcist—and not all are successful— is not only kind, yet firm, but is characterized by self-confidence and the absence of anxiety. Despite the provocations—and they are often outrageous and frightening—he does not lose control or his own sense of importance. In the relationship between patients and exorcists of this type one can observe, in an almost exaggerated form, that quality of positive transference which is such an important element in any type of psychotherapy.

A fourth psychotherapeutic element in the exorcistic ceremony is the opportunity it affords the patient for almost massive emotional abreaction of his conflict. While in trance, the patient not only articulates his unconscious wishes, but expresses his unconscious impulses. Thus, he shouts obscenities, mimics obscene sexual behavior, utters heresies, curses and insults the exorcist, and attempts physical assault against him and against anyone else in his immediate vicinity. At times it is difficult, if not impossible, to believe that this violent and obscene patient is the quiet, pious Buddhist one had known him to be only a short time before. These impulses, it must be emphasized, are expressed with enormous expenditures of affect and emotional energy. The writer has seen patients in trance whose violence could be restrained only by the power of as many as eight or nine men; violent episodes ending with the patient in a state of absolute fatigue; and recriminatory episodes ending with the patient bitterly sobbing, his body seized with trembling. In almost all cases, he is in a state of physical and emotional exhaustion when he comes out of trance.

Conclusion

Although this paper began with the observation that its data are based on village investigations, it would be erroneous to conclude that similar beliefs and practices are not to be found in the cities. In Burma (no more than anywhere else) urbanization, Westernization, and industrialization—some theorists to the contrary notwithstanding—have not been accompanied to any great extent by secularization. Since, then, the supernatural world-view upon which traditional Burmese medicine (as it relates to supernaturally-caused diseases) rests is as firmly entrenched in the cities as it is in the villages, there is good reason to believe that the traditional system described here is not confined to the villages. Rangoon and Mandalay abound in a variety of esoteric and occult sects (*gaing*), one of whose important activities consists of the prevention and healing of supernaturally caused illnesses, especially mental illness. Of course, since modern medicine—including modern physicians, clinics, and hospitals—is readily available in the cities, illnesses of obviously natural causation are typically treated by modern physicians. However, if the latter are not successful, or if, antecedently, the patient shows symptoms of supernatural possession or attack, it is a practitioner of one of these sects—in short, a practitioner of traditional medicine— who is most often consulted for treatment.

To be sure, the military regime that seized power in Burma in 1962 is committed, at least officially, to the secularization of Burmese culture, and it is possible that its expressed opposition to the occult (including beliefs in witchcraft, *nat,* ghosts, and so forth) and its expansion of medical schools and medical training (including the training of traditional herbal doctors) may have resulted in a gradual falling away from the consultation of shamans, astrologers, exorcists, and the numerous other masters of the occult (*hsaya*) found in the cities. Though possible, it is suspected that this is not the case. Admittedly the author has no firm evidence for this suspicion because the Revolutionary Council (the present government of Burma) has continuously, beginning with the 1962 *coup,* barred foreign researchers. Still, it is known that members of the Revolutionary Council themselves do not always practice what they preach. Even its chairman, General Ne Win, is known to have his favorite *hsaya,* although he also makes regular trips to London and Vienna for medical treatment.

But the author's skepticism concerning the gradual disappearance of traditional medicine as it relates to supernaturally caused illnesses is not based primarily on the fact that the members of the Revolutionary Council do not strictly adhere to their own ideology. In a recent trip to Rangoon it became evident that the belief in, and consultation of, *hsaya* are as prevalent as ever. Indeed, on the very first day of the writer's visit, the writer accompanied a Burmese friend (a tutor at the University of Rangoon) to the home of a (male) shaman—she was bringing him a secretary at the American Embassy, a young woman from Connecticut, for a consultation!—and that same evening, together with other friends, we attended an exorcism séance.

The persistence of this traditional system, a system which (if the argument implicit in the previous sections of this paper is correct) deals with various forms of psychogenic problems and complaints, should hardly come as a surprise to anyone who has been following the recent American scene. After all, Southern California is not the only section of the U.S. in which beliefs and practices similar (if not identical) to those described in this paper not only persist, but have enjoyed a rather dramatic surge in popularity over the past 7 or 8 years, and it is suggested that both cases, the Burmese and the American, are susceptible to similar social and psychological explanations—but that is a topic for another paper.

NOTES

1. Field work in Burma was made possible by a research grant from the National Science Foundation, for whose support the author wishes to express his appreciation.

2. For a detailed description and analysis of the materials presented in this paper, see Spiro (1967) and Spiro (1970:chs. 6, 11).

REFERENCES

SPIRO, M. E.
   1967   Burmese Supernaturalism: A Study in the Explanation and Reduction of Suffering. Englewood Cliffs, N.J.: Prentice-Hall.
SPIRO, M. E.
   1970   Buddhism and Society: A Great Tradition and Its Burmese Vicissitudes. New York: Harper & Row.

CHAPTER 11

PLURALISM AND INTEGRATION IN THE INDIAN AND CHINESE MEDICAL SYSTEMS

CHARLES LESLIE

The demand of laymen in Western countries for acupuncture and other Chinese medical treatments, and the desire of physicians to learn about them, have been stimulated by descriptions of traditional medicine in the People's Republic of China. The writer is skeptical about this Western enthusiasm for Chinese medicine. The economic and cultural reasons for the use of indigenous medicine in China should be distinguished from its potential contribution to medical science. Only fringe practitioners in Western countries hope to use theories of the Five Elements, of *yin* and *yang,* or the meridians. These theories belong in the domain of historians and cultural anthropologists. From this perspective, research in the PRC would provide valuable data to compare to the persistence of both humoral and magical theories of disease in Chinese communities outside the PRC described in essays in this volume and in other recent studies (Caudill 1974; Otsuka 1974; Topley 1970, 1974; Unschuld 1973, 1974). Although useful medications have been derived from the traditional Asian pharmacopoeias, few new discoveries are likely to come from this direction. Dr. Francisco Guerra writes:

> The value of the native systems of medicine lies in the cultural elements . . . a great mass population is tied down to the use of native pharmacopoeias chiefly for economic reasons, because native pharmacopoeias are cheaper than the products of the West (Guerra 1969: 252).

The sociology of Chinese medicine has greater potential value for the rest of the world than Chinese medical theories, acupuncture, or herbals. And this is particularly true because the PRC has provided a new model for the modernization of medical systems. Two main features of the model are the large-scale use of practitioners with little formal training, and the legitimization of indigenous traditions which from a scientific perspective were thought to be obsolete by giving them a major role in state-sanctioned medical bureaucracies. The model is most relevant, therefore, to societies with more limited resources than those of industrialized countries, and with dual systems of indigenous and cosmopolitan medicine. The countries of South Asia meet these criteria, and planners in these countries will surely compare their medical systems to the model of the PRC. The task of this paper is to describe a conceptual approach for making such comparisons, and to present relevant

235

data from India. This material should interest specialists in Chinese communities, for humoral traditions of considerable antiquity continue to be culturally important, and the institutions of cosmopolitan medicine have evolved in relationships where they were related to coexisting transformations of these traditions throughout Asia.

The common Western image of contemporary Asian medical systems pictures a small number of institutions for "Western medicine" as an alien enclave in an amorphous structure of indigenous folk curers whose practice is limited to traditional medications and shamanistic rites. Against this background the image of an extensive, bureaucratically rationalized system that integrates indigenous and cosmopolitan medicine in the PRC is enormously appealing. Both images should be treated as models rather than as descriptions of actual systems. It would be naive to assume that either one corresponds to social reality. The first model is based upon limited observation, and the second is an ideal of Chinese health planners. We lack systematic research on the social organization and health cultures of laymen and specialists in the PRC, but the papers on Taiwan, Hongkong, Malaya, Thailand and Burma in the present volume indicate the variety of practitioners and the diverse forms of therapy available to laymen in those societies. To discuss these papers during our conference we used concepts that contrasted sacred to secular medicine, Chinese to Western medicine, scientific to folk medicine, and the institutionalized medicine of specialists to the diffuse medicine of popular culture. These concepts divided phenomena in different ways but they all predicated the pluralistic character of the systems we were analyzing. For comparative purposes we must clarify different approaches to medical pluralism, and define the process that shapes its character in modern times.

The distinction that social scientists make between culture and society is useful for the comparative study of medical systems. As a cultural system medicine is an organization of concepts, theories and normative practices. It is a way of perceiving and thinking about health and illness coded in the traditions of a society.[1] As a social system medicine is a set of occupational roles, role relationships and institutional structures. It is part of the division of labor, more or less differentiated from other activities. From this perspective a medical system is a system of specialist roles. Laymen use the system but are outside it, and the primary desiderata for learning how a medical system works is to learn what access laymen have to it. In New York city, for example, Puerto-Rican laborers, Chinese shopkeepers, Jewish clerks and Christian Scientist school-teachers have different access to different kinds of curers.

Although the pluralistic health cultures of laymen are readily acknowledged in our own society, we ignore the corresponding pluralism of our medical system when we talk about it as if it were only the structure of hospitals, clinics, colleges and other agencies of "modern" or "scientific" medicine.[2] These institutions of cosmopolitan medicine dominate the prestige hierarchy and legal structure of practice. Their representatives brand other forms of curing as "irregular" or "fringe" medicine, thus putting them ideologically outside of *the* medical system. From a realistic sociological perspective, however, specialists in clinical psychology, yoga, chiropractic, homeopathy, espiritismo, curandismo, faith healing, health foods, or Chinese herbals, are part of the overall, pluralistic medical system of our society. Millions of people regularly consult these kinds of specialists, and at some points in their lives most American citizens probably resort to one or another of them.

The medical systems of all complex societies are socially and culturally pluralistic, but the professionalization of cosmopolitan medicine, which has progressed rapidly in this century, is an effort to reduce the degree and to govern the nature of medical pluralism. A struggle exists in the medical division of labor throughout the world in which advocates of cosmopolitan medicine attempt to standardize the curricula for training health specialists, to reserve the legal practice of medicine to individuals with the requisite training, to enforce a hierarchy of medical authority dominated by doctors who form a self-governing profession with the right to define and to supervise the work of paramedical specialists, to limit access of laymen or of other kinds of curers to the technology of cosmopolitan medicine, and to eliminate or narrowly restrict all other forms of medical practice.

The actual systems of different countries are compromise structures of cosmopolitan medical workers and of other kinds of health specialists, and the models of them projected by their critics or admirers are ideological tools in the struggle to gain or keep power, and to control their course of development. The ideological conflicts in modern medical systems have been extensively analyzed in the history and sociology of medical reform in the U.S. and other Western countries, but they are also an essential element in the lesser-known sociology of "Western" medical institutions in Asian societies. An American observer with long experience in India described a characteristic aspect of these conflicts in this manner:

> Medical education in India was based on the dogma that the early British educators were working in a complete vacuum of medical ignorance. British doctors essentially ignored or ridiculed the quackery of indigenous practitioners. . . . (Indian) doctors found security in accepting the professional culture of Western medicine *in toto*. As a result, it proved to be hard for Indian doctors to select and adapt those parts of the Western medical culture that were relevant to the country's needs while, at the same time, compensating for feelings of social inferiority imposed on them by representatives of the British Raj (Taylor 1968: 154).

As an organized professional group, cosmopolitan medical doctors in India have opposed governmental recognition and support of indigenous medical institutions. But this policy has never been fully successful, or fully supported by all members of the profession, and laymen from all social classes, religious communities, castes, ethnic and occupational groups resort to practitioners of indigenous medicine. Although the PRC has gained wide publicity for its extensive use of indigenous medicine, the scale of utilization of indigenous medicine in India is probably as great as that of China. Approximately 150,000 physicians now practice cosmopolitan medicine in India, but an estimated 400,000 physicians, many of them unregistered, practice indigenous medicine. The indigenous systems are Ayurveda, which is based upon Sanskrit texts, Yunani or Greek medicine, based upon Arabic and Persian texts, and Siddha, a tradition of humoral medicine in South India.

A dual system of professionalized indigenous and cosmopolitan medicine exists in India, with parallel institutions for research, education and practice. In 1972 the state boards of indigenous medicine had registered 257,000 practitioners, of which about 93,000 had at least 4 years of formal training.[3] There were 95 cosmopolitan medical colleges, compared to 99 Ayurvedic colleges, 15 Yunani colleges and 1 college for Siddha medicine. Many of the indigenous medical schools were small and ill-equipped, but 26 of them were affiliated with universities and 10 offered postgraduate training. Two research institutes for indigenous medicine awarded between 35 and 45 Ph.D. and D.A.M. (Doctor of Ayurvedic Medicine) degrees annually. Also, in 1972 the state and central governments supported entirely or in part 185 hospitals and 9,750 dispensaries for indigenous medicine. The Indian government allocated 160 million rupees for indigenous medical institutions in the fourth 5-year-plan, but in contrast to cosmopolitan medicine, where 75 percent of the physicians were in government service, more than one-half of the registered physicians of indigenous medicine were fee-for-service private practitioners.

Homeopathic medicine is also widely practiced in India, and for legislative purposes it is often associated with the indigenous systems. Dr. S. M. Bhardwaj has described a process that he calls "the naturalization of homeopathy" in India during the nineteenth century. He argues that homeopathy first appealed to the new urban elite as a "modern" system. Its basic ideas were readily understandable and were soon made accessible in Indian languages to "even moderately literate people." With the rise of nationalist sentiments, its German origin and the opposition to it by the British-dominated cosmopolitan medical profession prevented it from acquiring the stigma of colonialism. Unlike the advocates of cosmopolitan medicine, the advocates of homeopathy were sympathetic to indigenous medical practices and tried to show that the principles of Ayurveda were consistent with homeopathy. Finally, Bhardwaj writes:

> Although homeopathy was not an indigenous system, its practitioners were closely empathetic with the Indian ethos. Homeopathy ... had an aura of mysticism and spiritualism about it. Hahnemann speaks of energies such as "vital powers," "dynamic powers," and "moral powers." These beliefs were not lost on the Indian homeopathic physicians. Many of them consciously tried to bring religious ideas into homeopathy. Dr. A. C. Bhaduri claimed that according to the vedanta philosophy minute doses are best suited for the cure

of diseases . . . Whether the logic of harmonization between Hindu-
ism and homeopathy was faulty or not is not the issue. It is important
that the homeopaths saw no conflict between their system of medicine and their religious and cultural beliefs even though the system
was clearly imported from the West (Bhardwaj 1973: 292).

Most registered homeopathic practitioners are registered jointly with
practitioners of Ayurvedic and Yunani medicine, although separate state
Boards of Homeopathic Medicine are now being formed. The fourth
5-year-plan allocated 15 million rupees for this purpose, and 47 institutions offered homeopathic training in 1972 (Ministry of Information
1972). Even so, training is often acquired through correspondence
courses that thinly disguise the selling of credentials (Montgomery 1974).
   To describe the main area of fulltime professionalized medical practice in India we can imagine a continuum with one pole among the
highly-trained specialists who engage in scientific research and teaching
at the more prestigious cosmopolitan medical schools, and the other
pole among registered practitioners who may have a high-school education or a few years in college, and who have taken a correspondence
course in homeopathy, studied the brochures of companies that manufac-
ture indigenous and cosmopolitan medications, and perhaps served as an
apprentice to another physician with similar or more formal institutional
qualifications to practice Ayurvedic, Yunani or cosmopolitan medicine.
Most of the physicians who have completed full courses of training in
the colleges for indigenous and cosmopolitan medicine fall between these
poles. If we could measure their beliefs and practices I believe that they
would form a continuous series.
   The point that the writer wishes to make is that professionalized
indigenous medicine is not in practice isolated from cosmopolitan medicine, although separate colleges, hospitals, professional associations and
governmental agencies exist for the different systems. Ayurvedic and
Yunani concepts of health and illness are coded into the domestic culture, cuisine, religious ritual and popular culture of physicians trained
in cosmopolitan medicine, and indigenous medical practitioners often
use cosmopolitan medicines or instruments such as the thermometer and
stethoscope. Well known Ayurvedic and Yunani physicians will have
brothers, sons or other kinsmen who are cosmopolitan medical doctors—
or we could put this the other way around and say that many cosmopolitan medical practitioners have kinsmen who practice indigenous
medicine. Thus, despite the bureaucratic structure that the writer has
labeled a "dual system" of professionalized indigenous and cosmopolitan
medicine, a large measure of cultural syncretism and social integration
exists. In fact, different forms of medicine are sometimes brought together
in a single bureaucratic complex. For example, in Varanasi, a city on
the Ganges River midway between Delhi and Calcutta, the Institute for
Medical Science of Banaras Hindu University awards degrees in Ayurveda and in cosmopolitan medicine. Outpatient clinics and wards for
research and teaching both systems are located in the university hos-

pital. In the same city a large privately-endowed hospital has outpatient
clinics for homeopathy, Ayurveda and cosmopolitan medicine, along with
in-patient facilities for Ayurvedic and cosmopolitan medicine.

The described continuum between scientific specialists in India and
an amalgam of popular culture physicians more or less corresponds to
the distribution of practitioners from barefoot doctors to hospital specialists that recent visitors have described in the PRC (Sidel and Sidel
1973). But the essays on Taiwan, Hongkong and other Chinese communities in the present volume tell us about shamanistic and other kinds
of religious and folk medical practice that are not reported in the model
of the PRC. Since these forms of practice are an important dimension
of medical pluralism, we need to locate the described continuum in
relation to folk medicine and to religious curing. For this purpose the
writer uses a chart from another essay (Leslie 1973) (Figure 1) with one
axis to indicate a continuum between folk practices based upon the ways
of thought and traditional technology of illiterate rural and urban people,
and the popular culture medicine communicated through advertising,
school books and other mass media. A second axis diagonal to this one
has at opposite poles learned, secular scientific practice and learned
religious curing.

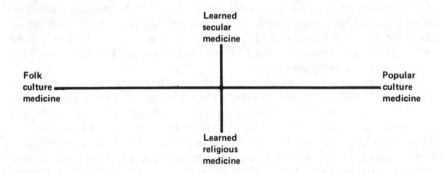

**Figure 1. Conceptual axes of folk and popular culture medicine, and of learned
secular and religious medicine.**

We can locate regions of practice in the conceptual space of such
a chart, marking the different regions with letters and, based upon
various studies of the Indian medical system, indicate the pattern of
full-time practitioners by dots. Also indicated in another chart is the
pattern of parttime practitioners, distinguishing full-time practice as one
that accounts for at least one-half of the practitioner's income. The continuum of full-time physicians who practice Ayurvedic, Yunani, homeopathic and cosmopolitan medicine, or some combination of these
traditions, is shown between regions (A) and (C) of Figure 2. These
physicians are employed in governmental health services and in private
practice, and form the majority of registered, institutionally trained

practitioners. But some physicians of this kind regularly practice in clinics attached to religious institutions, or themselves adopt forms of religious curing. They form a continuum with other kinds of practitioners such as astrologers, diviners, priests and holy men whom laymen consult for health problems, and who acquire some knowledge of indigenous medicine, homeopathy or cosmopolitan medicine which they use in association with their religious activities. Some of these specialists acquire considerable reputations for supernatural curing and become, by our definition, full-time medical practitioners. The pattern of their distribution is shown between regions (C) and (D). A similar continuum of priests, holy men, and astrologers who practice forms of shamanistic curing, links folk culture medicine to learned religious medical practice, and is shown between regions (D) and (E) of Figure 2.

Parttime practitioners far outnumber full-time practitioners in the Indian medical system. In 1965 a community development block in the Punjab with 80,000 people had 59 full-time and 300 parttime indigenous medical practitioners (Taylor 1974). In the same year a district in South India with a population of 120,000 had 6 doctors, 30 full-time practitioners of Ayurvedic and Yunani medicine, and 598 parttime practitioners (Neumann 1971). Almost all folk medicine is practiced as a parttime specialty by midwives, bone-setters and individuals who know a remedy for rashes, fever, diarrhea or other forms of indisposition. As these practitioners add aspirin, antibiotic ointments and commercially-prepared Ayurvedic and Yunani medicines to their repertory they form a continuum with numerous parttime practitioners of popular culture medicine. And as folk and popular culture practitioners deal with snake bites, or maladies attributed to supernatural causes, they form continua with learned religious medicine. These patterns are shown in Figure 3.

This way of looking at the Indian medical system does not emphasize the table of organization of professionalized medicine, beginning with the Ministry of Health and working down to the Primary Health Centers, nor does it start with the biomedical categories of pathology and epidemiology. These two approaches are the familiar ones of health planners, cosmopolitan medical specialists, and social scientists. They are essential for some purposes, but because they dominate our ways of thinking about medical systems they inhibit attention to the pluralistic structure of these systems and distort our understanding of the way they work. We characteristically look at our own and other medical systems from a statist perspective, and one biased by the categories and professional interests of cosmopolitan medicine.

Since parttime practitioners are rarely registered with state boards for indigenous or cosmopolitan medicine, they are not officially a part of the Indian medical system. Yet, if one superimposed the chart showing their distribution on the chart of full-time practitioners, and tried at the same time to represent their proportions, then one would have to show from 10 to 20 parttime practitioners for every full-time practitioner. And if one tried to distinguish registered from unregistered full-time practi-

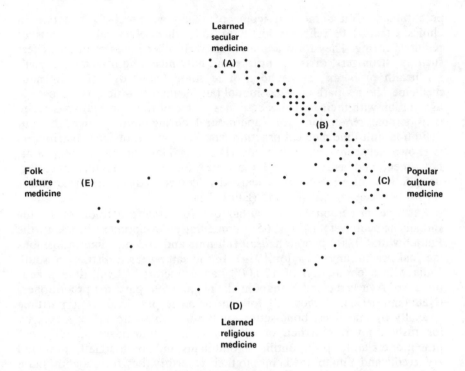

Figure 2. Regions of medical practice and the pattern of full-time practice in contemporary India.

(A) Physicians with M.D. and Ph.D. degrees engaged in advanced research and teaching at a prestigious cosmopolitan medical college.

(B) Physicians with degrees in indigenous medicine and with Bachelor or Licentiate degrees in cosmopolitan medicine, who teach at an Ayurvedic or Yunani medical college affiliated with a university.

(C) Physicians who have completed a correspondence course in homeopathic medicine, and have other limited training in indigenous or cosmopolitan medicine.

(D) Religious scholars or learned priests with reputations for unusual healing powers.

(E) Bone-setters, midwives and other individuals with reputations for traditional skills to handle common problems.

tioners, at least one-half of them would probably be unregistered. The survey already mentioned for a district in South India found three unregistered for every registered full-time practitioner (Neumann 1971). They, too, form a dimension of the medical system that a statist perspective frequently ignores, and that the professional ideology of cosmopolitan medicine relegates to the limbo of "quack medicine."

Indigenous and cosmopolitan medicine are not officially integrated in India as they are in China in a state-sponsored hierarchy of medical institutions, but the continua of practitioners that I have described indicate a substantial *de facto* integration between different regions of the Indian medical system. The integration of indigenous and cosmopolitan medicine is even more obvious when one adopts the perspective of laymen, for throughout Indian society they utilize whatever forms of medical knowledge and practice are available to them. They are less concerned with whether therapy is indigenous or foreign, traditional or modern, than with how much it will cost, whether or not it will work, how long it will take, and whether the physician will treat them in a sympathetic manner. They are also often concerned with the ways that different kinds of diagnosis and treatment attribute illness to a moral flaw of the patient or some other person, or to forces for which they are not responsible. In these respects laymen everywhere are pretty much alike. They differ in the knowledge they draw upon to resolve these issues, and the kinds of specialists they have access to.

Conflicts between indigenous and cosmopolitan medicine occur primarily between practitioners of these systems who compete for positions and legitimacy within state-sanctioned medical bureaucracies. Since the official integration of indigenous and cosmopolitan medicine in China has been achieved by denying the kind of professional autonomy that

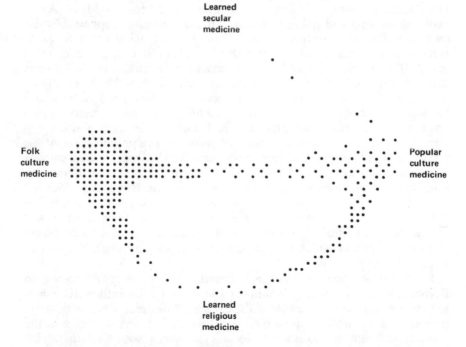

Figure 3. The pattern of parttime medical practice in contemporary India.

cosmopolitan medical practitioners have attained in India, it is unlikely that this aspect of the model presented by the People's Republic will appeal to them. But the *de facto* integration that already exists will continue to evolve. The patterns described are a momentary "compromise structure" that changes as the kind and number of practitioners change. Paul Brass, a political scientist, has analyzed the way that Ayurvedic and Yunani practitioners act as pressure groups to influence policies of the Indian government (Brass 1973), and this writer has argued in another essay that such activities bring these practitioners into an ambiguous paramedical relationship with cosmopolitan medicine (Leslie 1974).

A Cautionary Tale

The writer is sensitive to the fact that we hear a great deal lately about the accomplishments of the PRC, while visitors to India characteristically report the conflicts and failures of that society. Nevertheless, the writer concludes this essay with yet another narrative about conflict and failure drawn from the Indian scene. The Chinese revolution could only have occurred in China, and the events of this story are peculiar to their time and place, but the general is always embedded in the particular. This is a cautionary tale about one effort to integrate indigenous and cosmopolitan medicine.

The Aryan Medical School was founded in Bombay in 1896 by Prabhuram Jivanram, a traditional Ayurvedic physician, and his son, Dr. Popat Prabhuram Vaidya. The founders wrote that "vaidyas (Ayurvedic physicians) and hakims (Yunani physicians) have a sphere of their own in India, since people wanting their aid will never cease to exist. But there is a danger of the growth of irresponsible and incompetent men." To protect the public from quacks who practiced indigenous medicine they believed that "native medical science should be re-examined and revised in the light of Western science." Prabhuram Jivanram and his son were Prashnora Nagar Brahmins who in their native region would have used Vyas for a surname, but in Bombay they used Vaidya, the term for Ayurvedic physicians, for this purpose. Prabhuram brought his family to Bombay in 1870 from Probandar, in Gujarat. He had learned Ayurveda from the physician to the ruler of the princely state of Jamnagar, a member of his own caste and the father of Zandu Bhatt, who founded one of the most successful Ayurvedic pharmaceutical companies in present-day India. Prabhuram's elder brother, a religious teacher and priest, had earlier moved to Bombay and persuaded him of the advantages of that city, one of which was the opportunity to send one's children to English-language schools.

Dr. Popat was born in 1866 in Probandar. When the family moved to Bombay, he attended English schools and earned a Licentiate in cosmopolitan medicine from Grant Medical College. After receiving his diploma he took a government appointment in Gujarat, but was unhappy in the position and returned to Bombay to practice jointly with his father. This was a common pattern among physicians who worked to professionalize indigenous medicine by forming associations of practitioners, or by founding colleges and pharmaceutical companies. Young men trained in the cosmopolitan medical schools were also educated in indigenous medicine by kinsmen, and practiced both systems, or upon graduation from a medical college, established joint enterprises with relatives who were vaidyas or hakims.

Prabhuram and his son set out with good intentions to establish a school that would improve educational standards for Ayurvedic practitioners. Since proprietary medical schools were a common feature of professional medicine at that time, their scheme was a reasonable one. Dr. Popat and his father rented rooms for the school near their clinic, and supplied the institution with a small collection of books, charts and anatomical models. Dr. Popat's science courses at Grant Medical College had been taught without laboratories, so he could presume to teach in the same manner. Within a few years the school had 7 unpaid volunteer teachers, 4 with cosmopolitan medical training and 3 vaidyas. Five students graduated from its first class in 1901, and in that year nursing and midwifery courses were added to the curriculum. In 1903 the school opened a lying-in asylum, and in 1904 7 midwives and 77 nurses were awarded certificates. Twenty-eight students were enrolled in the 4-year medical course in 1906, and the faculty had grown to 16 teachers, including 6 vaidyas and 10 doctors. Khan Bahadur Chichgar, the convocation speaker that year, said:

> Let us follow in the footsteps of Europe and prepare the way for the great liberating movement for our country by introducing science with its accuracy in the medical art . . . To the newly initiated Vaidyas and others who had gone before them from this Institution, I have a word of caution . . . if they observe rightly they could see those who still look with suspicion on such institutions as theirs. As a word of warning, therefore, I would urge them to conduct themselves conscientiously . . . They should be careful not to give a handle to outsiders by stooping to quackery of any sort to please or to win over the ignorant mass about them . . . In proportion as this Institution seeks to raise the class of Vaidyas and Hakims from the state of ignorance and quackery it is a blessing to the masses among whom they find practice.

Thanking the speaker, one of the faculty said that institutions similar to the Aryan Medical School in other cities enjoyed the philanthropy of merchants and princes, and that their counterparts in Bombay should support this school. Indeed, one merchant had already contributed 40,000 rupees.

However legitimate the initial efforts of Prabhuram Vaidya and his son might have been, in the interval between the early 1880's, when Dr. Popat received his training, and the first decade of the twentieth century, the progressive development of medical knowledge and professional institutions made their small school inadequate for the purpose of integrating cosmopolitan and indigenous medicine. The faculty with diplomas in cosmopolitan medicine severed their connection with the Aryan Medical School when the first legislation to register qualified physicians was proposed for the Bombay Presidency in 1912. They were afraid that association with the institution would jeopardize their registration, and their fear was justified when Dr. Popat, who continued to run the school, was challenged in 1915 by the Medical Council to show why his name should not be removed from the registry. The charge was that his name appeared in an advertisement for the school, and that he aided unqualified persons to practice medicine. The ensuing dispute lasted for several years, and was reported in both the vernacular and English language press in other parts of India. A prominent politician, Vithalbhai Patel, introduced a bill in Dr. Popat's favor in the Bombay Legislative Council, and other well-known people indicated their support for him. The outcome was that he reorganized the curriculum on traditional lines, and renamed the school the Prabhuram Ayurvedic College in memory of his father, who died in 1902.

The new curriculum abandoned the order of subjects in the manner of cosmopolitan science—botany, anatomy, physiology, and so forth—and organized courses based upon Ayurvedic texts, beginning with "Sharangdhar, Madhavnidan and Bhavprakash, called the Laghu Trayi," and proceeding to "Charaka, Sushruta and Vagbhatta Ashtang Hridaya, called the Vrdha Trayi." Still, the school catalog promised that students would be taught the knowledge they would need to enter into consulting relationships with cosmopolitan medical practitioners, and to understand the treatments their patients might have received before resorting to a vaidya. Because students complained that the course, which had been lengthened to 5 years, was too long to study in a school that would not qualify them to become registered physicians, the new course of study was shortened to 3 years.

Dr. Popat began publishing a monthly journal in Gujarati and English in 1916. The journal included news about conflicts between organizations of Marathi and Gujarati speaking vaidyas, and criticism of a national association of practitioners, the All-India Ayurvedic Congress. One complaint was that leaders of the association used the annual meetings to promote medicines which they manufactured. Dr. Popat's son, Pratapkumar Popatbhai Vaidya, told me that his father lost money in an effort to establish his own pharmaceutical company. In reading Dr. Popat's publications, professional correspondence and scrapbooks, this writer was impressed by the fact that he continually accused other people of intrigue and mercenary interests, while they, apparently, felt that he had these vices. At any rate, he was exceedingly active, and maintained a large private practice while engaged in debates with other Ayurvedic practitioners, supervising his pharmaceutical company, publishing an Ayurvedic magazine, and managing the school he originated with his father.

Praburam Ayurvedic College became known among professionalized indigenous practitioners throughout India when the Bombay Medical

Council deprived Dr. Popat of his registration. Its reputation was also spread by publicity gained in conferring honorary Sanskritic titles on leaders in the movement to revive Ayurvedic medicine. The school awarded titles to the Maharaja of Gondal, the Ayurvedic physician to the Maharaja of Patiala, and to leading practitioners from Jaipur, Madras, Calcutta and other cities. Still, the school attracted few students and in 1928 its Board of Trustees established the Dr. Popat University of Ayurveda as an examining body, awarding Ayurvedic titles to individuals who had studied independently or by apprenticeship to a private practitioner. The precedents for this move were the universities the British founded in India, which also acted as examining bodies patterned after the University of London, and in 1911 the All-India Ayurvedic Congress organized a Vidyapath to administer periodic examinations for traditionally-trained practitioners throughout the country. The Dr. Popat University of Ayurveda offered examinations for the titles of Upavaidya, Rasavaidya, Bhishak, and Bhishagwar-and-Graduate of Prabhuram Ayurvedic College, with examining fees of 12, 18, 15, and 21 rupees. Students who offered proof that they had passed courses in anatomy and physiology in a cosmopolitan medical school could receive the title of Upavaidya without examination, by paying a 10-rupee registration fee. A few years later, for higher fees, people were invited to register for examinations to receive the titles of Acharya and Vaidyavara. Meanwhile, Prabhuram Ayurvedic College continued to operate, offering courses leading to the titles of Bhishak, or Bhishagwar-and-Graduate of Prabhuram Ayurvedic College, which could be written to resemble a regular college degree by using the initials G.P.A.C. after one's name.

The Bombay legislature in 1938 introduced a bill to establish a State Board of Indian Systems of Medicine. The Board would register practitioners, regulate the curricula of schools for indigenous medicine, and set examinations. This was a blow to Dr. Popat, and to his son, Pratapkumar Vaidya, who now helped manage the family enterprises. They organized practitioners to oppose the legislation and, when this failed, to influence the appointments to the Board. They advertised examinations to be given on five different dates during 1941, and 198 practitioners or would-be practitioners registered to take them with the expectation that this would help them meet the requirements to register with the new State Board of Indian Systems of Medicine. The Board had announced that 1941 would be the last year in which it would register practitioners who were not trained in the curriculum it had established for indigenous medical schools.

Dr. Popat died in January 1944 at the age of 78, but his son administered examinations that year, and again in 1946. According to the 1946 convocation program, 35 students registered for the Bhishak examination and 26 passed it. Those who passed were called Licentiates of Prabhuram Ayurvedic College, and Pratapkumar promised that he would continue to give examinations, even though the State Board refused to recognize them.

The writer talked to Pratapkumar Vaidya for many hours in 1963, at which time he published an Ayurvedic periodical in the Gujarati language, and practiced medicine in the clinic that had been attached to the now defunct school. He generously put the documents of the institution at the writer's disposal, translating some of them from Gujarati, though many were in English. He described his own and his father's careers with candor. As the writer listened, and studied the many documents Pratapkumar put at his disposal, it seemed that in undertaking to integrate indigenous and cosmopolitan medicine these men had been blinded by the virtue of their intentions. Yet they were not insensitive, or inexperienced, or ignorant men. Somehow or other they failed to imagine things that they knew. For example, it is believed that they knew the Dr. Popat University of Ayurveda was a bogus university, and the titles they awarded were fraudulent. Yet the writer does not think they imagined themselves to be engaged in fraud. Given their resources, the purposes of the Aryan Medical College were less feasible in 1896 than the similar purposes of the East India Company in 1822, when in Calcutta it had sponsored a school to integrate indigenous and cosmopolitan medicine. The gulf between indigenous and cosmopolitan medicine had grown larger during the course of the nineteenth century, and in the twentieth century the gulf became an ocean in which Dr. Popat, his father and his son, were shipwrecked. Having begun with the ideal of helping to eliminate quackery, they ended by promoting it.

NOTES

1. Arthur Kleinman's essay in the present volume (Chapter 17) develops a comprehensive theory for analyzing medicine as a cultural system.

2. The term cosmopolitan medicine is used in preference to "modern," "scientific" or "Western" medicine, following a suggestion by Fred Dunn. The Chinese, Hindu and Galenic medical traditions are also scientific in the sense that they use naturalistic theories to order empirical observations in a rational manner, and current forms of these traditions are "modern" in the sense that they differ from earlier practices. Since many aspects of cosmopolitan medicine are transcultural rather than "Western," and many aspects of medical practice are not "scientific," it seems wise to avoid referring to this system as Western or scientific medicine (Dunn, Chapter 7 in this volume).

3. The sources for the number of medical institutions reported in this paragraph arc a fact sheet prepared for me by Dr. P. N. V. Kurup, Director of the Central Council for Research in Indian Medicine, New Delhi, and the yearbook, *India: 1971–72* (Ministry of Information, New Delhi).

REFERENCES

BHARDWAJ, S. M.
1973   Early phase of homeopathy in India. Asian Profile 1:281-296.
BRASS, P.
1973   The politics of Ayurvedic education: a case study of revivalism and modernization in India. *In* Politics and Education in India, L. and S. Rudolph, eds. Cambridge: Harvard University Press.
CAUDILL, W.
1976   The culture and interpersonal context of everyday health and illness in Japan and America, *In* Asian Medical Systems, C. Leslie, ed. Berkeley: University of California Press.
GUERRA, F.
1969   Discussion, *In* Medicine and Culture, F. N. L. Poynter, ed. Publications of the Wellcome Institute of the History of Medicine XV (n.s.).
LESLIE, C.
1976   The ambiguities of medical revivalism in modern India, *In* Asian Medical Systems, C. Leslie, ed. Berkeley: University of California Press.
MINISTRY OF INFORMATION
1972   India: 1971-72. New Delhi: Ministry of Information.
MONTGOMERY, E.
1976   Systems and the medical practitioners of a Tamil town, *In* Asian Medical Systems, C. Leslie, ed. Berkeley: University of California Press.
NEUMANN, A., et al
1971   Role of indigenous medicine practitioners in two areas of India: Report of a study, Social Science and Medicine 5: 137-149.
OTSUKA, Y.
1976   Chinese traditional medicine in Japan, *In* Asian Medical Systems, C. Leslie, ed. Berkeley: University of California Press.
SIDEL, V. W. and R. SIDEL
1973   Serve the People, Observations on Medicine in the People's Republic of China. New York: Josiah Macy, Jr. Foundation.
TAYLOR, C. E.
1968   The health sciences and Indian village culture, *In* Science and The Human Condition in India and Pakistan, Ward Morehouse, ed. New York: Rockefeller University Press.
TAYLOR, C. E.
1976   The place of indigenous medical practitioners in the modernization of health services, *In* Asian Medical Systems, C. Leslie, ed. Berkeley: University of California Press.

TOPLEY, M.
  1970 Chinese traditional ideas and the treatment of disease: two examples from Hongkong. Man (n.s.) 5: 421-437.
  1976 Chinese traditional etiology and methods of cure in Hongkong, *In* Asian Medical Systems, C. Leslie, ed. Berkeley: University of California Press.

UNSCHULD, P.
  1973 Die Praxis des Traditionellen Chinesischen Heilsystems. Wiesbaden: Franz Steiner Verlag.
  1976 The social organization and ecology of medical practice in Taiwan, *In* Asian Medical Systems, C. Leslie, ed. Berkeley: University of California Press.

CHAPTER 12

ILLNESS, CULTURE, AND MEANING: SOME COMMENTS
ON THE NATURE OF TRADITIONAL MEDICINE

GANANATH OBEYESEKERE

Introduction

In this paper I shall attempt to describe some features of traditional medicine, confining most of my comments to the great tradition of Ayurvedic (Sanskrit) medicine. My own field experience is in Sri Lanka (Ceylon) which shared this tradition with India as well as other parts of Southern and Southeast Asia. However, I hope that my observations of Ayurveda will shed light on key features of traditional medicine in general, including the Chinese and Southeast Asian systems discussed in this volume. The main thrusts of my arguments are as follows:
(a) Traditional medicine is like Western or cosmopolitan medicine in at least one respect: it attempts to alleviate the suffering of the afflicted patient. The goal of the afflicted person is also to cure his illness, and it can be reasonably assumed that patients will resort to cures which they perceive can alleviate their distress. This has several implications for the relationship between Western and Ayurveda and other systems of traditional medicine. Peasants are bound to recognize the practical effectiveness of Western medicine for some illnesses, and will eventually patronize it, if these services are readily available.
(b) Nevertheless, it can also be demonstrated that Western medicine practiced in non-Western countries is inadequate to cope with other kinds of diseases. This does not refer simply to chronic diseases but to those I call "cultural diseases," as well as mental illnesses which are often implicated in complex personal experiences of the individual and defined in terms of a larger religious, or supernatural idiom. In dealing with these kinds of afflictions Western medicine, it can be shown, is hopelessly inadequate and Ayurvedic as well as religious therapies are both practically effective and comprehensible to the individual reared in his own (non-Western) culture.

The Relationship Between Ayurveda and Western Medicine

Charles Leslie, in his chapter (11) in this volume and in an earlier important paper (1974), shows that in spite of different historical antecedents and state policy Ayurvedic physicians perform a paramedical function very much like that in China. In both societies the indigenous tradition has an inferior paramedical and paraprofessional status vis-à-vis the dominant, implanted Western tradition. Leslie's paper has an excellent discussion of the development of modern Ayurvedic medicine which he appositely calls a professionalized Ayurvedic and Yunani (Arabic) medicine. Professionalized Ayurvedic medicine is based on the Western professional model, so that Ayurveda, emulating the Western model, has developed its own schools, research and degree-granting institutes, professional associations, journals and so forth. He shows that professionalized Ayurvedic medicine is quite different from traditional culture medicine (the great tradition of Ayurveda) and debunks incisively the ideology of revivalism. I suspect that the ambiguities in the ideology of revivalism in Ayurveda (e.g., the myth of its decline in modern times, its pristine purity, etc.) are probably true of revivalist ideologies in general.

He shows further that the avowed goals of revivalism—the resurrection of a pure, intimate, familial based system of Ayurveda—could not be realized. What *was* realized is a professionalized Ayurvedic and Yunani medicine. Pre-professionalized Ayurveda, which he calls traditional culture medicine, still exists, but it is being eroded by professionalized Ayurveda. My own experience in Sri Lanka confirms this. Here also the dominant Ayurvedic orientation is professionalized Ayurveda. Indeed traditional culture Ayurveda, i.e., village Ayurvedic practitioners and those trained in exclusive family traditions, are modeling themselves on the professionals turned out by Sri Lanka's "modern" Ayurvedic Colleges. Several other trends could also be noticed.

Ayurvedic physicians, as a village elite, have considerable influence in national politics and recently the government has given them the right to issue medical certificates to government employees seeking sick leave, a privilege that has been grossly abused by some Ayurvedic physicians. Thus, my Sri Lanka research indicates that the future of pre-professionalized Ayurveda is bleak; most of it will eventually wither away.

But what about the dominant contemporary *professionalized* Ayurveda, based on the Western professional model? Leslie has shown that the very adoption of this model by Ayurveda has willy-nilly relegated it into a paramedical profession in relation to its implanted Western prototype. This is true of both India and China, and according to my research, of Sri Lanka as well. At this point I have several questions to pose regarding the relationships between these two systems of medicine.

Charles Leslie in his paper on "The Modernization of Asian Medical Systems" (1974) has seen the adoption of the Western professional model as indicative of "modernization." Since I agree with his general view that modernization cannot be usefully seen in terms of specific criteria, generally based on modern Western societies like the U.S. or Sweden (Inkeles and Smith 1974; Myrdal 1968), but rather is a self-conception of a particular group as to what they perceive as being modern, I am reluctant to take issue with him. Nevertheless, I hesitate to call the emulation of the Western model by Ayurveda as a modernization process, since according to the self-conception of Ayurvedic practitioners they perceive their profession as inferior to the Western one. Politicians, planners, and elites may recognize the importance of Ayurveda and may stress its potentials, but the future of the Ayurvedic pharmacopoeia, in their view, depends on the test of its validity in modern laboratory conditions. The inferior and lower status of Ayurveda, I think, has several implications for the future of Ayurveda. Leslie notes that prominent Ayurvedic physicians send their sons to modern medical schools—this is exactly the case in Sri Lanka also. All this implies that the Western model is the ideal of emulation and aspiration. Ayurvedic physicians view themselves as inferior in status and some of the grandiose and exaggerated claims for the greatness of Ayurveda's past is an attempt at overcompensation. However, one of the advantages of the widespread professionalization of Ayurveda is that there are always members of low status groups ready to adopt the professional status of Ayurvedic physicians vacated by high status groups. I find this aspect of social mobility wholly desirable.

In discussing Ayurveda and its modernizing role it is useful to see it in relation to the Chinese example. Both perform crucial functions in contemporary life, but the Chinese is based on a deliberate modernizing strategy, or one might say following Weber, it employs a criterion of instrumental rationality, i.e., an attempt to solve practical medical problems in terms of realistic and instrumentally effective means. Also the Chinese case is part of a larger planned strategy of modernization whereas the Indian case is not. In Sri Lanka the Ayurvedic movement with its strong jingoistic overtones may have sometimes acted as an anti-modernizing force. The existence of *expressive paraphernalia* of modernity is no indicator of modernizing processes. For example, a shaman who packs his drum in the back seat of a chauffeur-driven limousine is less of a modern man than a villager who uses a bicycle wheel for winnowing his paddy. In India and Sri Lanka, Ayurvedic Research Institutes have the appearance of modernity but what in fact goes on there is not my idea of rational research.

If for a variety of antecedent historical reasons the two great indigenous medical traditions of India and China have developed into a contemporary paramedical and paraprofessional organization, we get some idea of the nature of cosmopolitan medicine. Cosmopolitan medicine erodes the sphere of traditional physical medicine, but how much of it? We will take this question up later but let us pose another. We social scientists like to think that the acceptance of Western medicine is due to government sponsorship, its prestige, as well as other historical and sociological reasons, but could it also not be due (partly at least) to an obvious and simple reason: its effectiveness? People go to medical practitioners to reduce pain and suffering; and cosmopolitan medicine is effective for some of the more serious ills they suffer from. Surely people are rational enough to recognize this—even if they are repelled by some of its impersonality. Anthropologists quite rightly stress the internal logic and rationality of indigenous medical systems and the sociocultural reasons why peasants shy away from Western medicine, e.g., its incomprehensibility and impersonality, lack of group support, etc. My experience in Sri Lanka suggests that while these views are true, it is also true that peasants can recognize simple instrumental rationality and visit Western practitioners simply because they have an effective medical system. I suspect Taiwanese peasants will very soon recognize this even if they don't do so now. Sometimes the praise we accord our informants (or the society we study) results in unintended dispraise, as for example when we do not grant peasants the capacity to make simple rational decisions on the basis of practical and instrumental efficacy. Sri Lanka is a clear example where peasants have learned to patronize Western medicine for some of their ills. Thus, for example, 99% of births are professionally supervised, mostly in government maternity wards and hospitals, or by trained midwives. The traditional midwife is practically non-existent today. Practically no one consults an Ayurvedic physician for malaria, and even if they do, the latter prescribes Western drugs.

The logic of the preceding discussion has several implications for the future of Ayurveda, or indeed of any similar medical system. If:

(a) Ayurveda is perceived by its practitioners to be inferior in status to the cosmopolitan system;

(b) people patronize cosmopolitan medicine for many of their ills;

(c) and modern cosmopolitan medical schools go churning out graduates—who eventually will be forced to move out of the towns and compete with indigenous practitioners—if so, what will eventually happen? Will Ayurveda (and other traditional systems of physical medicine) die out? The logic of the preceding argument may suggest that it will—but in fact it won't for a long time and for very good reasons. Not for reasons of group support, security, etc. that some have noted for sacred or ritual medicine, either, but for a much more complex reason which I shall now take up.

Traditional Physical Medicine and Cultural Diseases

Two fundamental features of any system of traditional physical medicine, like Ayurveda and Chinese, are relevant to the argument that follows. Firstly, a system of physical medicine entails a prior indigenous conception of the body (and mind) and its functions. Secondly, indigenous conceptions of body physiology and functions are in turn derived from the metaphysical and philosophical conceptions of a great tradition, or, as in all traditions, of an even larger cosmological or sacred world view. Thus, physical medicine has a *meta-medical* dimension: concepts used to define the body are consonant with a larger metaphysical or cosmological schema. This is clearly seen in Ayurveda which derived its basic principles from Saṃkya philosophy, and to a lesser extent from Nyaya-Vaisesika (see Dasgupta 1963, for a discussion of this problem, and Obeyesekere 1976b, for its applications to Ayurvedic practice). Thus the fundamental postulates *(mūla dharma)* of Ayurveda are meta-medical, based on the notion that the universe consists of five elements, ether *(ākāsa)*, wind *(vāyu)*, water *(ap)*, earth *(prthvi)* and fire *(agni)*. The five elements are constituents of all life, and as such also make up the three humors and the seven physical components of the body. As the five elements contained in food are "cooked" by fires in the body they are converted into a fine portion *(āhāra-prasāda)* and refuse *(kitta* or *mala)*. The body elements are produced by successive transformation of the refined food substance into food juice *(rasa)*, blood *(rakta)*, flesh *(mamsa)*, fat *(medas)*, bone *(asthi)*, marrow *(majja)*, and semen *(sukra)*. Semen is said to be the most highly refined element in the body, the "vital juice" that tones the whole organism.

Physical health is maintained when the three humors are in harmonic balance, but when they are upset they become *dosas*, or "troubles," of the organism. The universal element of wind appears in the body as a humor, also called wind *(vāyu)*; fire appears as bile *(pitta)*, and water as phlegm *(kapha or slesman)*. Illness is due to upsetting the homeostatic condition of these *tridosa*. The most serious condition is one in which all three humors are upset *(san-ni-pāta)*. When a *dosa* is "angry" or excited, it increases in proportion to the other humors. The aim of medication is to reduce or control this excess. The excited *dosa* also damages one or more *dhātu* (blood, flesh, fat, etc.), so that treatment must aim to restore the affected body substance.

Similar conceptions, most notably the ideas of *yin* and *yang*, and also humoral ideas, are present in Chinese medicine. These concepts of body physiology and function and their meta-medical extensions are coded through millenia into the thinking and cognitive orientations of South Asian and Chinese peoples, which in turn have considerable implications for their conceptions of illness as well as the persistence of such illnesses and their cures, in spite of the practical efficacy of Western medicine. Since indigenous ideas regarding the body are widely believed in and highly cathected by people, many people patronize cosmopolitan medicine because its technology is pragmatically effective and relieves pain, but that does not mean that they have revised their concepts of the body. I know of sophisticated patients who will go to a cosmopolitan physician for let us say a high fever, *based on belief in the practical efficacy of Western medicine*; but they will also follow a strict regimen of "cooling" foods, *based on traditional notions of body functioning*, i.e., fever is caused by excess of heat (bile) and therefore has to be cooled. Sometimes these cultural definitions of body functioning may result in indigenous disease classifications which may not even exist in Western nosology, so that for example a patient may go to a cosmopolitan physician with a set of symptoms that does not make sense at all in terms of the latter's Western training.

Nosological categories everywhere are not simply diseases but *conceptions* of diseases. I use the term "cultural diseases" to designate those maladies that are conceptualized in terms of indigenous ideas of body physiology and function. Consider the problem of body physiology. All cultures, including popular cultures in the West, have conceptions of the human body which from our contemporary scientific knowledge are false. Though objectively false from our viewpoint, they are subjectively true, from the point of view of the members of the culture. Physical illnesses exist within the organism, even if they are caused by external agents like supernatural beings (or germs). Thus the locus of illness, and very often their cause, are rooted in indigenous physiological theories. The matter may even be further complicated when an ethno-physiology may designate organs, or functions, that are not readily identifiable in terms of Western medical science. Thus ancient Sanskrit texts locate mind and its functions in the heart, much as popular and medieval Western culture considered the heart as the locus of emotion. These conceptions may produce "cultural diseases," which may defy, or be incomprehensible in terms of Western medicine. Ofttimes an indigenous disease may incorporate symptoms which according to Western diagnostic categories belong to different disease entities (complicating, I suspect, cross-cultural epidemiological studies). Not only are disease concepts formulated on the basis of the cultural definition of the body, but their cure is also based on these conceptions. Let me give some examples from my own work on Ayurveda.

Ayurveda, we noted, believes that the Universe consists of five elements, and three of these (fire, water, and wind) appear in the human body as bile, phlegm, and wind. These elements naturally are also present in the food we take, and Ayurveda describes in detail how foods get transformed into various bodily elements or *dhatus*.

According to this theory the most important of the body elements is semen, the very essence of vitality. Here we have a conception of body functioning which is radically at variance with our scientific knowledge. Nevertheless Sri Lanka people often act according to *their* definition of the body, so that you have a large class of patients who view loss of semen in dreams (and masturbation or even intercourse) with great anxiety and consult their indigenous doctors for what they may view as a disease. The patient may notice discoloration of the urine and view it as indicating pathology. Ayurvedic doctors have urine tests to diagnose this illness, which from the scientific point of view does not "objectively" exist. The matter is compounded further because semen is the essence of *human* vitality and consequently females may suffer from semen loss. Women who suffer from anorexia for instance may attribute their state to semen loss. Often vaginal discharges or even natural vaginal moistness or the lubrication of the vagina due to sexual fantasies may be interpreted as semen loss. In 1970 we examined 112,693 cases of patient visits to the free Ayurvedic clinics in Kandy (Sri Lanka) and found that 5,578 (4.95 percent) were women who came to be treated for "discharge from the vagina" due to semen loss! No wonder cosmopolitan doctors whom I interviewed were completely confounded by similar diseases, which of course are real for the afflicted individual. I am not of course suggesting that these kinds of cultural diseases cannot be understood scientifically. In the Sri Lanka case of semen loss there are underlying emotional factors like sexual anxiety and guilt and fears of impotence which could be understood in psychiatric and sociological terms. It should also be noted that an individual's awareness of the scientific knowledge of body physiology will not result in changes in such belief systems, implicated as they are in emotional problems. In order to study change we have to get behind ideology into personality. For example if the sexual liberation of the Sri Lanka female occurs, only then we may expect a change in the cultural disease of female semen loss.

Once a case is diagnosed in terms of "semen loss" then therapy must be directed towards (a) eliminating the causes that led to semen loss and (b) prescribing aphrodisiacs *(vajīkarana)* and semen fostering and vitalizing ingredients. Thus therapy is also ultimately related to concepts of body function and physiology (Obeyesekere 1976a).

My other example is from the Ayurveda theory of mental illness. We noted that classical Ayurveda theory based on Samkya philosophy locates the mind in the heart. However, contemporary practitioners in Sri Lanka, influenced perhaps by Buddhism, locate the mind primarily in the brain, and secondarily in the heart, the latter largely in deference to classic Sanskrit views. The cause of "mental illness" is basically physiological, i.e., owing to the upsetting of one or more of the three humors. Elaborate classifications of mental illness have been developed based on humoral nosology. A common form of mental illness occurs when excessive phlegm has been pushed upwards towards the region of the head, by currents of wind"; "heat" then may cause the phlegm to dry up, clogging the ducts and channels leading to the brain, thus upsetting the mind and producing symptoms of mental illness. In such a case therapy must be directed to loosening the phlegm and expelling it from the organism. A standard therapeutic device is the "head pack." Here the patient stands for two or three hours in the sun, with a pack containing cooling medications on his head. This is followed by a cold bath. These therapeutic actions loosen the phlegm which is then expectorated. Sometimes this therapy is followed by "nasal draining." The physician pours a pinch of medicinal substances, often containing white pepper, into a funnel and blows those substances into the patient's nose. After this somewhat painful experience, the patient goes outside and eliminates the loose phlegm through the nose. Here again both the conception of the disease and its cure are based on concepts of the body which simply cannot exist in Western science (Obeyesekere 1976b). Nevertheless, the illness is no fiction simply because it does not exist in Western medicine; it is a painfully experienced reality to the afflicted individual.

Meta-medical Extensions of Traditional Physical Medicine

The concepts used to define the body are derived from a body of meta-medical concepts, often used to describe the world, or the cosmos and its component elements. Thus bodily illness is paralleled by what Ahern (1975, and in her chapter (2) in this volume) appositely calls "cosmological disorder." In Ayurveda, fire and water are also constituent elements of the universe; ergo, excess of fire or water in the outer environment can lead to drought or flood, and these environmental conditions may in turn increase the incidence of bilious (fire) or phlegm (water) diseases among the human population. The physical health of the human population may be handled by either the Ayurveda physician, or a ritual specialist; but disturbances in the cosmos are more or less the preserve of magical or religious curing. Thus all over India and in Sri Lanka drought is believed to be caused by the anger of a Mother Goddess; the Goddess' anger must be calmed, or cooled in order to restore environmental homeostasis.

This is performed by priests in collective village rituals. Thus a study of traditional physical medicine may eventually lead us to larger cultural concepts of a cosmological, metaphysical or religious nature.

Traditional Sacred Medicine

It should be noted that while a consideration of traditional *physical* medicine of the great traditions must lead to wider meta-medical concepts pertaining to cosmological order and disorder, this must be distinguished from traditional *sacred* medicine that defines illness and its causes in religious terms. Ayurvedic and Chinese practitioners of traditional medicine are physicians like their Western counterparts. They deal with physical illnesses and treat the patient with medications that help restore physical health. While most, if not all cultures, have practitioners of physical medicine in this sense (herbalists, surgeons, bone-setters, etc.), some cultures may place greater stress on the religious definitions of illness and its symptoms, particularly in the realm of what we identify as mental illness. Ayurvedic physicians in Sri Lanka do not practice sacred medicine; yet, they recognize that some illness may be caused by supernatural agencies. There is no necessary conflict between sacred and non-sacred medicine either. For example, an Ayurvedic physician may recognize that a complicated illness may be due to the past sins of the individual, or caused by unfavorable planetary constellations, but these are outside his competence. Similarly, a ritual specialist may give Ayurvedic decoctions to a patient whose body humors have been upset owing to evil demonic possession. Nevertheless, it is important to make a distinction between traditional physical medicine based on ethno-physiological conceptions and traditional sacred medicine based on religious conceptions. The former produce what I have called "cultural diseases"; the latter have often been referred to in the literature as "culture-specific syndromes" (e.g., latah, amok, arctic hysteria, etc.). I shall not deal with sacred medicine or supernatural cures here except to highlight one central feature of sacred medicine parallel to that of physical medicine. Inasmuch as the indigenous definitions of the body and its functions produce disease conceptions we label "cultural diseases," what consequences flow from the definition of illness and its symptoms in a different cultural idiom, that of religion?

Let me start off with a simple (and unrealistic) example. If a peasant were to go to a Western trained MD for a consultation and the latter tells him "You have gastroenteritis" or "You are a paranoid-schizophrenic" (or any such technical label), it does not make a great deal of sense to my peasant, for such descriptions are outside of his range of experience and knowledge. Even if my peasant does understand them, nevertheless these terms from Western nosology refer to a specific, particularistic and localized experience. The position changes remarkably when illness is defined in a publicly intelligible idiom like religion. If someone tells my peasant, "You are ill because you have sinned," the experience of illness immediately becomes non-specific and generalized. The term "sin" (or any such term) articulates that specific experience of illness with the larger experiences of the individual—it extends to other contexts, which do not involve illness, in which he has committed "sin." Also the idiom in which illness is expressed is shared by ordinary people, and it is not the exclusive preserve of specialists. Healing may be the preserve of the specialist but not the idiom which defines it. It also follows that the individual by virtue of this shared idiom can relate his experience of illness with that of his fellows. Thus the *experience* of illness is existentially more "real" and relevant when it is defined in supernatural terms. Or once again following Weber one might argue that a religious idiom gives the experience of illness significance and "meaning." It is not surprising therefore that mental illness, which everywhere has a complicated experiential base, is most often defined in a supernatural idiom helping the patient to express that experience in a manner that makes sense to his group and is consonant with the rest of his culture.

Cosmopolitan and Traditional Medicine: The Division of Labour

After these somewhat discursive remarks we can come back to the point we made at the beginning of this paper: the relationship between traditional and cosmopolitan or Western medicine. Much of cosmopolitan medicine is practically effective, and non-Western peoples may patronize it for many of their ills, but it is at the same time culture-alien; its concepts are out of touch with those physiological-cosmological and religious concepts that help define illness and its experience in traditional societies. If so there are certain classes of diseases—cultural diseases and the so-called culture specific or religious syndromes—that elude the categories of Western medical thought, but are consonant with a particular society's view of both illness and its cultural setting. Gould-Martin (1975:121, and Chapter 3 above) has pointed out that a supernatural healing cult of Taiwan, the *Ong-ia-kong* cult, is doing remarkably well even in areas of Taiwan which are well provided with modern public health facilities, economic improvement, and rapid social progress. Similar examples can be advanced from almost all parts of the world with pluralistic medical systems (Leslie 1975). Sometimes the reasons for patronizing traditional medicine are also very practical, owing to chronic or incurable diseases, but it is also patronized for the reasons mentioned earlier.

The existence of "cultural diseases" (in conjunction with other factors) convinced us that through time there should evolve a division of labor between the two systems. To test this hypothesis effectively one has to have an urban sample where both kinds of medical facilities are readily available for all, free of cost. It is not possible to present our evidence here but we indeed found that in the Ayurvedic Hospital in Colombo and in the six free Ayurvedic clinics in Kandy most of the diseases treated were either "cultural" ones or incurable and chronic diseases. The indigenous doctors in the hospital were aware of this and often referred patients to cosmopolitan doctors for problems they could not tackle. When asked what kinds of diseases could be effectively treated by Ayurveda, students in the Ayurveda College in fact listed the diseases which they were familiar with in their hospital (Obeyesekere 1976a). Western doctors were more wary about formal referrals; but some of them gave "advice" to their patients about consulting Ayurvedic physicians for "cultural diseases." Many Western doctors, themselves products of their culture, did not interfere with the dietary habits of their patients based on hot-cold foods; indeed, some doctors personally believed in their efficacy. I suspect that an evolution of this kind of labor division is inevitable for perhaps all traditional societies confronted, and in competition, with the practically effective and high status system of Western medicine.

REFERENCES

AHERN, E.M.
1975 Sacred and Secular Medicine in a Taiwan Village: A Study of Cosmological Disorders. *In* Medicine in Chinese Cultures, A. Kleinman et al, eds., Bethesda, Md.: Fogarty International Center, N.I.H.; pp. 91-113.

DASGUPTA, S.N.
1963 The Kapila and Patanjali Samkya. *In* a History of Indian Philosophy, Vol. I. London: Routledge; pp. 274-366.

GOULD-MARTIN, K.
1975 Medical Systems in a Taiwan Village: Ong-ia-Kong, the Plague God as Modern Physician. *In* Medicine in Chinese Cultures, A. Kleinman et al, eds., Bethesda, Md.: Fogarty International Center, N.I.H.: pp. 91-113.

INKELES, A. and D. SMITH
1974 Becoming Modern. Cambridge: Harvard University Press.

LESLIE, C.
1974 The Modernization of Asian Medical Systems. *In* Rethinking Modernization: Anthropological Perspectives, J. Poggie, Jr. and R.N. Lynch, eds., Westport, Conn.: Greenwood Press.

1975 Pluralism and Integration in the Indian and Chinese Medical Systems. *In* Medicine in Chinese Cultures, A. Kleinman et al, eds., Bethesda, Md.: Fogarty International Center, N.I.H.; pp. 115-141.

MYRDAL, G.
1968 Asian Drama, 3 Vols. London, Allen Lane: The Penguin Press.

OBEYESEKERE, G.
1976a The Impact of Ayurvedic Ideas on the Culture and the Individual in Sri Lanka. *In* Asian Medical Systems: A Comparative Study, C. Leslie, ed., Berkeley and Los Angeles: University of California Press; pp. 201-226.

1976b The Theory and Practice of Psychological Medicine in the Ayurvedic Tradition. *In* Culture, Medicine and Psychiatry, Vol. I, in press.

CHAPTER 13

COMMENTS ON TRADITIONAL AND MODERN MEDICAL SYSTEMS IN EAST ASIA

JOHN C. PELZEL

The variety of these papers is warrant of the richness of materials and talents we have for the comparative study of medical systems. It is also, however, such as to discourage any attempt here to generalize about similarities and differences in the natures of the systems depicted, for each paper deals with a somewhat different aspect of its topic. Dunn provides a comprehensive survey of the professional services available to Malayan Chinese. Leslie treats modern alterations of medical theory in India. Spiro analyzes the treatment of illness believed to be caused by supernatural agents in Burma. Kunstadter creates a model of the process whereby individuals in tribal regions of Thailand choose from among the several alternative medical explanations and practices available in their culturally eclectic environment.

Nonetheless, the situations reported in all of these papers have one very important feature in common. Each author pictures a local medical system, the elements of which derive from distinct cultural sources. History has somehow brought it about that each local community today has at hand explanations, behaviors, roles and institutions relating to health and illness that are of varied origins. In most cases, the indigenous combines in some degree with the Western. In all cases, the indigenous elements of today represent an earlier fusion of what were then native and foreign elements. It is upon the subject of the extant medical system as a product of cultural history that this writer can perhaps most usefully comment.

These are all systems, then, that are eclectic in origin, and to a degree also in assumption and logic. At the same time, they are systems in which all elements, of whatever origin and nature, seem to operate with considerable vitality. Though Spiro has confined himself to what he notes is only a minor portion of the Burmese system, and a portion in which one would expect little evidence of Western influence, elements which were originally animistic and Buddhist are both at work. Kunstadter's peoples combine Western medicine with the features of several different indigenous systems. Leslie estimates that native medical systems, in contrast with the Western, provide 80 percent of all consultations in India, but the former are themselves a composite of Ayurvedic, Persian and Arabic elements.

When we turn to the Chinese cases, it is clear both that the indigenous Chinese elements are alive and very well indeed, and that features of Western medicine have been accepted into a vital eclecticism. The basically Western care provided Boston's Chinese must accommodate the many predilections of its clients, derived from Chinese medicine. As we know from these and other sources, Chinese and Western practices are available, in varying combinations, not only in metropolitan China, but also in regions as distant, and as long exposed to Western education, communications and medical services as Malaya and Hongkong. The mixture is evident not only where contemporary medicine has grown up under private aegis, but as well in the socialist atmosphere of the PRC. The indigenous Chinese portion of this amalgam, moreover, does not only survive, but exhibits as well a considerable capacity for qualitative growth, as is suggested by Dunn's remarks about training and advanced research in Malaya and, on other evidence, by reports out of the PRC.

This vital eclecticism—and for present purposes especially that in the Chinese areas—is to be remarked, since it is not the only possible result of the meeting of divergent medical systems. Our own Western systems long ago shrugged off humoral theories and supernatural etiologies, and have only recently and reluctantly come back to deal with such untitratable entities as the non-organic manifestations of the human mind. One may argue for unilineal evolution in these matters, and see the eclectic systems of East and South Asia today as at a way station along the same road taken by the West, but the case of Japan complicates this view. It will be the writer's task in the remainder of these comments to try and bring that case to bear on this question.

Certainly, what comes to be included into a medical system is everywhere a matter of the native definition of what is relevant to health and its disorders. I assume few would deny that among the major developments of the modern West, however, has been the growth of a radical esteem for systematized knowledge of the natural world and, with it, the appearance of an extreme degree of functional specialization in social roles. Professional specialists define what is relevant to their areas, and where a specialty touches life as intimately as does medicine, there is a tendency for the professionals' definition to dominate that of the laity. Health and its disorders in the modern West have come to be what doctors say they are. One recognizes that even among us there exist many beliefs and behaviors that in other cultures are defined as having to do with medicine—the laying-on of hands, astrology, massage, etc.—but professional medicine among us has forced these to be re-defined even by much of the public as "Religion," "Recreation," or worse, and in any event as "non-Medicine." It is in the contrast between this positivistic and narrow definition of medicine in the modern West, and its still eclectic and traditionalistic definition in Chinese areas, that the case of Japan may prove instructive.

Japan began with a system of medicine that seems to have been much influenced by animistic perceptions of nature.[1] From its first historical contacts with China after the middle of the first millenium A.D., however, and down to only a century ago, it borrowed continental medical theories and practices. The changing mixture of native Japanese and imported Chinese elements at varying points of time need not concern us here. Certainly medicine in Japan made much greater use than did that in China of shamanistic treatments, massage, hot spring baths and moxibustion, and less use of acupuncture. It is a fair hypothesis that, given the more persistent strength among them of organized Buddhism, Japanese also accorded Buddhist specifics, e.g. the healing power of the sutras, more attention than did Chinese.

Nonetheless, until the coming of the West, the Japanese system was not unlike that of China. The Japanese upper classes, at least, were cared for by professionals, normally inheriting their occupations and trained in public schools of medicine of Chinese type, and familiar with the latest Chinese texts. There seems little evidence that, until the variant Western model began to become available, Japanese were any more experimental in their approach than the Chinese. Both depended heavily upon an herbal *materia medica,* and Kaempfer in 1690 (Bowers 1970: 47) found Japanese physicians good at therapeutics. He also found them poor to the point of barbarism, even by seventeenth century European standards, at surgery. Neither country permitted dissection under conditions conducive to testing the deductive Chinese conceptions of anatomy and physiology, or a clinically-satisfactory method of examining patients (described in Chapter 4 of *Medicine in Chinese Cultures*). The theory and technique of Japanese medicine thus do not appear to have held within themselves the seed of any radical evolution away from the Chinese model.

It was in 1858 that the first official school of Western medicine was set up in Edo, and in 1862 that the first Japanese were permitted to go abroad for a Western medical education (Bowers 1970: 195). Yet in the century since, there has developed a professional medical establishment that is almost wholly Western in its orientation, and a governmental and popular definition of medicine that seems all but indistinguishable from that to be found in America or northwestern Europe. Treatments and practitioners deriving from native medicine persist, but are no longer recognized as "medical" by government or the majority of the population, and since 1875 no physicians not trained by Western standards have been permitted to practice. Indeed, one's impression is that such treatments of the sort as persist have lost much in quality—massage, for example, having been taken over by tarts and technicians less skilled even than their paramedical forebears of only a generation ago.

How is one to interpret so radical a change in Japanese medicine in what was no more than two or three generations? Why was there no way station of the sort that proponents of unilineal evolution might say has been the dallying ground of Chinese medicine for a 100 years now? Does the Japanese experience give us any assurance that the Chinese will also now rush to close the gap?

Japan, of course, embarked upon the importation of Western technologies at the time the medical milestones noted above were reached,
and thus much earlier than did China, but this difference of timing must
be explained by reference to factors other than opportunity. Western
missionaries and traders brought knowledge of their medicine to China
and Japan equally early, from the sixteenth century, and the full power of
the West was at the doors of both at the same time, in the early part
of the nineteenth century. It is also true that Japan incorporated Western
medicine as only one part of a massive reorientation of her culture, to a
degree that is only today perhaps occurring in continental China, but it
is difficult to argue that this was not the product of different choices by
Chinese and Japanese, to be explained by factors internal to the two
societies rather than by the chances of contact.

One must note that the massive reorientation initiated by the Meiji
Restoration had been preceded by certain events of intellectual, and
even social, preparation in Japan, events that do not seem to have
occurred in China. Chinese, for example, had easy access to Western
astronomy through the efforts of the Jesuits in Peking, but seemed
indifferent to the opportunity (Nakayama 1969: 230). On the other
hand, though the Japanese Shogunate after the seventeenth century imposed the strictest isolation upon foreigners in Japan, it was also alive
to the practical importance of certain areas of Western learning—
especially in medicine, agriculture and astronomy, the last to allow
correction of the all-important farming calendar. It therefore permitted,
and in cases required, the importation of foreign books on such subjects
and relaxed the ban against their study.

On this basis, some Japanese doctors discovered the inadequacies of
Chinese conceptions of anatomy and physiology, and in fact the whole
development of *Rangaku,* or "Dutch (Western) Learning," from the
mid-eighteenth century was intimately bound up with the importation of
Western medical knowledge and the development of a more experimental
clinical method. During the last century of the Tokugawa Period, 12
schools teaching Western medicine, and enrolling a not-insignificant
proportion of Japanese medical students, were established by Japanese
private physicians (Bowers 1970: 70–140). Nor was this Japanese interest
in the discovery of the facts of the case, and its application to practical
matters, limited to areas in which Western books supplied the initial
stimulus. Smith (1959: 87–107) has described the selfconscious development of agricultural technology during the same period, which also
saw rapid advances in handicraft and commercial technologies.

Clearly then, behind the stagnant facade of political autocracy, the
Tokugawa Period in Japan was one of a considerable intellectual fer-
ment that seems not to have occurred in contemporary Ch'ing China.
Indeed, there was also a social concomitant to this intellectual contrast.
Though it institutionalized social mobility through individual merit,
China could offer elite status only to those who would restrict their
training to the traditional and moralistic Confucian learning, and

practical rewards of any substance only to that infinitesimal portion of such persons who made it into the bureaucracy. By contrast, Japanese society at the time ascribed status by inheritance, but gave only small practical rewards to that vast majority of the rather large elite samurai class who did not hold hereditary bureaucratic posts. Perhaps 5 percent of Japanese must try and keep up an elite position, but find their own way to do so. There was thus much practical incentive for many Japanese of the period to go into new fields, inventing or co-opting new technologies in order to do so.

Yet one must not overestimate the degree to which Japanese were better-prepared than Chinese in 1868 to adopt Western culture on a wholesale basis. The adoption of a few Western techniques had not yet been accompanied by the development of anything like the deep philosophical underpinnings they had in their own homelands. The vast majority of techniques, even in areas most influenced by the kinds of change noted, were still thoroughly traditional. Social institutions were still predominately those of the past.

In this situation, it is tempting to explain the great difference in the reactions of China and Japan to the West in the middle of the nineteenth century in terms of the different historical precedents the two countries had before them of intercultural contact. China, long exposed to foreigners generally of an inferior culture, did not need to admit to having borrowed anything of importance from abroad prior to the development of her own original high culture. In fact, her leaders could point to the proscription of organized Buddhism in the ninth century as evidence that perhaps the major of such borrowings had turned sour. Japan, on the other hand, had frankly constructed most of her high culture out of borrowings from China and seemed content to have done so.

Nonetheless, these undoubted differences of precedent alone do not seem sufficient to explain the varying reactions of the two countries to the modern West. China had over the centuries suffered egregiously from her nomadic neighbors, time and again losing populations as large as those of many modern countries, draining her treasury for ransom, and seeing her governments captured. Yet, rather than borrow the dangerous nomad technologies of war and turn them, with some chance of success, against their inventors, China seemed to prefer to rely upon her ability to "manage the barbarian" in other ways, and to make good their ravages through her enormous reproductive potential. Quite by contrast, though Japan was physically well enough isolated that she might have felt secure, in fact on those rare occasions when the outside world posed a threat or offered an opportunity for aggrandizement, she to a man mobilized for the defense or the attack.

At every instance of foreign contact, in other words, Japanese have shown it to be their prime interest not to be bested as a people, militarily or culturally, by foreigners, even if to accomplish this end they must turn themselves, for a time and in every way but in their hearts, into those foreigners. As Nakayama (1969: 222) notes, when faced with the full strength of the modern West, China admitted only slowly, and has perhaps even today admitted only partially, that the Western threat rested upon a technology that grew out of a general background of science and learning that must be borrowed; Japan, on the other hand, grasped the entire logic, and accepted its conclusion, almost at once. The writer interprets this behavior as indicative of a basic evaluation of the ethnic and national group as *the* unit of welfare, and of culture as merely an instrument by the use of which the group maintains its successful adaptation to the changing conditions of life. By contrast, one is left with the distinct impression that China has usually been willing to pay almost any price in welfare for the preservation of her own culture.

If the writer is correct, the radically-different reactions of China and Japan—the eclectic and still heavily-traditional medicine of the one and the almost total adoption of Western medicine by the other—cannot of course be reduced to the contrast between idealism and pragmatism. The two peoples have merely idealized different things, and adopted different measures for their attainment. To Japan, its continued success as a people in a world of changed conditions was of paramount importance, and the new culture was the instrument for its attainment. To Chinese, some essential core of the old culture must be preserved, even at what to Japanese or to many of the rest of us would appear a terrifying cost. Nor need the decisions that led, and still lead, to these results have differed in the degree of conscious rationality applied. Japanese have long been used to leadership by a centralized and highly visible set of decision-making roles, Chinese to leadership by consensus among a diffuse and self-selected elite, most of whose members at any given time are not in formal posts of power.

The writer concludes this brief comparison of the recent histories of Chinese and Japanese medicine with the banal observation only that even so universal a problem as that of the most satisfactory way to maintain health will be solved on the basis of merits not immediately at issue. We may not have time to test the proposition that the "objective" value of Western conceptions about health and its disorders will in the long run result in a worldwide unilineal evolution, and indeed the Chinese and Japanese adaptations to date may prove to have no other relevance to the other cases presented in these papers.

NOTE

1. For brief English summaries of the history of Japanese medicine, see Ishihara (1962), and Steslicke (1972). For extended Japanese treatments, see Takahashi (1972) on traditional Chinese medicine in Japan and Kawakami (1961) on the modern medical establishment. Bowers (1970) is useful on the introduction of Western medicine before 1868.

REFERENCES

BOWERS, J. Z.
  1970   Western Medical Pioneers in Feudal Japan. Baltimore: Johns
         Hopkins University Press.
ISHIHARA, A.
  1962   *Kampō:* Japan's traditional medicine. Japan Quarterly 9:
         429–37
KAWAKAMI, T.
  1961   *Nihon no isha: Gendai iryō kōzō no bunseki* (The Japanese
         Doctor: An Analysis of Contemporary Treatment and Struc-
         ture). Tokyo: Keiso shobo.
NAKAYAMA, S.
  1969   A History of Japanese Astronomy: Chinese Background and
         Western Impact. Cambridge: Harvard University Press.
SMITH, T.
  1959   The Agrarian Origins of Modern Japan. Stanford: Stanford
         University Press.
STESLICKE, W. E.
  1972   Doctors, patients, and government in modern Japan. Asian
         Survey 12: 913–31.
TAKAHASHI, K.
  1972   *Kampō no ninshiki* (An Appreciation of Chinese Medicine).
         Nippon hōsō kyokai.

SECTION II
CROSS-CULTURAL PSYCHIATRIC
AND PUBLIC HEALTH STUDIES

CHAPTER 14

PATIENT AND PRACTITIONER ATTITUDES TOWARD TRADITIONAL AND WESTERN MEDICINE IN A CONTEMPORARY CHINESE SETTING

James L. Gale

Changes occurring in Taiwan during the past 25 years have affected virtually every aspect of life there. A variety of intellectual, social and economic influences from the West have been introduced as the country has become industrialized. The crude death rate has dropped from 18 per thousand in 1947 to 5 per thousand in 1970 as the birth rate has declined from 3.8 to 2.7 percent per year (Taiwan Provincial Government 1970: 87). The three leading causes of death in 1952, inflammation of the digestive tract, pneumonia, and tuberculosis have been replaced in 1970 by vascular lesions of the central nervous system, malignancies of all forms and accidents (ibid.). Although little of the decline in mortality can be ascribed directly to specific measures aimed at improving health, the format of health care has remained largely unchanged over this period. With the exception of certain services for prenatal care, tuberculosis care and immunizations, most illnesses are cared for on a fee-for-service basis. During this time, traditional Chinese medicine, whose practitioners are licensed by the government and which is almost entirely on a fee-for-service basis, has apparently flourished.

The studies described in this paper, consisting of a series of interviews conducted in the spring and summer of 1972 with practitioners of Western and traditional Chinese medicine and their patients examine the relationship between classic Chinese and Western practice.[1] In particular an attempt was made to see where the two systems overlap and where they are complementary, and what appeared to be the future of each. Throughout the island of Taiwan, 15 million annual patient visits were estimated to have been made to some 1500 licensed traditional practitioners in the early 1960's when the total population was about 12 million (Baker and Perlman 1967:71). At that time some 5450 Western-trained physicians were licensed island-wide. The official figures for both traditional Chinese and Western practitioners on Taiwan in 1970 were somewhat lower, 1106 and 4479 respectively (Taiwan Province 1970: 4, 6, 8). These figures should be interpreted with caution, however, for reasons discussed by Baker and Perlman.[2] At a time when many non-Western populations, including the Taiwanese, were striving to adopt many Western attitudes and patterns of behavior while undergoing a shift from an economy based on agriculture to one based on industry, the belief in and use of classical Chinese medical practices has remained widespread throughout all levels of Chinese society on Taiwan. The term "traditional Chinese medicine" in the following discussion refers to the formal body of knowledge in such works as the *Nei Ching* studied by classical scholars over the centuries.

Classical Chinese medicine was introduced to Taiwan following the expulsion of the Dutch by Koxinga in 1662.[3] Although education was largely by individual preceptors and apprenticeships to existing herbalists rather than through formal training, classical Chinese medicine continued without interruption even after the introduction of Western medicine to Taiwan by missionaries in the nineteenth century. According to Baker and Perlman, traditional medicine did suffer a decline following the signing of the Treaty of Shimonoseki and the assumption by Japan of political responsibility for Formosa. Taihoku University Medical School, an institution in which Western medicine was taught, and later to be known as the National Taiwan University College of Medicine, was established during this period.

Western medicine continued to flourish under the Nationalist government following their move to Taiwan after World War II. By 1963, four Western medical schools were established (Baker and Perlman 1967: 55–60). Although one institution, the China Medical College, was devoted to traditional Chinese medicine, it did not receive strong financial support. In Taiwan in 1962 the island-wide ratio of Western-trained physicians to licensed traditional Chinese practitioners was 3.6 to 1, using Baker's figures. This ratio was lower in the cities, however, since licensed herbalists had a greater tendency to practice in the cities than did Western trained physicians.[4]

Strong support for Western medicine has been a consistent position for the Nationalist government since 1929 (Croizier 1968:133). At that time Western medicine was regarded as modern and progressive by the Kuomentang. Classical Chinese medicine was looked on as reactionary, backward, and in general associated with the old order. Since World War II, the communists have turned back to traditional Chinese medicine, and their success in integrating traditional and Western medicine is discussed by Worth in *Medicine in Chinese Cultures* and by Wegman (1973). The Nationalist government until very recently showed very little interest in traditional Chinese medicine, and support for such institutions as the China Medical College probably has been as much for cultural and historical interest as out of any strong belief in the traditional medicine system per se. All physicians in the armed forces and in the government employees' insurance clinics are Western-trained. Five Western medical schools are presently (1973) in operation, with plans for a sixth, versus one traditional Chinese medical school. The Provincial Health Department which operates clinics throughout Taiwan, as well as the Taipei City Health Department, a separate entity, are staffed entirely with personnel trained in Western medical procedures.

Despite government support being given almost entirely for Western medical systems, the popularity of traditional Chinese medicine has remained high. Offices and clinics can be seen in all parts of Taipei. Pharmacies often sell both Western and traditional Chinese medicines. Although regulated by law to sell drugs by prescription only, most pharmacies sell any drugs except narcotics upon request.

The present data are drawn from (a) interviews with 33 practitioners of Western and traditional Chinese medicine, (b) direct observation of all patients seen and treated on 3, 2 and 5 clinic days of three traditional practitioners, respectively, (c) interviews with patients seen in the clinics of the same three practitioners and (d) a subsample of 25 of the same patients initially interviewed in the clinics with follow-up interviews made at their homes at intervals of from 1 to 2 months following their initial visits. Interviews and observations were conducted by three public health nurses and by a candidate for the master of public health degree from the National Taiwan University Institute of Public Health. All medical practitioners and patients were interviewed in Taipei, except for a group of 11 patients recently discharged from a Western insurance hospital in a small market town near Taipei. With few exceptions, interviews were conducted according to a standard form. Many of the questions were open-ended, however, and the interviewers were instructed to probe where they thought appropriate, recording all responses as closely as they could. Diagnoses were those of the attending practitioner, or of the patient himself based on previous visits to other practitioners. No attempts were made to verify these.

Interviews with Practitioners

Interviews were obtained from 15 practitioners of traditional Chinese medicine (Table 1). Eleven had been born on the Chinese mainland and four had lived all their life in Taiwan. All but two Taiwanese practitioners were over 50 years of age. Seven traditional Chinese practitioners had formal training outside of the medical field above the high school level. Two had degrees in Chinese literature, two were graduates of military academies, one was a graduate of the Peking National Law College, and one each had a Master of Science in engineering and a bachelor's degree in education. Five received their training in traditional Chinese medicine at colleges of Chinese medicine, seven received instruction from a tutor and three stated that they learned their art by self study from books. Only two doctors saw more than 20 patients per day and six saw fewer than 10 per day, reflecting the unhurried pace of most of their places of practice. According to Baker and Perlman, traditional Chinese practitioners see on an average, island-wide, more than 30 patients per day, 6 days per week, and see more persons who were born on the Chinese mainland in Taipei than are proportional to their representation in Taiwan. One might expect that patterns of medical practice, including the number of patients seen per day might be different in Taipei, for this and other reasons. No comparable figures are given for Western-trained doctors in Baker's study. However, Lee found that in Hongkong herbalists generally spent more time (12 minutes vs. 8 minutes) and saw fewer patients than did Western doctors.[5]

Of the 18 Western doctors interviewed in the present study, 14 were born in Taiwan and four had migrated from the Chinese mainland. Ten were under 50 years of age, and none had any other degrees. They tended to see more patients per day than did the Chinese medicine practitioners. Only two of the Western-trained doctors saw under 10 patients per day, and one of these was an army physician whose private clinic was open only in the evening. Eight saw 30 or more patients per day, and one of these said he often saw 150 patients each day. Both traditional Chinese and Western-trained practitioners said that 20-30 percent of their patients each week were new patients.

TABLE 1. NUMBER OF TRADITIONAL CHINESE AND WESTERN PRACTITIONERS INTERVIEWED BY AGE, BIRTHPLACE, AND NUMBER OF PATIENTS SEEN PER DAY

Pts. Seen/Day	Traditional Chinese Practitioners			Western Practitioners		
	less than 20	20 or more	unknown	less than 20	20 or more	unknown
Taiwanese						
Under 50	1	0	1	0	6	3
50 or older	1	1	0	0	4	1
Mainlander						
Under 50	0	0	0	1	0	0
50 or older	10	1	0	2	1	0
TOTALS		15			18	

When asked the question, "What is the most frequently diagnosed illness that you treat?" 14 Western-trained doctors who classified themselves as general practitioners, including two pediatricians, answered: "Upper respiratory infections, diarrhea, or both." A surgeon, an ophthalmologist and a gynecologist were the three specialists represented among the Western-trained group. Of the 15 traditional physicians interviewed, three said that gynecologic illness was their most frequently treated illness, and one said that skin diseases were seen most frequently by him. The remainder named a variety of common illnesses including respiratory infections, gynecologic disorders, rheumatism, and liver and kidney ailments as their most frequently diagnosed problems.

Practitioners were additionally asked whether, if patients with any of the following conditions appeared, they would treat them or refer them somewhere else: Acute trauma, fractures, high fever in young children, venereal disease, cerebral vascular accidents or acute myocardial infarctions. The responses were similar for both groups of doctors, with the exception of venereal disease which was treated more frequently by Western physicians (Table 2). Two practitioners of each type said they treated trauma and fractures. Only one traditional Chinese practitioner and the Western-trained ophthalmologist and gynecologist did not treat fever in children.

TABLE 2. PERCENT POSITIVE RESPONSES TO QUESTIONS ABOUT SPECIFIC ILLNESS TREATED BY TRADITIONAL CHINESE AND WESTERN PRACTITIONERS

	Traditional Chinese (n=13)	Western (n=14)
Fractures	17	20
Acute Trauma	17	7
High Fever in Children	92	87
Venereal Disease	33	73
Acute Cerebrovascular Accidents	50	40
Acute Myocardial Infarction	67	60

When asked about their policy regarding immunizations, all Western doctors, not surprisingly, either administered or recommended immunizations against smallpox, poliomyelitis, diphtheria, and tetanus. About three-fourths of the traditional Chinese practitioners recommended these immunizations also.

Relationships to other professionals were different in the two groups. Only two of 14 traditional practitioners indicated that they regularly referred patients to other medical facilities or colleagues, compared with seven of 10 Western trained doctors answering that question.

An attempt was made to evaluate the feeling of continuing responsibility of practitioners to their patients with or without continuing illness. Doctors were asked whether they recommended periodic checkups to healthy or asymptomatic patients. Additionally, they were asked whether they would visit a critically ill patient's house if the patient failed to return to the doctor's office as directed. Two of the 12 traditional Chinese and nine of 11 Western practitioners said they recommended regular, periodic examinations to their patients, regardless of the presence of symptoms. The second question failed to elicit information concerning the extent of responsibility practitioners might feel toward a patient well known to them in an extreme situation, since both groups of physicians stated that it would be bad luck for a doctor to visit a patient's house on professional business without being asked. However, when asked if they had ever made house calls to visit ill patients, 80 percent of each group said they did.

When asked about the future of traditional Chinese medicine on Taiwan neither group of practitioners was optimistic. Many of the traditionalists felt that the two systems would continue to coexist separately on Taiwan. One older traditional practitioner from the mainland felt that traditional Chinese medicine was dying out because the medicines themselves were getting too expensive.[6] Although few Western doctors condemned traditional medicine outright, several felt that it would continue in its present, subordinate relationship to Western medicine. A common opinion of both groups was that traditional medicine could not grow in stature on Taiwan unless the government supported schools and laboratories which could validate its effectiveness on a *scientific* basis in the Western sense of the word. The traditionalists and a few Western-trained doctors felt that the two systems could and should be merged into one system if such a "scientific" validity could be established.

It is interesting that evaluation of both groups of doctors by themselves was against a Western scientific standard. The implications of such a concession to Western standards by the traditionalists have been pointed out previously (Croizier 1968:99).

Although both groups practiced medicine within entirely different medical systems, both functioned the way urban general practitioners or non-university affiliated specialists do in the U.S. Both offer primary medical care on a fee-for-service basis, both see a substantial number of acute, self-limited diseases by their own estimates, and 20–30 percent of the patients of each group are new. Both groups regard themselves as professionals, both keep some sort of written records on their patients, and both appeared to limit their concern for their patients to the particular symptom which is presented in their office, rather than undertaking or recommending a comprehensive diagnostic or therapeutic regime. Some patients felt that traditional doctors treated the whole body and Western doctors only the affected part, however. This may reflect the degree to which the patient identified with a particular individual practitioner, or to a particular medical system. As will be seen from the patterns of usage presented below, many patients saw their doctors less as representatives of differing medical systems than as curers of their immediate problem. The patients were able to believe in each system to the extent necessary to accept treatment, but in general they were too pragmatic to continue fee payment to either type of practitioner without results.

Direct Observations of Patients of Three Traditional Chinese Practitioners

Observations were made of all patients seen by one Taiwanese and two mainland traditional Chinese practitioners for 3, 2 and 5 days, respectively. The Taiwanese doctor was self trained, had a master of science degree in engineering from National Taiwan University and saw an average of 20 patients from 5 to 82 years of age during the hours of

9:00 to 12:30, on these 3 days. Twenty-three percent of the 60 patients were seen for the first time, and 35 percent were foreigners, including 14 persons from Malagasy, two each from Tokyo, Korea, and Hawaii, and one person from the Philippines. The majority of patients received acupuncture for up to 40 minutes in addition to herb medicines. Complaints ranged from joint pain and headache (47 percent), partial or complete paralysis (10 percent), to corneal opacification with loss of vision, sterility, and irregular menses, 2 percent each. Many patients learned of this doctor through his advertisements in the newspapers and on the radio, and came to him after unsuccessful treatment elsewhere.

After an initial brief interview by an assistant and a reading from a machine to which was attached a galvanometer, patients were interviewed by the traditional practitioner. Treatment was usually started after a conversation of not more than 5 minutes. Patients returning for follow-up visits frequently engaged in little dialogue. The average patient's stay was 34 minutes as measured by the observing nurse. The patients could be seen seated around the edge of the large single room which served as an office in increasing numbers as the morning passed. The doctor moved around the room speaking to each patient quietly, adjusting or twirling individual needles, but offering little direct explanation of either the disease process or the mechanism of therapy. When asked, "What is the machine used at the registry?" the doctor replied, "It is a machine used to help the traditional Chinese doctor in diagnosis." A typical exchange was that recorded between the doctor and a 14-year-old boy with pain on the soles of his feet.

Doctor—"What is wrong?"
Patient—"I have pain here" (points to sole of one foot).
Doctor—"How long? A half year?"
Patient—Nods. The boy's mother explained that Western doctors had not been able to find anything wrong with the boy. The boy was given acupuncture for 25 minutes, told to take pills (which he was given) 3 times daily, and a second type of pill in the evening, and return in 2 days for more acupuncture.

In another instance, a 60-year-old woman patient known to the doctor came in and immediately lay down on a table. After the needles were inserted, the patient asked, "Why do I have pain in my left side?" "Because you have heart trouble," was the doctor's reply. A 22-year-old girl with dark blotches on her face being seen for the first time asked the doctor, "Why do I have these spots?" She was told, "These are caused by poor blood circulation. Don't worry, they will be cured. Take the pills I will give you. Your condition should be treated from inside the body." She was given pills and left, without acupuncture, after a 3 minute consultation, the shortest of the morning. In these examples and others like them, the patients either did not ask about the cause of their illnesses, or accepted an abbreviated explanation which possibly could have been placed in a context understood by both doctor and patient, but not stated by either. The explanations given would not have explained anything to someone who lacked a previous understanding of the doctor's reference system. An alternative explanation is that the patients chose to believe that if the doctor had an explanation for the cause of their illness, it was sufficient, particularly if they were cured. This interpretation requires no shared system of knowledge about illness between doctor and patient, only a confidence in the doctor and judgment by the results. This second interpretation would seem more consistent with the generally short-term relationship patients seen in this study appeared to maintain with either traditional Chinese or Western doctors, if their disease state wasn't stable or improving, as described in the next section.

Willingness to allow the doctor a second chance at treatment was also seen. A 40-year-old man had pain in his neck.

Doctor—"How is your neck?"

Patient—"Hasn't improved much, still aching."

Doctor—"Then the disease is not so simple. Let me change the medicine and try again."

Patient—"All right."

Thirty patients were seen by the second practitioner, who was originally from the Chinese mainland, during two half-day clinics. All but three patients were known to the clinic, and all but two received herb therapy only for a variety of complaints including bronchitis (nine patients), weakness, and malaise (nine patients), stomach pain or indigestion (three patients), a breast mass, nephritis, anemia, asthma, hepatitis, insomnia, a sore arm, urticaria and sequellae from an earlier stroke (one each). These patients ranged from 4 to 62 years of age, the median age being 32. Nine patients were born in Taiwan, 19 in mainland China and 2 were not recorded. No foreigners were seen by this doctor.

The last practitioner, also from the Chinese mainland, was observed to treat 22 patients in 5 clinic sessions over 5 days. He was the son of a traditional Chinese medicine practitioner, and in addition received formal training at a college of Chinese medicine. He held a bachelor's degree in education, and had the reputation of being a skilled acupuncturist. Eight patients were treated for neurologic disorders including numbness of varying severity and sequelae of a cerebrovascular accident, four for arthritis, two for gallbladder pain, and one each for headache, dysphagia, weakness, and upper respiratory infection. Except for four patients who were given only medication (two with gallstones, one with debility and one with an upper respiratory infection) all patients were treated with acupuncture. They ranged from 17 to 81 years old with a median age of 49.

Single Patient Interviews in the Doctors' Offices

Single interviews were conducted in a standard format with 30 patients who attended the clinics of these three practitioners. Eleven patients recently discharged from a labor insurance hospital were also interviewed according to the same format. The mean age of the first group was 43 years (range 24-73 years) and of the second group 64 years (range 15-78 years). The number of patients interviewed was almost equally divided by sex between the 17 patients interviewed at the Taiwanese traditional Chinese doctor's clinic (9 women, 8 men) and the 11 patients recently discharged from the hospital (6 women, 5 men). Eleven of the 13 interviews at the other two clinics were with men. Nineteen of the 30 patients were born on Taiwan and 11 on the mainland, although a majority of the patients interviewed at the clinics of the two mainlander practitioners were also born on the mainland. Five of the 26 patients responding to the question about occupation were classified as lower class, all at the Taiwanese practitioner's clinic, including a taxi-driver, a tailor, two farmers and a carpenter. One reason for the relatively small proportion of lower-class persons interviewed may have been the clinic fee, which ranged from U.S. $2.50 to $5.00 for all three practitioners. The remaining patients included businessmen, engineers, a Western drug salesman, a lawyer, and retired government workers of various sorts. Their ailments did not vary significantly from those described in the preceding section, and included respiratory infections, hypertension, weakness, shoulder and back pain and other chronic conditions for which Western medicine recognizes no single, specific cure. Many patients had sought help elsewhere for their conditions, some from more than 10 Western and traditional Chinese practitioners. This history was seen in patients of all three doctors and in lower- as well as middle-class patients. A mainland Chinese practitioner's three patients, interviewed once only, had previously seen an average of five doctors or clinics for the same condition for which they were receiving treatment at the time they were interviewed. These conditions included unsteady gait, rheumatism and general malaise for from 2 to 4 years. Thirteen patients consulting the Taiwanese traditional Chinese practitioner had collectively visited other traditional Chinese doctors and seven Western practitioners for the conditions for which they were now being seen.

Although many patients could not state the conditions under which they would prefer one type of doctor to another, many felt that both were competent, and their histories showed that they usually had tried both types of doctors in the past for a variety of conditions, including those for which they were presently receiving treatment.

In an effort to determine how patients thought they would behave in certain situations, they were questioned as to whether they would seek primary care with traditional Chinese or Western practitioners if they had the following conditions: (1) A simple fracture of one of the long bones in the arm, (2) cardiac arrhythmia, (3) thyroid disorder, (4) anemia and, (5) bursitis of the shoulder. Although preferences could not be elicited from all patients for all conditions, because some people had never heard of them, traditional Chinese practitioners were said to be preferred by the majority of those answering the question for fractures, anemia and by 9 to 12 persons answering about bursitis. Western physicians were overwhelmingly preferred for cardiac arrhythmias and by a majority for bursitis of the shoulder (Table 3). Preference for Western

TABLE 3. PREFERENCES FOR PRIMARY CARE OF 5 HYPOTHETICAL MEDICAL CONDITIONS ASKED OF PATIENTS

Preferred type of practitioner for initial treatment	Hypothetical Conditions				
	Fracture	Arrhythmia	Thyroid disorder	Anemia	Bursitis of shoulder
Traditional Chinese	10	2	5	8	9
Western	8	8	7	7	3

physicians for all five hypothetical conditions was expressed by a 59-year-old woman diabetic visiting a Chinese medical physician's office for the first time in her life because of diabetic neuropathy. A 44-year-old woman with psoriasis of 10 years' duration, who had initially sought care from a Western physician for her problem, was for traditional Chinese practitioners in all of her responses. Both women had chronic illnesses which were difficult to treat and were turning to the traditional Chinese physician almost because there was nothing else left to try. All patients were aware of the potent side effects of Western medicines, and often appeared to be turning to the traditional system to avoid these reactions, while still hoping for improvement, even if it took longer.

Patients With Whom Two Interviews Were Held

Twenty-five patients seen by the same three doctors were interviewed in depth a second time. A profile of these patients is seen in Table 4. All replied that they believed in both systems, but usually to a greater or lesser degree; answering that Western medicine was good for surgery, or for a "temporary cure," but not for permanent or long-term cures; for that one had to go to a traditional Chinese doctor. The term "scientific" is used frequently among patients. They go to Western doctors because they are "scientific," although their cures don't last so long. It is for this reason that patients said they often went to Western doctors first for a "fast" cure, and then went to the traditional doctor for the "permanent" cure. It is interesting that a Western doctor stated that all curable illnesses referred themselves to Western doctors. A traditional practitioner also said that most patients go first to Western, then to traditional doctors. Every patient was asked about the influence of their ancestors and ghosts on their health. All but two of 25 interviewed stated that ancestor worship either meant little to them or was to show respect only, but had no influence on health, nor did ghosts. Of the two responding affirmatively, one was a maid who was bringing the child of her house to a pediatrician because of longstanding congenital heart disease, who stated very strongly that both ancestor worship and ghosts could influence health. The child's mother later confirmed this belief. The other person expressing a strong belief in the influence of ghosts on health was the 41-year-old Taiwanese adopted daughter of an opera singer. She was the mother of nine children, and was married to a mainlander who made shoes for the Chinese opera troupe. However, she did not feel that their inability to properly care for her husband's deceased family members had had any adverse effect on her hypertension and facial nerve paralysis, for which she was receiving treatment.

TABLE 4. PROFILE OF 25 PATIENTS INTERVIEWED FOLLOWING TREATMENT BY TRADITIONAL CHINESE PRACTITIONER

1. *Chief complaint:*
   Rheumatic or chronic joint problem ⸻ 8
   Cardiovascular problems (CVA, hypertension,
      poor circulation) ⸻ 7
   Acute febrile illness ⸻ 2
   Other chronic illness (1 each) (Esophageal
      cancer, ptosis, chronic renal disease,
      menorrhagia, headache, tendonitis, gall-
      stones, congenital heart disease) ⸻ 8

2. *Patients with previous therapy from Western doctor* ⸻ 21

3. *Method of referral:*
   (a) Friend or relative ⸻ 17
   (b) Newspaper advertisement ⸻ 3
   (c) Previously known on Chinese mainland ⸻ 3
   (d) Referred by another practitioner ⸻ 1
   (e) Unclear ⸻ 1

4. *Evaluation of current therapy:*
   (a) Improved as a direct result of therapy ⸻ 15
   (b) Improved, unrelated to therapy ⸻ 0
   (c) Unchanged ⸻ 7
   (d) Worse ⸻ 1
   (e) No evaluation ⸻ 2

Interviews Summarized

When asked about Taiwan's greatest health needs, patients responded with a variety of answers, including pollution control, the need to integrate Western and traditional medicine, and environmental sanitation improvement. The most frequent response was "better doctors" as distinguished from "more doctors." Many people said they felt "more comfortable" with traditional Chinese doctors, but that they wished that a single system would emerge from the best elements of traditional and Western medicine. This wish was expressed by both types of physicians as well, although none seemed optimistic about ever seeing such a single system coming to pass.

In summary, interviews with 33 Western and traditional Chinese doctors and 55 patients were conducted in Taipei over a 3-month period in 1972. An attempt was made to standardize the questions in a fashion which would allow some quantitative analysis. The traditional practitioners were largely more than 50 years of age, came from the Chinese mainland, and often held a degree in a non-medical field. The Western doctors were younger, came largely from Taiwan, and tended to see more patients per day. According to their interview responses, both groups saw acute self-limited illness most frequently. During direct observation of 10 clinic days with three traditional practitioners, chronic illnesses associated with joint pain or vascular insufficiency were the most frequent illnesses treated. Fifty-five patients of traditional practitioners were interviewed, 25 on two occasions. The patients interviewed were largely from the middle class. Although expressing about equal preference for traditional Chinese and Western practitioners for primary care in five arbitrarily chosen conditions, almost all had initially sought care from Western physicians for their present illnesses, which were mainly chronic. Of the 25 patients interviewed twice, 15 felt better as a direct result of therapy. Only two persons from this group who were interviewed expressed concern with the influence of ghosts on their illnesses, although 4 of 11 recently treated persons interviewed in a small market town near Taipei did express such concern. Most patients expressed a need for the upgrading of the quality of medical practice, and hoped that traditional and Western medical systems could be joined in a single system in the near future.

NOTES

1. Many of the ideas for the study design came out of discussions with E. Russell Alexander and Arthur Kleinman. I also acknowledge the suggestions of Emily Ahern, whose comments were particularly helpful at the time the interviews were being conducted.

2. Baker and Perlman obtained their figures by a census of all physicians on Taiwan. They (1967) stated that official counts of licensed practitioners of both Western and traditional Chinese medicine available in the Provincial Health Department were not accurate, because no provision was made to remove the names of physicians who had died or emigrated.

3. This historical account is given by Baker and Perlman (1967), who cite no other sources.

4. In 1962, 5450 Western-trained physicians included 825 "Grade B" doctors with up to only 2 years of training. He estimated that an additional 3600 unlicensed Western and herbalist practitioners were giving medical care, largely in rural areas of Taiwan.

5. In discussing the duration of patient contact with physicians (Western-trained) and herbalists (traditional Chinese practitioners) Lee states that: "Most physicians spend 5 minutes or less, while herbalists spend more than 15 minutes" (Lee 1972:16).

6. Elsewhere in this volume (Chap. 15), Lee states that traditional Chinese medicines have become more expensive than Western medicines.

REFERENCES

BAKER, T. D. and M. PERLMAN
  1967   Health Manpower in a Developing Economy: Taiwan, a Case
         Study in Planning. Baltimore: The Johns Hopkins Press.

CROIZIER, R. C.
  1968   Traditional Medicine in Modern China: Science, Nationalism,
         and the Tensions of Cultural Change. Cambridge: Harvard
         University Press.

LEE, R. P. L.
  1972   Study of Health Systems in Kwun Tong. Hongkong, Social
         Research Centre, The Chinese University of Hongkong. Pre-
         liminary Research Report No. III: Organizations and attitudes
         of the Western-trained and the traditional Chinese personnel
         in an industrial community of Hongkong.

TAIWAN PROVINCIAL GOVERNMENT,
  DEPARTMENT OF HEALTH
  1970   Health Statistical Abstract, Taiwan Province. Taipei: Depart-
         ment of Health.

WEGMAN, M. E., T. Y. LIN, and E. F. PURCELL, eds.
  1973   Public Health in the People's Republic of China. New York:
         The Josiah Macy Jr. Foundation.

WORTH, R.M.
  1975   The impact of new health programs on disease control and
         illness patterns in China. In Medicine in Chinese Cultures:
         Comparative Studies of Health Care in Chinese and Other
         Societies, A. Kleinman, P. Kunstadter, E. R. Alexander, and
         J. L. Gale, eds.: Bethesda, Md.: Fogarty International Center,
         N.I.H. DHEW Publications No. (N.I.H.) 75-653

CHAPTER 15

INTERACTION BETWEEN CHINESE AND WESTERN MEDICINE IN HONGKONG: MODERNIZATION AND PROFESSIONAL INEQUALITY [1]

RANCE P. L. LEE

Classical medicine in China, based upon the cosmological concept of *yin-yang* and the Five Elements, has been developed and accumulated for more than 3000 years. It has been well-documented by scholars and supported by governing regimes throughout Chinese history. *Nei Ching* (The Classic of Internal Medicine), *Mo-Ching* (The Pulse Classic), *Shang-han Lun* (Treatise of Fevers, and *Pen-ts'ao Kang-mu* (General Compendium of Materia Medica) represent some of the major literature in classical Chinese medicine. Although there existed a great many folk remedies and religious-medical practices in the various localities of China, it was classical medicine that dominated the entire sector of medical and health care services, and became the "Great Tradition" of medicine in the history of China. As Croizier (1968: 14–19) has observed, the great tradition is established on the basis of naturalistic and relationalistic principles, but it is neither scientific, magical, nor superstitious.

The introduction of Western scientific medicine into China in the late nineteenth century, however, began to put the great tradition under critical challenge. Although there were serious debates among intellectuals and the public concerning the relative merits of Chinese and Western medicine and the possible integration of both approaches, the remarkable success of Western military force and the outstanding achievement of the scientific technology developed in Western countries gradually made the Chinese people abandon their heritage in favor of Western medical science (Croizier 1968: 14–19). During the first half of the twentieth century, the realm of medical and health services in China was dominated by Western, rather than Chinese, medicine. Chinese medical practice was criticized as being unscientific and, therefore, "backward, superstitious, and unreliable."

Since the communist takeover of the mainland, a revivalist movement has emerged. Responding to Chairman Mao's call for "maintaining independence and keeping the initiative in our own hands and relying on our own efforts" and his assertion that "Chinese medicine and pharmacology are a great treasure-house; efforts should be made to explore them and raise them to a higher level," medical and health workers in China have been struggling hard, since 1958, to restore and revive their own medical tradition (Hou 1970). They constantly seek to re-examine its techniques and theoretical rationale, to upgrade its quality, to widen its utilization by citizens, and to integrate it with modern Western medicine. Their devoted and persistent hard work over the last 20 years has made notable contributions not only to the advancement of medical knowledge and skills, but also to an increase in the quantity of medical care. A larger volume and a greater variety of both preventive and curative health services are now available to the PRC's 800 million inhabitants.

In view of the medical revivalism and the subsequent achievements in contemporary China, we should ask: In what way is traditional Chinese medicine related to modern Western medicine in other Chinese societies, especially those which are not under the control of the communist regime? To provide an answer to this broad question, this writer has chosen the Chinese society of Hongkong as the area of study. However, before commenting on the pattern of interaction between Chinese and Western medicine—a few remarks about Hongkong's general socio-economic context.

Hongkong is situated in the southern coast of mainland China. It has been a colony under the British Crown since the late nineteenth century, and at present has a total area of about 1045 square kilometers. Ever since the mainland was taken over by the communist regime in 1949, Hongkong has been undergoing rapid demographic, social, and economic transformations (Hongkong Social and Economic Trends 1968–1972; Hongkong Statistics, 1947–67.)[4]

Because of the great influx of refugees from China, the population grew from an estimated 600,000 in 1945 to 3.95 million in 1971, an increase of nearly sevenfold over one quarter of a century. The very great majority of local residents are Chinese, and according to the census of March 1971, about 98.3 percent of the total population can be classified as Chinese by place of origin.

The population is not equally distributed in the various areas of Hongkong. The 1971 census indicates that approximately 90 percent of the total residents are concentrated in the urban area of about 184 square kilometers, with the remaining 10 percent living in the rural area of about 861 square kilometers. The urban population density is about 18,831 persons per square kilometer, as compared to 462 persons per square kilometer in the rural area. Apparently, Hongkong is a highly urbanized Chinese society.

Concomitant with population growth and urbanization is industrial and economic expansion. The proportion of the working population engaged in manufacturing increased from less than 10 percent in 1948 to about 50 percent in 1972. In the last 5 years, the electricity consumption rose from 3,449 to 5,412 million kilowatt-hours, and the gas consumption from 7,252 to 10,759 thousand Therms. The per capita expenditure on Gross Domestic Product at market prices increased from HK$3000 in 1966 to HK$4517 in 1970.

Hongkong obviously has become an industrialized metropolitan city that is still ruled by the British minority but densely populated by the Chinese majority. Like many other industrial-urban societies, Hongkong inevitably has been moving toward modernity. Various aspects of the society have been mobilized and transformed 'from traditional patterns into those types of technological and social-organizational systems characteristic of advanced Western nations. A striking example of the modernization process can be found in the realm of medical and health services. Over the last several decades, there have been downward trends in the incidence of various kinds of infectious diseases including typhoid, bacillary dysentery, tuberculosis, chickenpox, diphtheria, and whooping cough. Infectious diseases have been replaced as major causes of death by chronic illnesses such as malignant neoplasms and heart diseases. Infant and maternal mortality rates have also been substantially reduced (Annual Departmental Report 1971–72; Bowman et al 1970). These changes in disease-patterns might be partly due to rising educational and income levels. However, the contribution of advancement in medical technology cannot be overstated. A striking phenomenon in the modernizing society of Hongkong is the increasing utilization and expansion of the medical science and technology developed in advanced Western countries. Some questions then arise: How does the Western medical system operate in a modern Chinese society which is politically dominated by Western power? In what ways does it come to displace the traditional medical practices which have been held by the indigenous population for several thousand years? How does the traditional Chinese medical system persist and react to the growth of Western medicine in Hongkong? To delimit the scope of discussion in this paper, the writer focuses on (1) the personal medical care system, rather than public or environmental health services, and (2) Western scientific and classical Chinese medicine, rather than home remedies and religious-medical practices.[5]

Western Medical Dominance

There exists a wide spectrum of Chinese and Western, public and private health services in Hongkong. In the Western medical sector, for instance, there are general and psychiatric hospitals, outpatient clinics for general and specialty services, maternity and child health care services, nursing homes, immunization services, medical laboratories, and rehabilitation centers. Traditional Chinese medical practitioners can be grouped into three major types: (1) herbalists, specializing in the use of herbs for internal medical care, (2) acupuncturists, treating illness by inserting needles into certain points of the body, and (3) bone-setters, specializing in the treatment of sprains and contusions.[6]

Over the last two decades, the role of government in the provision and subvention of health care services has been increasingly important. It has been estimated that government expenditure on health services increased from 15 million Hongkong dollars (about 6.2 percent of the total expenditure for the colony) in 1951 to 304 million dollars (about 10.5 percent of the total expenditure) in 1972 (Annual Departmental Report 1971–72:70). Nevertheless, the center of gravity of medical care in Hongkong remains in private practice. Unlike in Great Britain, there is no national health scheme in Hongkong, though the government has been financing a comprehensive School Medical Service for a small fraction of the student population.[7] The government employs about one-fourth of all Western-trained doctors,[8] and none of the Chinese medical practitioners. In other words, all the Chinese medical practitioners and three-fourths of the Western-trained doctors are in private practice. Furthermore, there are slightly more than 10,000 general hospital beds in Hongkong, of which over 60 percent are provided by non-governmental hospitals (Report of Medical Development 1973). The health sector in Hongkong thus can be characterized as pluralistic and entrepreneurial. The emphasis of the entire sector is on an "individual, fee-for-service" mode of compensation and "free choice" of medical practitioners. Both Western-trained and Chinese medical practitioners have a great deal of control over their economic terms of service.

In the pluralistic health context of Hongkong, there coexist two major systems of professional services with different technical orientations and social-organizational patterns; they are the classical Chinese and the modern Western medicine. Instead of coexisting in a coordinated fashion, the two systems are competitive on an unequal basis. Western-scientific doctors constitute the dominant profession of medicine in Hongkong, while Chinese medical practitioners work in a subordinate and disadvantaged manner.

It is explained that the Medical Council of Hongkong, established by the government, plays the most crucial role in the legitimization and supervision of medical practice. The council, chaired by the Director of Government's Department of Medical and Health Services, consists of representatives from the armed forces, government health services, university medical school, and the two major medical professional associations in Hongkong (Fang 1970). All the council members, however, have to be qualified Western-trained doctors.

The council has been granted by the government a mandate to register medical practitioners and to regulate their practices through the setting of minimum and uniform standards. Only those Western-trained doctors holding a diploma granted by the Hongkong University or any other diploma which is recognized by the General Medical Council of the United Kingdom are registrable with the council, and are then recognized by law as qualified medical doctors. Chinese medical practitioners are thereby excluded from the council, and their services are not recognized by the legal authority as duly qualified. They are denied certain privileges granted to the registered Western-trained doctors. For instance, Chinese practitioners are not permitted to issue death cerificates or to undertake surgical operations.

With expert authority granted by the government in the realm of health, the profession of Western medicine has the greatest influence on the social organization of medical care in the colony as a whole. In the formulation of major policies dealing with health, the government normally consults with representatives from two major medical professional associations: The Hongkong Medical Association and the Hongkong Branch of the British Medical Association; both associations are oriented to Western medicine. The government rarely seeks advice from Chinese practitioners and, furthermore, there is no Chinese practitioner working in the government's Department of Medical and Health Services. All doctors in public service are trained in Western medicine. It is thus not surprising to see that though the government has provided and subvented an increasing volume of different kinds of medical and health programs, none of them is involved with Chinese medicine. With regard to the future development of health care services, the Governor, in early 1973, appointed a Medical Development Advisory Committee to make recommendations appropriate for the next 10 years. Some of the Committee members are Western-trained doctors, but none is a Chinese medical practitioner. The plans recommended by the Committee are primarily concerned with the provision of hospital beds and increasing the number of doctors and nurses in Western medicine (Report of Medical Development 1973). There is no discussion about the development of Chinese medicine. Apparently the social organization of medical care in Hongkong has been under the influence of the Western medical profession, rather than the Chinese medical practitioners.

The profession of Western medicine controls not only the social-organizational terms of service, but also the technical content of its work. As suggested by the previous discussion concerning the structure and functioning of the Medical Council of Hongkong, the profession has acquired an officially approved monopoly of the right to determine how and by whom the work of healing should be done and evaluated. Members of the profession are free to practice with very few formal constraints which are not made by their own professional colleagues. Relative to the profession of Western medicine, Chinese medical practitioners have a lower degree of technical autonomy, and their practices are constrained by the legal authority in many ways. For example, Chinese medical practitioners are not permitted to practice surgery, to undertake the treatment of eye-diseases, to possess antibiotics and dangerous drugs, or to make use of certain Western medical equipment such as X-ray machines and inoculation instruments.

The profession of Western medicine is obviously superior to that of Chinese medicine regarding their relative control over the social and technical terms of work in Hongkong.[9] This pattern of "professional inequality," which results mainly from government's differential support of the two professions, has been reinforced by the system of medical education. Hongkong has only one University medical school, producing about 100 graduates each year. These graduates are entitled to be registered with the Medical Council of Hongkong. However, the training program concentrates entirely on Western medical science, giving no attention to Chinese medicine. If one wishes to learn Chinese medicine, he may do it either by becoming a disciple of a Chinese medical practitioner or by enrolling in one of the organized training programs in Chinese medicine. None of these educational channels in Chinese medicine is financially supported or recognized by the government and the Medical Council. Up to the present, there has been no way in which a person may obtain a university diploma in Chinese medicine. With its academic authority the university has passed on the technical competence of Western medical science but not that of traditional Chinese medicine.

The above discussion suggests that the profession of Chinese medicine is subordinate to its Western counterpart. Western medical dominance, however, has by no means wiped out the widespread existence of traditional services in Hongkong. It was estimated that the colony had a total of 2,317 Western-trained doctors in 1969 (Hongkong's Medical and Health Services 1970). The ratio of Western-trained doctors to the total population is about 1 : 1720. But according to a survey by the Hongkong Medical Association in cooperation with the government's Census and Statistics Department in 1969, there were then 4,506 Chinese practitioners of various kinds. The Chinese medical practitioners to population ratio is about 1 : 1161. Thus there are considerably more Chinese- than Western-trained medical practitioners in Hongkong. Why is it so? It may be due to the differing patterns of control over licensing procedures.

The profession of Western medicine has been granted by government the power to define the minimum standards for the training and licensing of its own practitioners. This professional control results in there not being a very large number of registered doctors in Western medicine. In fact, the colony has for many years had a shortage of Western-trained doctors. The ratio of registered Western-trained doctors to the population was estimated in 1972 as 1:1747, which is considerably lower than the ratios in Great Britain and the United States. And, according to a 1973 estimate of the Medical Development Advisory Committee, a shortage of about 100 Western-trained doctors would ensue for about 10 years.

The government's attitude toward Chinese medicine, however, can be described as "conditional tolerance." Because of its colonial policy of minimal interference with local customs, the government has been tolerant, though not supportive, of the existence of Chinese medical practice, and the Medical Ordinance in Hongkong primarily regulates Western medical practice. The government has set no standard examinations or licensing procedures for qualifying practitioners in Chinese medicine. In fact, anyone can practice Chinese medicine without interference from legal authority. What is required is a payment of 25 Hongkong dollars for commercial registration. As a result, it is easy to have a situation where there exists a very large number of Chinese medical men. It should, however, be noted that the government's tolerance of Chinese medical practice is not unconditional. As earlier mentioned, a person practicing

Chinese medicine is subject to certain technical constraints imposed by the government, and he is prohibited by law from using any name or title which may induce belief that he is qualified to practice according to modern scientific methods. These legal constraints serve to prevent traditional practitioners from misusing Western techniques, but also serve to protect the economic interest and medical dominance · the Western medical practitioners.

Since both Western and Chinese services coexist widely in the pluralistic health context of Hongkong, one might be concerned with the implications of Western medical dominance for (1) the ecological distribution and organizational structure, (2) the professional evaluation of medical quality, and (3) the public's evaluation and utilization of both types of medical care services. To shed light on these issues, the writer will utilize some empirical data gathered in 1971-72 on medical organizations and health behavior in the district of Kwun Tong, Hongkong.

The district of Kwun Tong is located on the east coast of the Kowloon peninsula of Hongkong, covering about 32 acres. Over the last two decades, it has developed into one of the largest industrial and residential satellite towns in Hongkong. Currently there are about 2000 industrial undertakings and some half million Chinese residents in the community. Most live in various kinds of public housing. About 14 percent reside in private apartments and tenement buildings. Residents are therefore largely in the middle and lower income groups. (For a more comprehensive description of Kwun Tong see Wong 1970.) Kwun Tong is by no means a self-contained community. As a colleague of this author has empirically demonstrated, the social, economic and political life in the community is to a large extent connected with, and thus in many ways similar to, Hongkong society as a whole (King 1973).

The author undertook three health surveys in Kwun Tong in 1971-72. The first was a complete enumeration of the health care units in various subdistricts of Kwun Tong. The second survey focused on the organizational structures of all Western general outpatient clinics as well as Chinese herbalist services.[10] Health-related attitudes of their medical practitioners were also assessed. The third survey was a random sample of 702 household heads for the purpose of understanding their health concepts and their utilization of health services. The data collected in these three surveys is used in the following discussion (Lee 1972a, b and c; Lee 1973). Since Kwun Tong is an integral part of, rather than separated from, the larger society, it is believed that the survey findings are generally applicable to the colony as a whole.

Ecological Distribution and Organizational Structure

There were 174 Chinese and 101 Western health care units in the entire district of Kwun Tong in 1971-72. Both types of service were found to be unevenly distributed in the 11 administrative subdistricts of Kwun Tong. Western services were more unevenly distributed than

Chinese services. The standard deviation of the distribution of Western units among the 11 areas was 17.3, while that of Chinese units was 14.1. Nevertheless, the distributions of both types of service were strongly associated. The correlation coefficient was .55, indicating that the larger the number of Chinese services in a paritcular area, the larger would be the number of Western services; or vice versa. There exists a significant pattern of ecological convergence between Chinese and Western health services. Why is it so?

The distribution of health services may be dependent upon either "effective demand" or "medical need." The demand for medical care is largely conditioned by economic factors and popular beliefs about health and illness. The real need for medical care is, however, a medical concept; it is mainly defined in terms of the physical and psychic conditions of the individual. It can be hypothesized that in a pluralistic and entrepreneurial health context, the distribution of health services is more likely to be dependent upon the demand, than the need, for medical care. The primary concern of a medical practitioner in the provision of medical service is whether the people want it and how much they are willing to pay for it. Is this the case in Kwun Tong?

The data suggest that the distribution of both Chinese and Western services is greatly dependent upon the population size and the socioeconomic status (as measured by the quality of residential housing) of particular subdistricts. The relationships of Chinese services to population size and socioeconomic status were .90 and .54, respectively; while the relationships of Western services to population size and socioeconomic status were .65 and .68, respectively. Hence, the larger the population size and the higher the socioeconomic status of a subdistrict, the more the Western (as well as the Chinese) medical services in that subdistrict.

If it is assumed that a larger population size would increase the demand as well as need for medical care and that a higher socioeconomic status would lead to a greater demand but less need for medical services, then two major conclusions can be suggested. First, in the pluralistic context of Hongkong, the distribution of both Chinese and Western medical care is more likely to be determined by the medical demand than the need of the people. This is obvious as the relationships of Chinese and Western services to both population size and socioeconomic status are consistently positive. If health services are dependent upon medical need, then they should be negatively associated with socioeconomic status.

Second, relatively speaking, Chinese services seemed to be more responsive to medical need than were Western services, while Western services were more sensitive to medical demand than were Chinese services. As shown by the above correlation coefficients, the availability of Chinese units has a relatively stronger association with population size, but a weaker association with socioeconomic status, than that of Western units.

The responsiveness of Chinese services to the medical need may not be based on the "good will" of the practitioners. Instead, they may be forced to be responsive. The number of Chinese practitioners was found to be much larger than that of Western doctors but, as is reported later in this paper, Western services were more likely to be utilized by the public than are Chinese services. To avoid or reduce competition with other medical professionals, Chinese practitioners have to move into poor areas, and cannot afford to be as choosey as Western-trained doctors.

As reported, there appears to be a general tendency for both Chinese and Western units to converge in the same areas. Their organizational structures and operations, however, are different in many ways. Some of their major differences are described below, based on data collected for Western outpatient clinics and Chinese herbalists' offices.

First, Western units are in general larger in size than Chinese units. The average number of medical personnel among Western units is 4.8 persons, but that of Chinese units is only 1.8. About one-fifth of the Western units employ two or more doctors, while 98 percent of the Chinese units have a single practitioner. Hence, a Western outpatient clinic typically consists of one doctor or sometimes two, together with two to four nurses and technicians. In a herbalist's office, however, normally a medical practitioner is found working there alone.

Second, as compared to the Western units, Chinese units generally provide a greater number of service hours and spend more time for each consultation, but have a smaller number of patient contacts. On the average, the total number of service hours provided by Western units is about 31 hours per week, while that by Chinese units is about 37. The average duration of each outpatient consultation among Western-trained doctors is about 8 minutes, while that among Chinese practitioners is 12. The average number of patient contacts among Western units is about 244 contacts per week, while that among Chinese units is about 100.

Third, Western-trained doctors are more likely than Chinese practitioners to work for more than one health unit. About one-half of the Western doctors work for two or more units, while over 90 percent of the Chinese practitioners work for a single unit.

Fourth, Western-trained doctors are both technically and socially more cohesive to each other than are Chinese practitioners. Both Chinese and Western practitioners are more likely to maintain close friendship ties with those practicing in the same medical tradition. However, the friendship cohesion among Western doctors is relatively stronger than that among Chinese practitioners. About 76 percent of the Western doctors reported that they maintain informal social contacts with friends of their own profession, while about 67 percent of the Chinese practitioners so reported.

Western doctors are not only socially but also technically more cohesive among themselves than are Chinese practitioners. More than three-fourths of the Western doctors referred patients to their own professional colleagues, while fewer than one-fourth of the Chinese practitioners did so. Unlike among the Western doctors, the network of patient-referrals among Chinese practitioners is rather weak. The question arises: Do Chinese and Western-trained medical practitioners refer patients to each other? Over one-half of the Chinese practitioners have referred patients to Western-trained doctors, especially those working in hospitals. The referral of patients from Western doctors to Chinese practitioners is a rarity: only 2 percent of the Western-trained doctors had so referred patients. Apparently there exists an asymmetric process of patient-referral between Western-trained and Chinese practitioners. Such referrals are likely to go from Chinese to Western-trained practitioners, but not the other way around. The above data also suggest that Chinese practitioners are even more likely to refer patients to Western-trained doctors than to colleagues of their own profession.

The above analysis of social and technical cohesion shows little interaction between the two professions, and that even if interaction occurs, it is likely to be asymmetrical. Does this mean that the two professions distrust each other with regard to the quality of medical performance?

Professional Evaluation of Medical Quality

The writer found that most Western-trained doctors (84 percent) believed their own colleagues medically more competent than those in Chinese medicine, while most Chinese practitioners (73 percent) felt that there was no significant difference in competence between the two groups. Hence, Western-trained doctors are more distrustful of their counterparts than are Chinese practitioners. The distrust in Chinese practitioners by Western-trained doctors could be a barrier to interaction between the two professional groups.

Since there are three major types of Chinese practitioners (i.e., herbalists, acupuncturists, and bone-setters) in Hongkong, which type do Western-trained doctors trust the most? The data show that about 16 percent of Western-trained doctors trust herbalists, 23 percent trust bone-setters, and 30 percent trust acupuncturists. Thus, Western-trained doctors tend to trust acupuncturists the most, relatively speaking, and are most skeptical of herbalists.

The focus of the above analysis is on the quality of the Chinese *practitioner* in Hongkong. However, a distinction should be made between the competency of practitioners and the efficacy of medical *knowledge* itself. Since there is no uniform control over Chinese medical practice in Hongkong, it could be that Western-trained doctors have some trust in the traditional approach to medical care but not in the training and qualifications of the existing Chinese practitioners. There is some evidence to support this hypothesis. Most Western-trained doctors (67 percent) agreed that hospitals in Hongkong should set up a Chinese medical division. A number of them (56 percent) suggested that a government-recognized Chinese Medical College should be established for the training of qualified practitioners. Moreover, most Western-trained doctors (61 percent) believed that the convergence of Chinese and Western medical traditions could be realized.

The author has presented some findings about the evaluation of medical quality by practitioners themselves. In short, Chinese practitioners are quite receptive to Western medical practice, while Western-trained doctors are skeptical of the technical competence of Chinese practitioners in Hongkong but tend to have trust in the efficacy of Chinese medical knowledge itself. We now shift attention to evaluation by the lay population.

Lay Evaluation and Utilization

According to the author's sample survey of 702 adults in Kwun Tong, most people (67 percent) perceive Western-trained doctors to be *in general* technically more competent than Chinese practitioners. However, they seem to have differential evaluations of different aspects of medical practice.

Most people (84 percent) believe that Western medicine is more effective than Chinese medicine in the prevention of infectious diseases. With regard to tonic care, i.e., the promotion and maintenance of good health, more people believe in Chinese herbs (18 percent) than in Western drugs (11 percent).

For the treatment of illnesses, a greater number of people are more confident in Western medicine (65 percent) than in Chinese medicine (10 percent). To be more specific, most people (about 60 to 80 percent) suggest that in the treatment of most diseases (1) Western medical care works faster than Chinese medicine, but (2) Chinese herbs are less likely to produce side-effects, and (3) Western medicine is good for the treatment of symptoms while Chinese medicine is more effective in the curing of disease.

The evaluation of the effectiveness of medical treatment may be dependent upon the specific types of disease in question. Respondents were given a list of illnesses and asked to make comparison between the two medical approaches. The responses are percentaged below:

	Western Better	Chinese Better	About the Same
(1) Tuberculosis	91.2%	1.4%	7.4%
(2) Fever	90.5	5.7	3.8
(3) Heart diseases	84.9	0.9	14.2
(4) Stomach-ache	84.3	3.4	12.3
(5) Mental illness	84.0	0.4	15.5
(6) Skin diseases	83.6	6.6	10.4
(7) Throbbing and diarrhea	78.3	13.4	8.3
(8) Whooping cough	76.9	14.0	9.1
(9) Dysmenorrhea	65.0	17.5	17.4
(10) Anemia	55.0	29.1	16.0
(11) Measles	47.9	47.0	9.1
(12) Rheumatism	24.2	54.1	21.7
(13) Sprains and fractures	8.2	86.5	5.3

The data suggest that most people prefer Western to Chinese services for the treatment of most diseases, particularly tuberculosis and fever. Opinions are evenly split in respect to measles. Chinese medicine is considered to be more effective than the Western approach in treating rheumatism, sprains and fractures.

All the above findings suggest that in general the lay population is more trustful of Western than Chinese medical care. Nevertheless, Chinese medicine is still trusted in some specific ways, such as for tonic care, producing fewer side-effects, curing diseases rather than symptoms, and in the treatment of certain illnesses such as measles, rheumatism, sprains and fractures. In light of these findings, it could be expected that Western services are more widely utilized by the people than Chinese services. This is in fact the case.

Among the various types of Western services, private physicians are most often visited by the people (70 percent). Among the three major kinds of Chinese services, herbalists are most often consulted by the people (36 percent), while acupuncturists are visited by a very small fraction of the population (2 percent).

Concerning the relative utilization of Chinese versus Western services, it is noted that (1) among those respondents who consulted doctors during the previous 3 years, 83 percent reported that they visited Western-trained doctors more often, while 11 percent consulted Chinese practitioners more often; (2) among those whose parents used medical services during the previous 3 years, 68 percent reported that their parents visited Western-trained doctors more often, while 20 percent preferred Chinese practitioners; (3) among those whose children used medical services in the previous 3 years, 92 percent reported that their children consulted Western-trained doctors more often, while 5 percent preferred Chinese services. These findings suggest that Western services are more widely utilized by the people than Chinese services. Moreover, it seems that the younger the generation, the more extensive is the use of Western medical care in comparison to Chinese services.

Although Western services are more widely utilized, there are combined uses of Chinese and Western medical care by the local population. A number of people (42 percent) made attempts to shift between the two types of medical care for the treatment of the same illness.

In investigating the process of seeking medical help, it is noted that most people begin with self-medication. If it fails, then they consult Western-trained doctors. When the second step does not seem to be successful, they shift to seeking help from Chinese practitioners. This process of seeking medical help reconfirms the fact that most people prefer to make use of Western services, but it does not mean that they do not contact Chinese practitioners. For many individuals, the use of Chinese services is a "second alternative" or even the "last resort."

Since most people (58 percent) self-medicate in the initial stage of illness, what kinds of medicines do they use? Many people keep Chinese medical herbs, pills and ointments at home for possible self-medication.

The use of Chinese medications is thus quite pervasive, though the professional services of Chinese practitioners are not so widely utilized.

Medical Revivalism and Integration

The above discussion indicates that there is a pattern of professional inequality in the dual system of medical and health care services in Hongkong. Compared to Chinese medical practitioners, the profession of Western medicine enjoys greater support from the political and educational authorities. As a result, the Western-medical profession is both socially and technically more autonomous than its counterpart in Chinese medicine. Although both Chinese and Western services generally tend to concentrate in areas with greater demand for medical care, a relatively greater proportion of Chinese than Western-trained practitioners have to practice in poverty areas. Relative to the Chinese services, the professional services of Western-trained doctors are structurally more complex, and are more favorably evaluated and extensively utilized by the lay population. Western-trained doctors are also both socially and technically more cohesive with each other than Chinese practitioners. Relationships between the two professions are asymmetric: Western-trained doctors are more medically skeptical of, and are less likely to make patient-referrals to, Chinese practitioners than the other way around.

The question arises: Why is the profession of Western medicine given greater support by the government, and the lay public, as well as by the medical practitioners themselves? The "good results" of Western-scientific medical care may be an important source of its dominance. However, it is the writer's impression that this may also result from ideological forces.

Moving toward modernity is a great temptation to many people in developing societies. To these people, however, modernization in effect means adoption of the Western way of life and the use of scientific technology. As a result, anything which is developed in advanced Western nations and is connected with science will be accepted with little resistance. This ideological complex of "learning from the West and making use of scientific procedures" emerged in China during the late nineteenth century and was rapidly accepted by most people. As Hongkong is a modernizing city largely populated by immigrants from China but governed by a *Western* regime, these ideological forces have increasingly penetrated into the colony's social life. The fact that Hongkong is a British colony is important. First, it has greatly reinforced the West-oriented ideology in the mind of the public. In fact, there exists a clear-cut racial stratification in Hongkong. Westerners are widely perceived as superior to the indigenous Chinese. Second, because of cultural consciousness, the government is more sympathetic to the use of Western ideas and technology than to indigenous practice. It is thus logical that since the knowledge and skills of Western medicine were originally developed in the West through the use of scientific procedures, Western medicine has replaced traditional Chinese medicine as the dominant system of medical beliefs and practices, both in China shortly before the communist revolution and in the contemporary Chinese society of Hongkong. It commands a higher prestige, more income, and greater power in the dual system of professional health services.

Western medical dominance, however, has not entirely displaced the system of Chinese medical care. As reported, possibly because of the lack of legal control over registration, there are a great many Chinese practitioners in Hongkong. More important, in many specific ways the local population remains trustful of and dependent on Chinese medicine. Chinese and Western medicine are also used by many people in combination. Why?

Perhaps because illness is so threatening to one's life, one has to be pragmatic about the use of medical care. In the view of the Chinese resident in Hongkong, Chinese and Western approaches represent alternative responses to illness, and he uses each of them to the extent that they may appear to produce positive effects. Although Western medicine is defined by the government and the university as a better alternative to illness, it is a deep-rooted belief that since the body of knowledge and skills in Chinese medicine has been developed from, and has been tested by, the empirical experience of countless people over several thousand years, it ought to have a reasonable degree of medical validity.

The efficacy of Chinese medicine has been reconfirmed and advanced by medical and health workers in the People's Republic of China in recent years. No less important is that its knowledge and skills have been systematically integrated with Western medical science. The Chinese approach (or its combination with Western techniques) has been found to be more efficient than Western methods alone in the treatment of some diseases. For, it is not only more effective, but is also safer, simpler, and more economical. The effect of acupuncture anesthesia for surgical operations is a well-known example (Acupuncture Anesthesia 1972). Others include notable successes in treating extensive burns covering over 80 percent of the body surface, in rejoining severed limbs even 10 or 18 hours after injury, and in dealing with such chronic diseases as neuralgia, arthritis, neurasthenia, and the sequelae of infantile paralysis (Revolutionary Committee of the Chinese Academy of Medical Science 1970). These medical successes in China have perceivably affected the state of health affairs in its next-door neighbor, Hongkong.

In recent years there has emerged a revivalist movement in the colony's health-care sector. Both medical professionals and the lay public have been increasingly interested in re-examining and reviving the use of Chinese medical skills. Some evidence follows:

As reported, the author's survey results reveal that most Chinese and Western practitioners tend to believe in the convergence of Chinese and Western medical approaches. Moreover, the writer observed an increasing number of medical "elites" publicly advocating the unification of

Western and Chinese medicine and the improvement of the social-organizational and technical content of Chinese medical practice in Hongkong. These elites included not only leaders of some major professional associations in Chinese medicine, but also several renowned Western-trained doctors, such as the medical director of one of the largest welfare programs in the colony, the medical superintendent of a large community hospital, and the President of the Hongkong Medical Association. More striking, a group of Western medical elite has taken the initiative to establish a Chinese Medical Research Center as a beginning step toward integration. The Center plans to cover both acupuncture and herbal medicine, although it is currently focusing on the former and has given training to over 100 Western-trained doctors. Some months ago, the Hongkong Medical Association, which is the largest and most influential Western medical association in Hongkong, offered an 8-week training program on the theoretical rationale and technical application of acupuncture. The program was attended by some 150 members of the Association.

Medical revivalism also appeared on the university campus. As mentioned, students in the University Medical School are given formal training only in Western medicine. The Medical Society of the University Student Union, however, recently sponsored a public exhibition of Chinese medical herbs and techniques. Several articles, published in the official newspaper of the medical society, accused the School for its policy of excluding Chinese medicine from the teaching program. It was reported that some faculty members in Physiology and Anatomy have begun to undertake scientific research on the medical effects of acupuncture.

Also rising is public concern with Chinese medicine. The author has been deeply impressed that in recent years most local newspapers and magazines have devoted much space for the discussion of Chinese medical skills and pharmacy, and for the reporting of medical achievements in the PRC. Increased utilization of Chinese services, however, remains hindered by at least three major obstacles.

The first and most serious problem faced by Chinese medicine in Hongkong today is the lack of minimum and uniform control over education, licensing and practice. Some practitioners may be well-qualified; others may be quacks. The public is much less certain about the possible results of seeking help from a Chinese practitioner than from a Western-trained doctor. In this state of uncertainty, people are hesistant to make use of Chinese services.

The second obstacle is that, because of the rising cost of Chinese medical herbs, it has become more expensive to use Chinese than Western services for the treatment of many diseases. Moreover, the government and many voluntary agencies in Hongkong have provided an increasing number of low-cost medical care services to the public, but none of them is in Chinese medicine. Consequently, the use of Chinese medicine is gradually becoming a privilege of the well-to-do, rather than a service available to the poor.

The third obstacle is the amount of time and effort required for preparing Chinese medical herbs for consumption. Most herbs are in the form of preserved roots and brews, and it takes special effort and time to prepare them. As life is busy in a metropolitan city such as Hongkong, people have to think twice before they utilize Chinese medical care.

However, these obstacles can be overcome. What is most needed is the modernization of both the *technical* and the *social-organizational* aspects of Chinese medicine. To upgrade its technical quality, the use of scientific methods seems important. Medical workers in China have remarkably demonstrated that, with the application of scientific procedures, the efficacy of Chinese medicine or its combination with Western skills can be greatly improved. No less important is that by means of scientific methods of extraction, pharmaceutical workers in China have made a substantial contribution to the transformation of Chinese medical herbs into patent medicines, such as medicated liquors, inoculations, tablets and pills. To name a few examples, these include medicines used in treating schistosomiasis, tumors and fulminating epidemic cerebrospinal meningitis, in dealing with snake venom, and in treating septic shock resulting from toxic dysentery (Chinese patent medicine 1972; Revolutionary Committee of Chinese Academy of Medical Science 1970). A great variety of patent medicines, imported from China, is available in the markets of Hongkong. These patent medicines are not only cheaper, but also easier to use than the preserved roots and brews.

To modernize the organization of work, the most important and immediate task is to introduce into the Chinese medical profession minimum and uniform standards for training and practice. Traditional knowledge and skills should be taught in university classrooms with standard textbooks. Professional coordination in the form of mutual consultation or patient-referrals should be encouraged. With its rich amount of financial and technological resources and with its great variety of patients and disease-patterns, the hospital should include Chinese medical practice in its research and service programs. Government and voluntary agencies should also provide accessible, low-cost, high-quality Chinese services to the public.

With its political and financial resources, the government has been playing a major role in the modernization of medical services in Hongkong. However, its efforts have led to "partial" rather than "total" modernization in medicine. The government concentrates on the development of Western medical science at the expense of Chinese medicine. In spite of rapid modernization of the system of Western medical care, the technical quality and social organization of Chinese services remain in a traditional state.

The strategy of medical modernization in the PRC is "to walk on two legs." Both Chinese and Western medical resources are mobilized by the government, and are increasingly being integrated into a single unity. In the view of the PRC regime, medical modernization means not only increased availability of health services of higher quality, but also organizational as well as technical integration of both Chinese and Western medical approaches. Unlike the PRC, however, the Hongkong Government's strategy of medical modernization is "to walk on a single leg." Although from the impact of medical successes in China there has emerged a revivalist movement in the health context of Hongkong, the government still has no plans for the development of Chinese medical care services. Up to now, Chinese medical services have been neither organizationally nor technically incorporated into the mainstream of health affairs in Hongkong. To what extent and in what ways the medical revivalism will challenge and change the existing pattern of professional inequality in the realm of health remains to be seen.

NOTES

1. This paper makes use of part of the data from the author's survey study of the health system of Kwun Tong (Lee 1972a,b,c) which was carried out under the auspices of the Social Research Center of the Chinese University of Hongkong and was financed by the Harvard-Yenching Institute, the Lotteries Fund of the Hongkong Government, and the Chinese University of Hongkong. For helpful suggestions, I am indebted to S. L. Wong of the Chinese University of Hongkong. For a comprehensive description of the research procedures and statistical findings of this study, see Lee (1972a,b,c; Lee 1973).

2. For an elaborated social-scientific analysis of the role of political ideology in the development of China's health-care system, see Geoffrey Gibson (1971). Gibson argues that the thoughts of Mao serve as a guide to treatment priorities, basis for diagnosis and therapy, explanation of health care failures, rationale for health delivery systems, channel for patient gratitude, justification for health, sensitivity training for health workers, basis for health ethnocentrism, and also as motivational devices for health workers and patients. Robert Chin (1972) has also explicitly pointed out that health behavior in the People's Republic of China is more accurately described as health "conduct," because it is moral and political.

3. It is not the intention of this paper to engage in a comprehensive description of the dynamics in the People's Republic of China's health-care system. Nevertheless, a few concise and relevant articles are suggested: Chien (1964), Rifkin and Kaplinsky (1973), and China: Revolution and Health (1972).

4. For some discussion of these changes see the articles by Podmore (1971) and Brown (1971) cited below.

5. Home remedies remain pervasive among Chinese people in Hongkong (Choa 1967; Chung 1973). Religious-medical practices, however, seem to have declined. According to the author's recent survey of adults in Hongkong, only 2 percent of respondents reported that they had received medical treatment from religious institutions (Lee 1972b).

6. It has been estimated that a great majority of the Chinese practitioners are herbalists (about 70 percent), followed by bone-setters (about 20 percent) and acupuncturists (about 10 percent).

7. It was reported by the School Medical Service Board that a total of 70,758 students took part in the Service during the academic year 1972–1973, constituting less than 10 percent of those eligible. These students were attended by 181 Western-trained doctors in private practice.

8. The total number is approximately 2800, including doctors registered with the Medical Council of Hongkong and unregistrable doctors who are permitted to work in government institutions or charity clinics.

9. For an excellent discussion on these three dimensions of professional autonomy in a pluralistic health system, see Friedson (1972).

10. These two specific types of services were chosen for the study because both together constitute the majority of medical practitioners and provide the health services which are most widely utilized by the public.

REFERENCES

ACUPUNCTURE ANESTHESIA
  1972   Peking: Foreign Languages Press.

ANNUAL DEPARTMENTAL REPORT
  1972   Director of Medical and Health Services. Hongkong: Hong-
         kong Government.

BOWMAN, R. K., F. I. FORBES, and J. D. F. LOCKART
  1970   Trends in notifiable infectious diseases in Hongkong Island
         1961–1965. Far Eastern Medical Journal 6:223–29.

BROWN, E. E. P.
  1971   The Hongkong economy: Achievements and prospects. *In*
         Hongkong: the Industrial Colony, K. Hopkins, ed. London:
         Oxford University Press.

CHIEN, H. C.
  1964   Chinese medicine: Progress and achievements. Peking Review
         February: 16–19.

CHIN, R.
  1973   Changing health conduct of the New Man in China. *In* Public
         Health in the People's Republic of China, M. Wegman and
         T. Y. Lin, eds. New York: Josiah Macy, Jr. Foundation.

CHINA: REVOLUTION AND HEALTH
  1972   The Health-PAC Bulletin 47. New York: The Health Policy
         Advisory Center.

CHINESE PATENT MEDICINE
  1972   Hongkong: Patent Medicine and Medicated Liquor Exhibition.

CHOA, G.
  1967   Some ideas concerning food and diet among Hongkong Chinese.
         In Some Traditional Chinese Ideas and Conceptions in Hong-
         kong Social Life Today, M. Topley, ed. Hongkong: Hongkong
         Branch of the Royal Asiatic Society.

CHUNG, Y.
  1973   Food Therapy, 4 Volumes. Hongkong: Tak Lee Book
         Company.

CROIZIER, R. C.
  1968   Traditional Medicine in Modern China. Cambridge: Harvard
         University Press.

FANG, H. S. Y., ed.
  1970   Medical Directory of Hongkong. Hongkong: The Federation
         of Medical Societies.

FRIEDSON, E.
  1972   Profession of Medicine. New York: Dodd, Mead and Company.

GIBSON, G.
   1972   Chinese medical practice and the thoughts of Chairman Mao.
          Social Science and Medicine 6:67–93.
HONGKONG SOCIAL AND ECONOMIC TRENDS
   1972   Hongkong: Census and Statistics Department, Hongkong
          Government.
HONGKONG STATISTICS
   1967   Hongkong: Census and Statistics Department, Hongkong
          Government.
HONGKONG'S MEDICAL AND HEALTH SERVICES
   1970   Hongkong: Hongkong Information Services.
HOU, C. W.
   1970   Mao Tse-tung thought lights up the way for the advance of
          China's medical science. Peking Review 13, 25:23–27.
KING, A.
   1973   A Theoretical and Operational Definition of Community: the
          Case of Kwun Tong. Hongkong: Social Research Center Paper,
          the Chinese University of Hongkong.
LEE, R. P. L.
   1972a Spatial Distributions of Modern Western and Traditional
          Chinese Medical Practitioners in an Industrializing Chinese
          Town. Hongkong: Social Research Center, The Chinese Uni-
          versity of Hongkong.
   1972b Study of Health Systems in Kwun Tong: Health Attitudes and
          Behavior of Chinese Residents. Hongkong: Social Research
          Center, The Chinese University of Hongkong.
   1972c Study of Health Systems in Kwun Tong: Organizations and
          Attitudes of the Western-trained and the Traditional Chinese
          Personnel in an Industrial Community of Hongkong. Hong-
          kong: Social Research Center, the Chinese University of
          Hongkong.
   1973   Population, housing and the availability of medical and health
          services in an industrializing Chinese community. Journal of
          the Chinese University of Hongkong 1:191–208.
PODMORE, D.
   1971   The population of Hongkong. In Hopkins, op. cit.
REPORT OF THE MEDICAL DEVELOPMENT
BY THE ADVISORY COMMITTEE
   1973   Hongkong: Hongkong Government.
REVOLUTIONARY COMMITTEE OF THE CHINESE
ACADEMY OF MEDICAL SCIENCE
   1970   Developing China's medical science independently and self-
          reliantly. Peking Review 13, 1:24–30.

RIFKIN, S. B. and R. KAPLINSKY
  1973   Health strategy and development planning: Lessons from the People's Republic of China. Journal of Developmental Studies 9:213–32.
WONG, S.
  1970   A Preliminary Ecological Analysis of the Development of Kwun Tong, 1954–70. Hongkong: Social Research Center, the Chinese University of Hongkong.

CHAPTER 16

TRADITIONAL AND MODERN PSYCHIATRIC CARE IN TAIWAN

WEN-SHING TSENG

Introduction

For the purposes of a comparative study of medical systems, it is interesting and challenging to examine psychiatric care, since psychiatry, as a discipline of medicine, is unique in that (1) it is oriented extensively by biomedical, psychological, and sociocultural concepts; (2) it is concerned with a wide scope of problems, not only in the area of clinical pathology but also in general life, and (3) various forms of psychiatric care are to be found, such as traditional or modern, folk or classic, professional or paraprofessional; so divergent in theory and practice that they are pertinent for comparative study.

In this paper I attempt to describe the various forms of traditional and modern psychiatric care that exist in contemporary Taiwan, and to compare reference systems, styles of approach, and problems cared for, with the aim of understanding these psychiatric care systems from professional, sociological, and cultural points of view. Psychiatric problems are defined broadly in this paper as any psychologically-related problems, regardless of whether they are manifested by clinical pathology or by trivial daily-life difficulties. Psychiatric care is considered to be any formalized professional attempt to solve such psychologically-related problems.

A brief sketch of the mental health situation in contemporary Taiwan will provide a background for further discussion. A census survey of a sample population carried out in the past revealed that 10 out of every 1000 persons in the sample population manifested mental illness (mainly minor psychiatric disorders) requiring some degree of psychiatric care, of which the great majority (over 95 percent) of cases were untreated by modern psychiatry (Lin 1953). Fewer than 100 physicians are presently functioning as modern psychiatrists among the total population of 16 million, and due to the fact that most of the modern psychiatrists are practicing in the large cities, they are unavailable to the majority of the people who live in the rural areas.

Thus, theoretically and practically it is important to ask what other kinds of psychiatric care, in broad terms, are available and utilized so that the mental health of the people is well maintained and there is no malfunctioning of society. Anthropological studies (Gallin 1966; Jordan 1972; Diamond 1969), sociological surveys (Chai 1968), and medical experiences indicate that in Taiwan, beside modern psychiatry and counselling, there exist numerous kinds of folk psychiatric care in the forms of shamanism, divination, fortune-telling and physiognomy, as well as traditional herbal medicine, all of which are utilized by the people to deal with their psychologically-related problems. Comparative description and analyses will be made of these forms of psychiatric care, and an attempt made to understand how they function simultaneously to maintain the mental health of the people as a whole.

Description and Analysis of Various Forms of Psychiatric Care

Healing practice—shamanism as psychiatric care

Shamanism as a religion-related healing practice still exists in contemporary Taiwan and is one of the important healing systems available in most of the rural areas (Tseng 1972). According to recorded history, a shaman was originally called *wu* in China. Today in Taiwan a shaman is called *dang-gi* by local people, which literally means a "divining youth."

A *dang-gi* is a person supposed to have special powers to communicate with gods. When he is in a state of trance, he will speak and behave as if he is possessed by a god and, supposedly, when in such state he is able to help people by providing interpretations and suggestions for solving their problems. Thus, shamanism is characterized by a basic belief in supernatural powers.

A *dang-gi* may be attached to a certain temple, but he may practice at his own home. He usually holds a job during the day and practices shamanism at night. In the past, during the Japanese occupation, shamanism was forbidden, but after the war there was no pressure from the government, thus it became prevalent again. There is no island-wide sociological or epidemiological data to indicate how many *dang-gi* now exist in Taiwan. However, from a census survey of a fishing village, 10 *dang-gi* were found among the total population of approximately 7,000. This supports the general impression that *dang-gi* are more prevalent in fishing villages than in farm villages. It can also be said that at least one or two *dang-gi* may be found in any village or town throughout most of the rural areas.

A *dang-gi* candidate may be chosen through a selection ceremony, by a *dang-gi,* or by the temple elders. A *dang-gi* candidate usually goes through a training ceremony at which time religious and traditional medical knowledge are taught in a secret manner by temple elders or an experienced *dang-gi*. Usually an initiation ceremony is needed for him to perform his special skills, demonstrating that he will not be seriously injured by sword or fire, etc., so that the people will have confidence in him.

Ordinarily, from 10 to 20 clients may visit a *dang-gi* in one evening. The majority of the clients are women, although men are frequently found among them. They usually come from the nearby neighborhoods, but some will come from far if the *dang-gi* is a well-known healer. Since *dang-gi* were forbidden to practice and were arrested by the police before the war, they still are cautious about performing their practice, and avoid the public and outsiders. Nevertheless, a *dang-gi* usually is respected by the local people and regarded as a savior for providing such service. A *dang-gi* never charges any money, since practice is considered to be a divine service; however, clients will customarily donate money to worship the gods associated with the *dang-gi*. Thus, a *dang-gi* gains both honor and material reward.

The clients visiting a *dang-gi* usually present various kinds of problems, relating to health, social concern, or fate in general. The problem may be how to cure insomnia, how to invest money, or how to raise cattle; indicating that a *dang-gi* serves multiple functions, as if he were priest, physician and counsellor for the local community. This is based partly on the assumption that a *dang-gi* is omnipotent and knows answers for every kind of problem, and partly on the practical ground that since there is no other source of service available, a *dang-gi* has to perform multiple functions for the community.

Analyses of problems presented by clients indicate that more than one-fifth of them are psychiatric in nature. They include, for example, a child who cries fearfully at night, a client who can't sleep well, a student who worries too much about college examinations, a married person who does not get along with an in-law or is deserted by his wife, a client unable to keep a job, or has frequent attacks of dizziness, or is afraid to go outside in the evening, and so on. Many clients present somatic symptoms which may be either medical or psychosomatic in nature. Occasionally a person who suffers from a hysterical neurosis in the form of a dissociative state (or possession) or mild acute psychosis may be brought in for treatment. In general, a *dang-gi* is reluctant to treat chronic psychotic cases, because they seldom respond to such healing practices.

Besides supernatural interpretations of illness, such as a disturbance made by the devil or an ancestor's spirit, loss of soul, violation of taboo, etc., which are related to ancient animism and Taoism, a *dang-gi's* interpretation is frequently influenced by traditional herbal medicine. Thus, the concept of *yin* and *yang* disharmony of humors, as well as other medical terms and concepts, are utilized by a *dang-gi* in his practice. As for treatment, besides the supernatural methods of keeping taboo, praying, the use of charm-paper and exorcism, herbal medicine is also prescribed by many *dang-gi*.

As Chinese culture is characterized by great concern with the family system, in the practice of shamanism many mental disturbances are frequently attributed to an ancestor spirit's influence. In an anthropological survey (Li 1972), it was found that nearly one-half of such problems were interpreted by a single *dang-gi* as being caused by disturbance of the family's spirit. Consequently, family-related therapeutic activities such as worshipping ancestors, changing the location of an ancestor's tomb, or performing a "spirit wedding" (marrying a deceased girl's spirit as a bride in order to solve the problem) may be suggested as aiming to restore the proper family functions within the cultural setting.

The folk interpretation made by a *dang-gi* has its therapeutic implications. The message in folk-terms is more concrete, compact, and familiar to the client, and thus is more easily understood and accepted. Although the interpretation may be "supernatural" and not "rational" from a modern scientific point of view, it is more meaningful and useful to the client. Also, there is psychological significance in citing a supernatural power as the cause of the client's problem. A devil or a ghost can merely be the external aspect of any person in a real-life situation. However, such an interpretation is more easily tolerated and accepted by people who live in a society where close relationships between family members are maintained and overt conflict between persons is prohibited. A successful shaman knows how to make use of his sensitive perception to discern the client's problems, and also knows how to give advice relevant to his client's cultural background.

However, from the clinical point of view, the usefulness of shamanism as a psychiatric therapeutic practice should be carefully evaluated and criticized. If an inexperienced *dang-gi* is so ambitious as to pretend that he is powerful enough to solve all problems presented by his clients, there is always the danger that he may be harmful to a client by not only wasting the client's money and time but also by delaying the opportunity for him to obtain proper treatment if the problems are beyond the *dang-gi's* ability to help.

Folk Counselling Practices—Divination, Fortune-Telling, and Physiognomy

Divination

Divination by drawing bamboo sticks is called *chou-chien* in Chinese, which literally means "drawing a divine stick." The practice of divination has existed in China since prehistoric times. However, the contemporary method has become popular since the Sung Dynasty.

In nearly every temple in Taiwan there is a bamboo pipe placed near the altar. When someone wants divine instruction for solving his problems, he goes to the temple. After worshipping and presenting his problem to the god, he goes to the bamboo pipe and takes from it one stick randomly. According to a number on the stick he gets a divine paper of corresponding number. On each divine paper there is written a Chinese poem, together with answers to various problems. Because of their limited education, the diviners often find the poem too difficult to understand, so there is usually at the temple an old man experienced in the service of providing an interpretation of the poem and the accompanying instructions. After the diviner presents the problems for which he is seeking an answer, the old man provides an appropriate interpretation and advice. He may ask the diviner several questions and suggest customary ways of coping with his problem, as if these were given by the divine paper.

According to one sociological survey, more than 700 persons visited three temples in a city during a period of 1 week. Approximately 70 to 80 percent of these were women. Nearly one-half of the diviners are illiterate and the rest have at best a grade-school education. This indicates that the diviners are primarily from the middle and lower social class backgrounds. Surprisingly, all age groups are involved, including both young and old, with the peak at around 30 to 40 years of age. Many kinds of problems are presented, including concerns about health and disease, wealth, business, marriage, moving, travelling, childbirth, academic examinations, and fate in general. These items are listed on each divine paper so that specific answers can be given regarding corresponding items. According to this survey, health and disease, business, and fate in general are the most frequent areas of consultation.

From a psychotherapeutic point of view, the intrepretations given through this practice not only provide hope for the client and eliminate anxiety due to lack of knowledge about the future, but also reinforce adaptive social behavior. An analysis of the comments made on the divine paper indicates that they are characterized by suggestions to be conservative; that is, not to be too aggressive or ambitious, and not to do things which are inappropriate for one's social role and status (Hsu 1974). One is frequently encouraged to be patient, to endure, and to make an effort to cultivate oneself. Such suggestions reflect the socio-culturally-sanctioned value system, and such folk-counselling practices reinforce socioculturally-sanctioned behavior.

Fortune-telling

Fortune-telling is called *suan-ming* in Chinese, meaning "the calculation of fortune." It is another form of folk counselling often utilized by the people of Taiwan. The fortune-teller usually opens his stall near a market, inside a temple, or in a park, enabling people to visit him easily. There is no need for god worshipping. The client is supposed to reveal the time, day, month, and year of his birth, so that the fortune-teller can calculate his fortune based on these four sets of numbers.

Theoretically, the basis of fortune-telling rests upon the idea that there exist certain universal principles which rule nature. According to the *I Ching,* or *Oracle of Change,* changes arise from the interaction of the two primal forces, *yang* and *yin.* The complex interplay of energy between these two poles results in the perpetual creation and transmutation of all things, including human matter. The purpose of fortune-telling is to calculate the changes constantly operating throughout all levels of the universe.

The fortune-teller in Taiwan is usually a man of middle or old age. There is no special process of training required to become a fortune-teller. A candidate usually reads books on fortune-telling to obtain the necessary knowledge for practice, or occasionally he may be tutored by an experienced fortune-teller. The client is supposed to pay a certain fee to the fortune-teller for the service. The fee varies according to the status of the fortune-teller and the intensity of the fortune he is asked to calculate. Generally speaking, however, the fee is low enough to enable a person to consult a fortune-teller if he feels the need to do so.

The problems presented by clients are personal matters relating to fate, business, marriage, health, wealth, the future, and so on. The clients consult the fortune-teller at times when they encounter difficulties and there is a need for advice. The fortune-teller interprets the nature of the problems in terms of something being wrong with a person's predisposition; things are not being done according to the cycle of change in nature or the principle of balance and harmony, and so forth. The fortune-teller not only interprets but also suggests how to cope with problems.

The clients consulting the fortune-teller are, in general, middle-class people. Both men and women are interested in fortune-telling, but in contrast to divination in the temple, fortune-telling is utilized more by men than by women. Perhaps this is because fortune-telling is performed in a relatively private situation, making it easier for men to ask for help.

Physiognomy

Physiognomy is called *k'an-hsiang* in Chinese, which means "the examining of features." It is based on the theory that there is a close correlation between body and mind, thus enabling one to read your character, behavior pattern, and life adjustment by examining your physical features. Physiognomy is theoretically different from fortune-telling in that it is not concerned with the principles that rule nature, but is interested in the person himself; nevertheless, many people practice physiognomy and fortune-telling in combination, while others specialize in one or the other.

A physiognomist can be readily found by the people in Taiwan, as he will have his stall in the street or near the market just as the fortune-teller does. The clients consulting a physiognomist are similar to those visiting a fortune-teller in regard to age, sex distribution, and social background. The physiognomist examines the client's features, interprets the client's personality, behavior pattern, and past and future life, and gives advice on how to deal with problems the client may encounter in the areas of business, family, marriage, love-affairs, and so on. The basic concept of such practice is to encourage a person to acknowledge his own assets and develop them for maximal use and, at the same time, to be aware of shortcomings and the need to minimize such defects.

From the standpoint of psychiatric care, the practices of divination, fortune-telling, and physiognomy are useful as folk counselling. When a person is facing a serious problem he always wants to know why he has been so afflicted and what he should do to solve the problem. A successful folk counsellor is skillful enough to provide the client with a clear and convincing explanation for his problems, so that he can help him to make a decision in a time of difficulty and so that the client can actively do something to solve his problems.

The limitations of such practice are found in the fact that, by definition, the folk practitioner is supposedly superior in that he knows the answer for every problem. In practice, he can only make use of his sensitive perception to speculate about the client and he is not supposed to obtain information about him through direct inquiry. This naturally limits his ability to obtain information about the client necessary for an appropriate suggestion as to how he should solve his problems. From the professional point of view, there is no adequate training provided for these practitioners, and there is no way to determine the quality of the individual practitioner except by the judgments of his clients.

Psychiatric Care in Traditional Chinese Medicine

Traditional Chinese medicine has evolved in China over the past 25 centuries. Theoretically, it is based on the concept of *yin* and *yang,* the Theory of Five Elements, and the idea of correspondence between microcosm and macrocosm. From the viewpoint of medical development, it is heavily characterized by natural philosophy and the transition from humoral to visceral organ-oriented pathology. Although traditional medicine has been replaced by modern medicine in the past several decades, it is still popular in Taiwan and is frequently relied on by clients of various backgrounds, regardless of their social class.

Although traditional Chinese medicine recognizes a wide range of illnesses, as a medical practice it functions primarily as internal medicine with close relation to pharmacy. There was no early differentiation into several sub-branches such as surgery, pediatrics, gynecology, etc., as in today's modern medicine. In reviewing the description of psychiatric maladies appearing in Chinese medical documents of various periods, I have found that various kinds of mental illness have been described sporadically, following the order of organic mental illness, excited psychosis, hysteria, depression, and minor psychiatric illness, indicating that rather remarkable progress in the area of psychiatric knowledge was developed in the past (Tseng 1973a). However, such knowledge was not organized systematically, and no independent branch of psychiatry was developed.

In spite of the fact that since the beginning of Chinese medicine emotional factors have been considered to be one of the internal causes for developing illness, and that improvement of the emotional condition was emphasized as a means of improving illness, particularly in disorders such as nausea, palpitation, sweating, sexual impotence, and so forth, in actual practice the treatments for such disorders are characterized by herb-oriented therapy, which is the principal form of treatment in Chinese medicine.

Psychiatric care in traditional Chinese medicine is characterized by the tendency to interpret disturbance of the system of balance, invasion by natural agents, imbalance of the humors and vital forces, and unfulfilled desire or excessive worry as the reasons for becoming mentally ill. Very little blame is placed upon the patient himself, and no significant responsibility for achieving self-improvement is given the patient.

The basic attitude is that the patient is "sick" and is in need of rest, care, nourishment and recuperation so that he can regain a state of harmony and normality. This is a different approach than that of modern psychiatry, in which "improvement" and "growth" are emphasized to obtain the ideal condition of "adjustment.")

Based on the concept of organ-pathology and the emphasis on herbal therapy in traditional medicine, psychiatric practice is characterized by the fact that Chinese patients frequently describe their problems somatically, that is in terms of body organs, even when the underlying problems are emotional in nature. "Elevated liver fire," "insufficiency of kidney power," and "exercised heart" are examples of the terms used by patients to describe their problems of agitated anxiety, sexual impotence, and apprehension, respectively.

The study of Chinese personality development indicates that oral gratification is very much permitted in the early stages of life and is continuously emphasized even in later life (Tseng and Hsu 1970). Parallel to the traditional medical practice of herbal treatment, Chinese patients are oriented to drug therapy even for emotional problems. Many so-called neurasthenic or hypochondriacal patients, as well as psychosomatic cases, consult traditional medical practitioners when oriented by the concepts of weakness, insufficiency, and exhaustion, are concerned about their somatic conditions, and anxious to obtain drugs for fulfillment. Thus, psychiatric care in traditional Chinese medicine is characterized by a biomedical orientation and approach that is the combined result of the traditional medical system, Chinese personality, and Chinese culture.

Although in the past traditional medical schools existed for training herbal doctors, such institutions have vanished in Taiwan concurrent with the processes of modernization and the development of modern medicine. The majority of herbal doctors today obtain their knowledge and skill from self-study and personal experience; however, some of them are tutored by experienced doctors. Although there is a formal organization for traditional medical doctors, there is no formalized and standardized process of determining professional qualifications. The degree of sophistication varies remarkably among herbal doctors, and there is no way of standardizing it. In spite of this situation, and the availability of modern medical facilities, particularly in the urban areas, traditional medicine is still prevalent and frequently utilized by some groups of people in Taiwan, regardless of whether or not they are educated. For this, there are several reasons. If a person is accustomed since his youth to rely on traditional herbal medicine, then he is likely to depend on it continuously thereafter, even if other facilities are available. Chinese tend to value anything old and traditional. Such a tendency is reinforced by the belief that traditional medicine is effective "gently" but "radically," aiming to deal with the primary cause, while the effect of modern medicine is "rapid" and "dramatic," but is good only for treating the symptoms or signs of illness. Such a view is supported by the less-frequent occurrence of side-effects from herbal drugs in contrast to the more frequent side-effects accompanying modern medicine. Herbal doctors always emphasize that the prescription has been transmitted secretly from ancient times through many generations. The mysterious nature of such prescriptions is very appealing to some people, particularly many patients suffering chronic illnesses who are looking for magical improvement. From a sociopolitical point of view, traditional medicine is used as a symbol of tradition in a defense against modernization. The recent sudden increase of interest in the study of acupuncture is an example of how traditional medicine is emphasized as a special national excellence, and is used to support racial self-confidence. For the above-described reasons, the effectiveness of traditional medicine may be over-emphasized beyond its true medical efficacy, therefore necessitating careful evaluation.

From the clinical point of view, psychiatric patients with minor disorders, particularly psychosomatic problems, may be helped to some extent by traditional medical care through the mechanisms of (1) its actual medical effectiveness or (2) non-specific psychological support. As for major psychiatric disorders, there is no convincing evidence indicating that they are benefited by traditional care.

The study of the history of Chinese medicine reveals that although it has shown continuous development in many aspects, it has not shown any radical change in its basic theory in the past 20 centuries. The Chinese in general are oriented toward the past and tradition, particularly in regard to learning. A student was expected to learn how to translate and interpret what had been said by scholars in the past rather than to search out new ideas of his own. The process of medical development has been influenced by this way of learning.

In training and practice, herbal doctors have emphasized tutorship and the private transmission of secret prescriptions. Since knowledge and skill were not subject to public transmission, this became an obstacle for continuous development. The future of traditional medicine will also be limited unless this obstacle can be removed.

Modern Psychiatric Care and Counselling

Modern psychiatric care in Taiwan evolved almost from a vacuum after the war, when Taiwan was returned to China from Japanese occupation (Lin 1961). All Japanese psychiatrists had been repatriated, and there was no single Chinese psychiatrist sufficiently trained in this field. In association with the reorganization of political, social, economic, and educational systems, the government was burdened by many important cares. The medical and public-health professions were busy in their immediate tasks of combating the acute infectious diseases and restoring health services to prewar level. The general attitude of the medical profession, as well as the lay public, to modern psychiatry was characterized by indifference, ignorance and prejudice. However, it did not discourage the development of a psychiatric program. A psychiatric center was established at the university hospital in order to develop a nucleus of staff psychiatrists, to intensify the training of personnel, and to provide modern psychiatric service to the public.

Although theory and practice were oriented to descriptive psychiatry in the prewar stage, emphasizing biological predisposition and viewing mental illness as a manifestation of "defect" and "sickness," after the postwar turnover of the medical system in general, the system of modern psychiatry in Taiwan became a dynamically-oriented one. (The nature of emotional illness is now seen as a reaction to stress or a maladjustment to the environment, and an attempt is made to understand the mechanism of illness through a dynamic and sociopsychological approach. In spite of this, there is some difficulty in absorbing and digesting some psycho-analytic theories, because it is not clear whether they should be rejected or modified to meet this very different sociocultural setting. In practice, the availability of somatic treatments such as shock therapy and the newly-developed psychopharmacological therapy certainly facilitates the progress of psychiatric care, particularly for the major disorders (psychoses). A large proportion of psychotic patients now can be improved in a short period, and long-term custodial care can be avoided.

The image of psychiatric care has changed remarkably among the medical profession and the lay public. After the first 10 years the clinics began to be flooded with patients seeking both in-patient and out-patient psychiatric care.

In the process of psychiatric training, neurological knowledge and skill are required as well as psychiatry. Since the medical differentiation between neurology (brain-nerve disorders) and psychiatry (mind disorders) is not clear among some of the medical staff and patients, it is useful to have training for both at this stage of development, even though the separation of these two fields will be both necessary and unavoidable in the near future.

A review of the psychiatric problems initially presented by out-patients in Taiwan reveals that nearly 80 percent of patients complain of somatic symptoms to psychiatrists, including educated and psychologically-sophisticated patients. The majority of these patients have no difficulty in focusing on their psychological problems later on, if these problems are their primary concern. However, a large proportion of patients still expect to receive drug treatment. This does not necessarily mean that they will resist a psychotherapeutic approach; on the contrary, most of them appreciate this approach to their problems.

(The emotional problems presented by patients are, as everywhere, variable. However, in contrast to patients in other cultures, such as in Western societies, the problems are frequently centered around the theme of intra-family conflict, pressure for achievement in education, pressure to conform to a given situation, and the like. These themes reflect the stresses that tend to be encountered in contemporary Taiwan. The problems of loneliness, sexual competition, the identity crisis of youth, and so on, are not the major issues among Chinese patients.)

The mental-health idea and mental-health movement are accepted and welcomed by the people, particularly the intellectuals, as if mental health were a familiar concept to them. Today, many modern counselling systems have been developed in the large cities by psychologists and educators, focusing on the issues of youth psychology, mate-selection, occupational guidance, and suicidal crisis. Counselling is free and is welcomed by most of the people, particularly the youth, indicating a great need for such services and a readiness to utilize them.

Although psychiatric care and mental-health programs are rapidly progressing, from a realistic point of view, no matter how many psychiatric personnel are trained in the near future, there will still be a great shortage of such professionals, even in several of the cities, not to mention rural areas. Many chronic psychotic patients are still likely to receive custodial care from insufficiently trained personnel, and many clients will still rely on folk counselling.

Fortunately, the problems current among Western youth such as alcoholism and drug abuse are not prevalent in Taiwan. Dyssocial behavior among the youth in the form of a "hippy" movement has not occurred in Taiwan. This is due partially to the Chinese people's negative attitude toward such phenomena and partially to the government's active efforts to suppress such tendencies. The government learned a bitter lesson in the past with respect to the opium problem and the youth-riot movement, and thus is sensitive and guarded concerning such psychiatric problems and wastes no time in dealing with them.

Although the history of modern psychiatry in Taiwan is very short—only about three decades—and it is too early for it to have developed any unique theory of its own, in the area of practice, particularly of psychotherapy, psychiatrists have learned that special concern is needed in treating Chinese patients so that psychotherapeutic practice will be culturally relevant (Hsu and Tseng 1972) Chinese are taught not to openly and directly express their personal feelings in public, particularly such negative feelings as hostility or aggression, or sexual desire. Therefore, in the process of psychotherapy, even though its aim may be to reveal the client's repressed feelings and desires in the initial stage of treatment, it is wise not to encourage the patient to express his feelings too soon.

The Chinese response to parental authority is traditionally expected to be submissive, obedient, and compliant (Tseng and Hsu 1972). Thus, even if a client suffers from such social demands, he is not to be guided toward behaving rebelliously and antagonistically toward his parental authority, as this may increase rather than resolve his problems. For a Chinese person to obtain social independence is a gradual and delayed process. Harmony between generations is more valued than individual independence. It is the modern psychiatrist's task to devote more study to the sociocultural aspects of psychiatric care among Chinese patients so that such services can be more useful and meaningful to Chinese people.

Discussion

Comparison of referential systems

Comparative analyses of these various forms of psychiatric care in Taiwan indicate that the basic difference among them relates to their systems of reference (Tseng 1974).

Shamanism is based upon the belief that a devil or a spirit is the interfering power, and clients are taught how to cope with such *supernatural* power through exorcism or counter-magic. Divination is still based on the assumption that such supernatural power exists, and the client is supposed to learn how to live compatibly with nature, which is ruled by this supernatural power. Fortune-telling interprets an underlying principle of *nature* that presumably rules human beings. Thus, a client is instructed how to adjust his nature by following the principles of nature in order to set a matter in the right direction. Physiognomy takes the view that a *person* is predisposed to problems, and a client is taught to make good use of himself. Traditional Chinese medicine tends to interpret disharmony of internal forces or *humors* and the intrusion of external (natural) agents as the causes of emotional disturbance, and the aim of treatment is to regain a balanced condition through recuperation and the supplementation and regulation of internal forces. Modern psychiatry takes the view that human behavior is a mixture of biological, psychological, and sociocultural factors. Mental disorders are conceived to be reactions to stress, or a phenomena of *maladjustment* to the environment, and treatment is focused on how to change and/or correct a person's behavior so that the problem can be solved.

It appears that the theory and means of mental treatment have evolved historically from *supernatural, natural,* and *biomedical* ones to *sociopsychological* ones, in that sequence. It is remarkable to find these various care systems co-existing and functioning together in a contemporary society.

Comparison of service-functions

Clinical and sociological analyses of these various forms of psychiatric care in Taiwan indicate a certain pattern of distribution among them regarding service-function. This is illustrated conceptually by Figure 1. In this illustration, psychiatric problems are grouped as *major disorders,* which include various forms of psychoses; *minor disorders,* which include neuroses and psychophysiological disorders and which are subdivided into groups—*somatic*-complaint dominating and *psychological*-complaint dominating; and *psychological problems in general,* which refers to any problems commonly occurring in daily life and relating to family, marriage, business, or other social affairs.

Shamanism, as a primitive form of healing practice, serves a wide scope of psychiatric problems, except the area of major disorders. The client served is primarily one from a lower social class who still believes

PSYCHIATRIC PROBLEMS

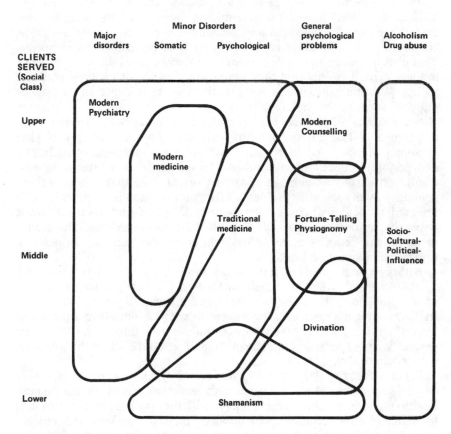

Figure 1. Distribution of service-function among various forms of psychiatric care in Taiwan.

in supernatural power and for whom shamanism is a part of familiar daily life activities. Divination functions mainly for general psychological problems and for the middle and lower social classes, while fortune-telling and physiognomy function for middle and upper social classes. Traditional medicine as well as modern medicine (internal medicine) mainly treat minor psychiatric disorders with predominant somatic complaints. Modern medicine is utilized by the upper and middle social classes, while traditional medicine is used primarily by the middle and lower social classes, although this division is not absolute. Modern psychiatry provides care mainly for major disorders and various types of minor disorders, while modern counselling provides care for general psychological problems. Care is available only for those who live in the city. As for the problems of alcoholism and drug abuse, sociocultural and political forces have prevented them from becoming prevalent in contemporary Taiwan.

The distribution of service-functions among various forms of care in Taiwan is related to several determining factors. In the remote rural areas where modern medical and psychiatric facilities are not available, shamanism and divination are the only services accessible to the people. This does not mean that people from such remote areas do not appreciate modern care; it is only that they have to rely on the one source available to them—a shaman who, in his part-time work, is expected to provide multiple services for the community.

Some forms of service are specialized in some areas so that they function only for certain kinds of problems. Fortune telling and physiognomy are confined to common psychological problems of daily life, and perform counselling rather than healing functions. In the same way, traditional herbal medicine is pharmacy-oriented so that it is concerned primarily with somatic problems. In contrast, modern psychiatry is oriented to deal with major psychiatric disorders and severe neurotic cases, but is not used for advising on daily life problems. Thus, each form of care remains more or less within its own territory because of this function specialization.

Although many kinds of services are available, a client has a tendency to choose a particular one based on his belief in that service, the nature of his problem, and the benefit that can be obtained from that service. In Taiwan it is not necessary for a client to commit himself to a particular kind of service. He may take the opportunities available to him to contact several kinds of service simultaneously and to utilize all of the available care syncretically.

From a functional point of view, various types of care do not have any interrelations. Modern psychiatrists are concerned with the mental-health situation of the whole society, and they usually make an effort to maintain close relations with modern medical workers and modern counsellors. However, there is no extension of contact to the folk care system. Among folk practitioners every person performs individually and there is no organization within this system. The general attitude is one of ignorance of each other, almost of suspicion, and cooperation between practitioners is not attempted.

Sociocultural aspects of psychiatric care

Although the various forms of psychiatric care available in contemporary Taiwan are so divergent in respect to systems of reference and different styles of approach, nevertheless, a close examination gives the general impression that all share some common elements related to the underlying Chinese culture and manifested in the basic philosophy of each system of care (Kleinman 1973).

Throughout all forms of care there is a common tendency to emphasize compliance, harmonization and regulation as the means for obtaining a condition of normality. There is relatively less emphasis on conquest, mastery, or improvement, which may be stressed in other societies. The Chinese form of psychiatric care is oriented to the concepts of Taoist thought which values the meaning of harmony and regulation in the natural world.

There is strong concern for the family as the basic and essential social unit, and efforts are demanded to maintain this central structure. In China there is a familial organization of society; thus, the destruction of family organization and relationships, in the forms of rebellious youth, divorce, or inter-generational conflict, is discouraged in psychiatric care and is seldom suggested as a means of solving problems.

Influenced by Confucian mental health concepts, the main goal of treatment defined by these various forms of care is to obtain internal satisfaction (Tseng 1973b). A person is encouraged to make use of his potentiality, to develop his talent, and to cultivate his own personality. Above all, he is advised to be ready to accept any kind of outcome with equanimity. Such a philosophical view of mental health is presented in all forms of psychiatric care in Taiwan, regardless of whether it is modern or traditional, classic or folk. This suggests that the principles and strategies of psychiatric care are strongly influenced by cultural factors, either explicitly or implicitly.

Implications for the future

Psychiatric problems are wide in scope and psychiatric care can be served in divergent ways. Although the mental health of the whole society is the major concern of modern psychiatry, in practice today's psychiatric workers can deal with only a limited panoply of problems and serve a limited number of clients, while many clients have to rely on other care systems for psychiatric services.

Although it is necessary to be critical and to evaluate the practicality of folk and traditional forms of care, unless obvious hazards exist from such folk or traditional services, it is wise not to take a negative attitude toward these care systems, nor to be too anxious to destroy them before other sources of service are made available. Proper attention and support should be given to various forms of care so that maximum service can be provided for the whole society. However, it would be foolish to believe that magical answers can be found in folk or traditional methods.

An overall review of the mental health situation in Taiwan suggests that due to the limited service-functions of other forms of care, the problems of major psychiatric disorders should be left in the hands of modern psychiatry. This does not mean that the care of major psychiatric disorders is the modern psychiatrist's main concern and only interest. It is simply a fact that other forms of care cannot therapeutically help cases of major psychiatric disorders, which often are manifested as psychoses.

A modern psychiatrist is advised to study the various forms of psychiatric care, and to learn the nature of psychiatric care from professional, sociological, and cultural points of view, so that he can understand his responsibility in a broad sense and know how to function properly for his society.

REFERENCES

CHAI, W. H.
1968 A study of divination in a Chinese temple in Taiwan. Thought and Word 6:19–22. (in Chinese)

DIAMOND, N. J.
1969 K'un Shen: A Taiwan Village. New York: Holt, Rinehart and Winston.

GALLIN, B.
1966 Hsin Hsing, Taiwan: A Chinese Village in Change. Berkeley: University of California Press.

HSU, J.
1974 Counseling in the Chinese temple: Psychological study of divination by "Chien" drawing. In Culture and Mental Health Research in Asia and the Pacific, Volume 4, W. Lebra, ed. Honolulu: University of Hawaii Press.

HSU, J. and W. S. TSENG
1972 Intercultural psychotherapy. Archives of General Psychiatry 27:700–05.

JORDAN, D. K.
1972 Gods, Ghosts, and Ancestors: The Folk Religion of a Taiwanese Village. Berkeley: University of California Press.

KLEINMAN, A. M.
1973 Some issues for a comparative study of medical healing. International Journal of Social Psychiatry 19:159–65.

LI, Y. Y.
Aspects of the Chinese character as viewed from some ritual behaviors. In Symposium on the Character of the Chinese: An Interdisciplinary Approach, Y. Y. Li and K. S. Yang, eds. Taipei: Institute of Ethnology, Academia Sinica.

LIN, T. Y.
1953 A study of the incidence of mental disorders in Chinese and other cultures. Psychiatry 16:313–36.
1961 Evolution of mental health programs in Taiwan. American Journal of Psychiatry 117:961–71.

TSENG, W. S. and J. HSU
1970 Chinese culture, personality formation, and mental illness. International Journal of Social Psychiatry 16:5–14.
1972 The Chinese attitude toward parental authority as expressed in Chinese children's stories. Archives of General Psychiatry 26:28–34.

TSENG, W. S.
1972 Psychiatric study of shamanism in Taiwan. Archives of General Psychiatry 26:561–65.
1973a The development of psychiatric concepts in traditional Chinese medicine. Archives of General Psychiatry 29:569–575.

TSENG, W.S. (continued)

1973b The concept of personality in Confucian thought. Psychiatry 36:191–202.

1974 Folk psychotherapy in Taiwan: Comparative study of shamanism, "chien" drawing, fortune-telling, and physiognomy as ways of folk psychotherapy. *In* Lebra, op. cit.

CHAPTER 17

COMPARISONS OF PRACTITIONER-PATIENT
INTERACTIONS IN TAIWAN:
THE CULTURAL CONSTRUCTION OF
CLINICAL REALITY

ARTHUR KLEINMAN

Orientations

Clinical practice (traditional and modern) occurs in and creates particular social worlds.[1] These worlds are cultural constructions. That is, not just beliefs about illness but the behavior of a sick person and the response of family and practitioners are cultural realities, shaped distinctly in different societies and in different social settings within those societies. Amongst other aspects of health care, practitioner-patient relationships are part of these special forms of social reality. This is not a remarkable insight for anthropologists and sociologists, and it is appreciated at present by surprising numbers of educated lay people in our society; but it is still something of a radical notion amongst health scientists and clinicians.

For health scientists and clinicians the most fundamental reality is biological. Everything else is somehow less "real." This ideological bias is an artifact of socialization into biomedical science and the modern medical profession. It is a very powerful ideology, however; one on which behavioral and social science teaching in medical schools has had little impact. If there is a single concept in social science which challenges this ideology it is the idea of the social construction of reality. Not surprisingly then, this is a concept that you find few medical people hold, and it is extremely difficult to teach it to them. Part of the problem is that the concept of social reality like certain other excellent social science notions in the health field—the sick role, illness behavior, cultural labeling of illness, professional socialization—is usually taught (if it is taught at all) in the pre-clinical years of medical school and in such an "academic" manner that it is isolated from clinical experience. The clinical reality that medical students and house officers incorporate, negotiate, and help create is, of course, one of the special forms of social reality (indeed a most strange version) mentioned above, but they do not see it that way because they are not taught to see it that way. That is, social reality is simply not taught to clinicians or made relevant to clinical problems and practice. To my mind, this is the single greatest failure of social science teaching in schools of medicine and public health. It is more precisely a failure to translate from social science to clinical science. It will be corrected only when cadres of physicians trained in social science (or social scientists trained in clinical skills) make their presence felt in patient care. Although physicians resist the concept of social reality, my personal experience is that when this seminal perspective is translated into a useful approach to an individual case and the clinical problems it presents, clinicians are quick to appreciate and effectively use it. In fact, even though there is no agreed-upon method for systematically applying the concept of social reality to clinical cases, it is so frequently at issue as a major contributor to clinical problems that (in my experience) such clinically relevant translations are frequently not difficult.

Cross-cultural experiences in medicine and psychiatry often (but not always) sensitize researchers and practitioners to the cultural construction of clinical reality. However this has not yet led to much research on basic clinical issues. Unfortunately, anthropological research frequently is irrelevant to these issues, since it is understandably motivated by intellectual concerns usually quite different from those motivating medical people. The emergence of medical anthropology as a full-fledged subdiscipline in anthropology has begun to correct this situation. But practitioner-patient relationships and the core tasks of clinical care are for some reason not a major focus of medical anthropological research, at least not yet. This is an area of research, however, that should become one of the chief concerns of medical anthropology, and especially of physicians and psychiatrists who do cross-cultural studies. With this in mind, I shall use the idea of the cultural construction of clinical reality to examine materials that I gathered in Taiwan. I do so to point up both cultural differences and universals.

In Taiwan, and perhaps in all developing and developed societies, one can distinguish three separate domains of health care. These are the professional, folk (non-professional, and usually non-licensed, specialists), and popular (largely family-based) domains. For the areas in Taipei where we conducted our field research, the professional domain consisted of both Western-style and Chinese-style doctors; the folk domain included shamans (*tâng-ki*s), fortune-tellers, temple-based interpreters of *ch'ien* (fortune) paper, physiognomists, herbalists, and numerous other specialists. The popular domain principally comprised the family context of care, but also included at times the social network and even some community groups.

Each of these health care settings constructed a distinct type of social reality. These patterns of expectations, behavioral norms, and communicative transactions I shall refer to as special forms of *clinical reality*. Not only do these clinical realities differ for the different domains of care, but each practitioner-patient transaction involves separate views of clinical reality. These may be isomorphic, but more usually, as we shall see below, are quite distinct. Tseng (Chapter 16 above) compares the psychotherapeutic functions of some of the same types of Taiwanese systems of healing we shall examine.

After briefly describing the setting of the field research in Taiwan, I shall compare the clinical reality established in four distinct types of practitioner-patient interactions in this Chinese society. I shall present actual case illustrations in order to illuminate these social worlds. We shall enter the shrines of several shamans, the temples where *chien* interpreters work, the offices of Chinese-style doctors, and the offices of Western-style doctors. In a final section, the implications of this tour for research, teaching, and clinical practice are discussed. Even though we shall examine four types of practitioner-patient relationships, the reader is cautioned that we are not considering the most important form of clinical reality in Taiwan, or in the U.S. for that matter: health care problems, transactions, and practices in the context of the *family*. That is an entire subject in itself, best left for a subsequent paper.

One cautionary note is in order. The paradigm I apply in this field study is a medical one; i.e., I speak of practitioner-patient relationships, illness, health care choices, etc. While facilitating cross-cultural comparisons, this medical paradigm may distort the reality I describe. For example, this model presumes that practitioner-patient transactions are dyads as is most common in the West at present. But in Taiwan, and many other non-Western societies, the practitioner-patient interaction usually involves the family as well as the sick person. It is most often not a dyad. Similarly, the label illness may be attached to more than just the sick person. In Taiwan, not infrequently the entire family may be labeled as sick or inharmonious. And accordingly, treatment will be directed at the entire family or at key (usually female) members, not merely at the patient. In folk practice, as we shall see, sometimes the affected individual is not the focus of clinical care; on some occasions he may not even be present. Perhaps a close relative will come with some of the sick person's clothing; or relatives and friends will give the fortune-teller that individual's eight characters (*pa-tzu*) specifying his exact time of birth in order to inquire about his fate, the course of his illness, and treatment alternatives. In most situations of this kind which I have witnessed, the healer deals with his clients as if they were the patient. He explains matters to them and for them. He performs rituals which are specifically meaningful to them. That is, he gives his care to people other than the sick person: advice, support, and technical and symbolic therapies, in order to treat them for their concern about the sick person. The folk healers I studied seemed to view illness, in such cases, as directly influencing family and social relationships. They responded by treating those relationships and family members.

Since most clients in folk practice are females, folk healers often are asked to treat the problems of other (usually male) family members. But they know that their patient is actually the woman before them. They know her problem is her concern for the sick person. Even when the sick person is present, it is not uncommon to see the folk healer direct most of his attention to that person's mother or other female relatives who have accompanied him. The folk healer seems to recognize that his therapy is principally meaningful for the female relation who is with the sick person, not for the sick person. In fact I have often found this to be the case. When I have made follow-up visits in such cases, it has usually been that "other" person for whom the treatment has had the greatest impact. For example, mothers frequently told me *they* felt better and even that the patient was better, when in fact the patient reported virtually no symptom improvement. In such cases mothers evaluated the folk healing practices as effective, while the sick person often refused to do so, or stated that they were ineffective. This was particularly evident in cases where the patient was better educated and significantly more modern in his orientation than his relatives who had participated in the folk healing.

Here is an example of differences in the way clinical reality is constructed in the West and in Taiwan, and amongst M.D.s and folk practitioners. The danger arises from the use of concepts (e.g., doctor-patient interaction) which tend to impose our own Western medical views of clinical reality on the other types.

Setting[2]

Taiwan presently has about thirteen thousand licensed Western-style doctors (*hsi-i-sheng*), three thousand licensed Chinese-style doctors (*chung-i-sheng*) not including licensed bone setters for whom no figure is available, nine thousand professional nurses, nine thousand modern midwives, and five thousand licensed pharmacists (Western-style). Public health services and government-sponsored health care services are dispensed from 346 rural township and urban district health stations, each of which is staffed by a medical team consisting of public health nurse, midwife, sanitation expert, and either full-time or part-time doctor. Besides licensed practitioners there are large numbers of unlicensed practitioners of both Western-style and Chinese style medicine. Both Western-style and Chinese-style doctors have their own licensing examinations, professional bureaucratic organizations, and systems of training, but only Western-style medicine receives direct financial support from the government (see Baker and Perlman 1967, and chapters by Gale (14), Ahern (2, 5), and Gould-Martin (3) in this volume).

In addition to these practitioners, there are various sorts of practitioners of secular and sacred folk medicine, including: herbalists, itinerant drug peddlers, unlicensed specialists in skin and eye disorders, experts in massage and systems of calisthenics (e.g., *kung-fu* and *t'ai chi ch'uan*), fortune-tellers, physiognomists, traditional midwives, priests of the local folk religion (a syncretic mixture of Taoism and Buddhism), shamans, temple-based interpreters of *ch'ien* and ritual experts, and numerous other folk specialists besides. Most folk practitioners are unlicensed and illegal, but they have been tolerated by the authorities, at least until September 1975 when the government began to enforce some of the rules concerning medical practice.

Although drugs are by law only to be distributed by doctors' prescriptions from licensed pharmacies, in fact all Western and Chinese medicines, except narcotics, can be readily obtained from pharmacies and drug stores without prescriptions. Pharmacists frequently diagnose and prescribe, at a lower fee than most doctors. Western and Chinese medicines are now roughly equally expensive, and patent medicines of both kinds are very widely available. There is no regulation of advertising, and bill-boards, signs on doors, radio and television are filled with commercial advertising by all sorts of practitioners and on behalf of every available type of therapy, especially medicinal agents.

In a survey I conducted of health beliefs and practices of 115 families in Taipei, more than 90 percent of responding individuals stated that they first treated adult illnesses by self-treatment with Western or Chinese medicines, along with diet, special foods, tonics, and balancing foods considered to be symbolically hot or cold. Patients will as frequently use antibiotics and other major medicines on their own as patent medi-cines. Thus, patients in Taipei have greater autonomy in choosing a type of practitioner and type of treatment than they do in the U.S. Medical legal suits, which are frequent, quite commonly involve Western-style doctors, rarely involve Chinese-style doctors, and almost never involve folk doctors. Medical fees vary greatly as we shall see in other sections of this chapter. Patients, practitioners and public health authorities regard the family (rather than the doctor) as chiefly responsible for the care of the patient.

The research reported in this Chapter was part of studies that I conducted in three districts of Taipei City (Yen-Ping, Lung-Shan, and Swang-Yuan). All the practitioners described below practice in these three districts, which are the oldest in Taipei. They are noted for being inhabited primarily by Taiwanese, for being the most culturally traditional sections of the city, and for housing some of the poorest people in Taipei, along with middle-class residents. Swang-Yuan is probably the poorest district in all of Taipei, and also has many recent migrants from rural areas. The 1972 figures for population and *licensed* private medical practitioners in these three districts are summarized in Table 1. Note that Swang-Yuan has more than twice the population but substantially fewer Western-style and Chinese-style practitioners (counting bone setters) than the other districts.

Only the very poorest families in Taipei receive social welfare assistance and free medical care at local health stations. Some families, including most mainland families, have access to virtually free medical care at military hospitals and clinics. Some workers and government employees have health insurance but most people do not. Each district has a health station run by the Taipei City Health Department, in which public health work (vaccination, sanitation, etc.), medical education, and some health care services are provided. Health care services include treatment at relatively low cost of tuberculosis, hypertension and stroke, and a variety of maternal and child health problems. There are also public and private hospitals in each district. But the shops and shrines of traditional healers far outnumber those of modern medical care. Note also that only one district has private psychiatrists. In fact, these are not trained psychiatrists but general practitioners who specialize in treating major psychiatric disorders with drugs and E.C.T., and who own and run their own mental hospitals. These hospitals, unfortunately, are more like prisons than hospitals and reflect the same ills that have afflicted state mental hospitals in the past in the U.S.; but the University and City psychiatric hospitals

TABLE 1

Licensed Private Medical Practitioners in 3 Districts of Taipei City

	Yen-Ping District	Lung-Shan District	Swang-Yuan District
Total Population	58,263	67,933	142,961
Western Pharmacists	68	76	84
Chinese Pharmacy Owners	86	39	37
Western Patent Drug Stores	16	13	15
Chinese-style Doctors	16	43	17
Bone Setters	7	4	0
Modern Midwives (private)	8	8	13
Western-style Doctors*			
Total	66	81	45
Pediatricians	6	6	2
Internists	35	56	36
Ob-Gyn	3	3	2
Surgeons	11	4	2
ENT	3	3	1
Ophthalmologists	2	2	0
Psychiatrists	0	0	2

* Specialties listed for practitioners do not reflect particular specialty training, since Western-style and Chinese-style doctors can advertise as specialists as they desire regardless of qualifications.

are comparable to their modern American counterparts. There is virtually no psychotherapy available in Taipei (or Taiwan). The psychiatric clinics of the National Taiwan University Hospital, the Military Hospitals, and the Taipei City Psychiatric Hospital are far from these three districts and only treat the most severe psychiatric problems and former inpatients. Therefore, it comes as no surprise that traditional healing agencies provide most of the psychiatric care (at least for the less severe forms of mental illness) as well as a good deal of the general medical care in these areas. Since this care goes unrecorded, however, it is not reported in local or national statistics, and is virtually disregarded in reports by public health officials, except where they make negative remarks about it. Obviously such reports and statistics, as in many other societies, seriously distort the true picture of health care.

The vicissitudes of Chinese and Western medicine in China (and Taiwan) are reviewed by Croizier (1968) and in Kleinman et al (1976). Both Chinese-style and Western-style medicine flourish in Taiwan at present (as does folk medicine), but only Western-style medicine receives financial support from the government. Since 90 percent of Chinese-style

herbal medicines come from the mainland, these are about the only mainland products the government allows official entry into Taiwan via
Hongkong. The China Medical College in Taichung gives training in
both Chinese-style and Western-style medicine, although most students
study only the latter. Recently, it has graduated practitioners who are
qualified to practice both kinds of medicine, but in fact almost all limit
their practice to Western-style medicine. In the family-based surveys of
health beliefs and attitudes I conducted, there was considerable sentiment
in favor of integrating the two types of practice into one unified system,
but there is no evidence that this will occur. The Western-style medical
profession and the government health bureaucracy which it controls are
against this happening. Thus the situations in Taiwan and the People's
Republic are quite different. There are many other interesting and
relevant aspects of the relationship between these two forms of professional
medical practice, but these go beyond the limited scope of this Chapter
(see Kleinman et al 1976).

Our family-based survey also reveals that, as in other rapidly modernizing societies, people frequently hold odd combinations of traditional
and modern beliefs about illness and treatment. Similarly, treatment
choices frequently involve recourse to both modern and traditional
practitioners. There is a basically pragmatic use of treatment facilities
such that several treatment alternatives are employed in rapid succession
or simultaneously until there is demonstrated symptom relief. Folk
religion and healing practices are thriving as never before, and at the
same time the latest fads in Western and Chinese medicine are widely
used. Indeed, modern hospitals and clinics, traditional Chinese pharmacies, and small shrines where healing rituals occur are often located
on the same street. In the rest of the chapter I shall focus solely on the
patterns of social reality found in these places and within which these
different types of clinical practice occur.

Practitioner-Patient Interactions 1:
Shamans

Taiwan's shamans are part of a great Asian tradition of shamanism
that includes Japan, Korea, and Okinawa, and that in the past extended
across the enormity of China, through various central Asian peoples into
what is now the Soviet Union, and connected up with similar traditions
in Tibet. Ancient Chinese texts contain frequent mention of *wu*, shaman,
and that tradition seems to have been part of Chinese culture in all areas
of the State. But in modern times it seems to have been an especially
active tradition in Fukien province, where most Taiwanese trace their
ancestry. Probably at no time in the past have there been as many shamans
as now. This is attributed to both an upsurge of folk religion as the
only tolerated expression of Taiwanese nationalism and the financial
success of shamanism in present day Taiwan. Of course it it not possible
to accurately calculate their number—they are not registered. But based
on estimates that I made in the field there must be at the very least eight
hundred practicing shamans in Taipei alone. This is an incredible figure

when you realize that for years people in Taiwan claimed shamans could only be found in rural villages. Informants have estimated that Swang-Yuan District's oldest section may have as many as fifty shamans in fairly close proximity to one another.

The word for shaman in Taiwan is the Hokkien term *tâng-ķi*, which means literally "divining youth." There are no mainland shamans in Taiwan as far as I can tell, and mainlanders are not frequently seen in the small shrines where most *tâng-ki*s practice. The popular ideology has it that young men or women are chosen by gods to manifest the gods' wish to "save the world." This is revealed via trance, at which time the god "speaks through" the entranced shaman. The ideology also states that a shaman is poor, and usually illiterate; that he is often cured of an otherwise incurable illness (usually physical illness) by his god, who thereafter establishes a Confucian style master-disciple relationship with him which the shaman cannot end by himself if he wishes to keep his health; and that the shaman remains ignorant of what happens when he is in trance. The shaman does not "charge" a fee, but the client "donates" a gift to the shaman for the god.

It is not the shaman who heals, but the god. And healing is in fact his dominant activity (see Gould-Martin's Chapter 3 above). Half to three quarters of all shamanistic consultations deal with health problems. The rest of the problems include personal, family, and business concerns. In each the god is asked to be instrumental in resolving problems. Revealing one's fate and treating bad fate are other important activities, but most frequently shamans in Taiwan see acute disruptive interpersonal problems requiring immediate intervention. Illness which occurs out of the family context of control is precisely such a problem. Thus, from a biased medical and psychiatric perspective shamans function as traditional emergency room and crisis intervention experts. Shocking as it may sound to ethno-scientists, at least five of the dozens of shamans I have had the privilege to study agreed with this description once I had replaced the "person" with the "god" as active force. That is, the god is seen as a healer. The *tâng-ki* recognizes illness as the most common and often the most difficult problem he treats.

We studied shamans by obtaining introductions to their shrines, and thereafter attending faithfully for several sessions of observation before asking permission to interview them, their assistants, and clients. We then systematically interviewed clients before they consulted the shaman, observed their interaction with the shaman, and later visited them at home, at which time we asked them to evaluate the care they had received. Many shamans are quite suspicious of visitors, especially mainlanders or foreigners. They fear publicity, which is almost always negative. Shamanism is a cultural metaphor that Taiwan's elite class does not believe is consonant with the image of social development, just as traditional Confucian scholars in China over the centuries felt it was inconsistent with Confucian values, and just as the People's Republic sees it as a superstitious vestige of capitalistic feudalism incompatable with Maoist socialism. Moreover, now that they make a considerable amount of money, *tâng-ki*s rightly fear the tax people and the police. Only on one occasion was I denied permission to enter a shrine. Otherwise shamans generally went along with any inconvenience my methods caused. In several cases, shamans took an active part in the research: they allowed us to put our tape recorders on the altar table; they encouraged clients to cooperate and permit us to perform follow-up home visits; and they had their assistants make sure that we did not misinterpret their words and actions. But in no case did a shaman provide us with a "real" life history. What we obtained were stylized accounts which followed all the key points of the popular ideology concerning what shamans should be like.

Of the many shamans I observed, I had the opportunity to personally interview and evaluate the mental status of ten. None exhibited any evidence of major psychopathology, nor gave any history of psychiatric problems. Most were rather remarkable individuals, and were recognized as such by neighbors and clients. As we shall see shamanistic healing clearly demands personal strengths and sensitivities which are incompatable with major psychopathology, especially chronic psychosis. What is of interest is my impression that shamans in Taiwan frequently come from quite poor families, sometimes with a history that one or both parents died when the shaman was still young. They subsequently were identified as helpful, "good", understanding individuals by neighbors and people in the community; but were seen not to have a direction open for their advancement nor to have much family support. Then through a variety of circumstances, this particular activity was made available to them by their social network as a means to succeed—as a gift which the shaman repays through his service to the community or network. If this pattern is true, then achievement orientation should be a common characteristic of practicing shamans, who always seem to be in the process of building a new and bigger shrine (or home). This orientation also appears to be an important part of their "healing powers."

Most shamans obtain training from older and quite experienced Taoist priests or other shamans. They are taught how to control trance behavior, and about herbs and Chinese medicine, which they frequently prescribe. They are taught how to perform seemingly (and at times actually) dangerous activities at festivals: cutting themselves with swords, sitting on a bed of nails, walking over fires of coals or spirit money, climbing up sword ladders, holding boiling oil in their mouths, burning themselves with incense sticks, etc. Those activities frequently involve "tricks of the trade", but some are frenzied performances of self-mutilation, e.g., when tâng-kis slice open their scalps or tongues in order to obtain blood for rituals. But shamans also learn, especially by observing other shamans, how to speak to clients and how to respond to common problems, including different kinds of illnesses. They learn, for example, not to treat acute trauma, or any other acute health problem that looks like it might eventuate in death; or if they do treat these they also refer the patient for appropriate medical attention. Nor will they treat violent psychotic behavior or psychotic disorders. Yet they learn to extricate themselves from these situations without damaging the popular ideology that the gods are powerful therapists. They can do this in a number of ways, the simplest of which is to define an illness as from "within the body," rather than from "gods, ghosts, or ancestors", and therefore outside the boundaries of sacred healing. A more systematic discussion of Taiwan's shamans will be presented in a book I am preparing: *Patients and Healers in the Context of Culture.*

We now shall visit the shrines of several Taipei *tâng-ki*s. Instead of focusing on the *tâng-ki*, we shall examine the interaction between *tâng-ki* and client. That should give us a sense of the social reality the patient participates in when he visits the *tâng-ki*.

The first shrine is rather typical of the settings where *tâng-ki*s practice: it is a small room, attached to a temple, poorly ventilated, almost airless, hot, packed with ten to thirty clients (including children and infants). Most of the clients are middle-aged women and young mothers from the lower class. In the center of the room is a large, impressive altar upon which are placed the small painted wooden figures that represent the shrine's gods. The chief god in this shrine is *Ong-ia-kong* (the plague god; see Gould-Martin, Chapter 3 above). It is late afternoon. Most shamanistic séances occur at this time or in the evening.

The *tâng-ki*, a middle-aged man with a red sash tied around his waist and a prominent scarred area on his scalp where he has performed ritualistic self-laceration, now possessed by his god, is singing in a falsetto copied from Taiwanese folk opera. He has spent five to ten minutes with each of several cases. The assistant announces the next case: a middle-aged man, poorly dressed, unshaven, appearing deeply troubled and surrounded by his family members. The *tâng-ki* does not know this man or his family, as is true of most of his cases and many of those of urban as opposed to rural village *tâng-ki*s, but like me he had an opportunity to observe this client before the séance began and to hear his family talking to other people in the shrine about his problem. The man looks deeply depressed, and the family has told people in the shrine that he has been this way ever since he suffered severe business losses several months ago. The patient tells the *tâng-ki* that he has many physical complaints: he lists nonspecific symptoms, including lethargy, insomnia, weight loss, headache, palpitations, dry mouth and difficulty swallowing, and many gastrointestinal symptoms including constipation. He also briefly mentions his business reverses, and admits to feeling anxious (*fan-tsao*) about them. At no times does he mention any word for depression, nor do his family members, but in the background people are whispering *mên* (depressed).

The *tâng-ki* speaks: "You have too many symptoms. Don't worry about them and your health so much. You are certainly depressed, since you have had bad fate in your business and lost much money. That is caused by your younger brother's ghost who is giving you trouble now." The *tâng-ki* had asked the patient in detail about his family and had learned that two family members, including this younger brother who died in a fire, had died without leaving descendents who could worship them.

The *tâng-ki* tells the man the ghost is "hungry" and must be appeased by being "fed" with ritual foods and worshipped at the family altar. He talks with this man in a supportive way, encouraging him to get back to his work and family responsibilities. Twice he tells jokes. The second time, the patient smiles. (It is the first time his troubled expression has changed since he arrived.) The *tâng-ki* prescribes Chinese medicine, and tells the patient's wife that she must prepare this medicine by steaming it with a specially prepared chicken dish, which is to be given to the patient several days per week. Now the *tâng-ki*'s tone has changed from a supportive one to an authoritarian voice that sounds stern and commanding: "Surely if you do what I tell you, if you take the medicine and appease the ghost, you will get better! You will have no more symptoms!" The *tâng-ki* finishes by writing charms for the patient and by performing a very brief ritual to treat ("patch") the patient's bad fate.

The assistant tells the patient his fate will no longer be bad. He reexplains much of what the *tâng-ki* has said to the patient and his family. They pass on to another assistant who gives them a prescription for Chinese medicine based on the words the *tâng-ki* sang. (They are also told where they can purchase this medicine—a Chinese pharmacy not very close to the shrine but one owned by the *tâng-ki*'s cousin.) Before the family leaves the shrine, and while the *tâng-ki* goes on to treat several other cases, they talk with other clients for more than thirty minutes. They receive additional support and encouragement. Someone tells them: "Now you know what should be done. The god has made it clear. You shall soon be better. Surely your fortune will change." Although the shaman-patient encounter lasted only twenty minutes, the patient and his family spent several hours in the shrine. Before leaving the patient retold his story several times—each time he referred to himself as "depressed." This profoundly depressed man looked so much better when he left that I could not recall any case that I had treated or observed treated which had such a noticeable and immediate effect. Nor did I encounter others like this in this shrine.

Unfortunately this case was lost to follow-up, and I do not know if his affect steadily improved or worsened. Since the patient had all the biological symptoms of the depressive syndrome, I would not be surprised if the treatment response did not last. But even if it did not last, that should not diminish our respect for the skilled way that this therapist treated this case, and for the contribution made by the cultural ethos in the shrine to the patient's care.

There are many ways to interpret what happened in this case. We could invoke, and properly so, the nonspecific psychotherapeutic factors which obtain in practitioner-patient interactions. We also might stress the healer's warmth, empathy, supportive techniques, or his authoritarian approach. I purposefully have not detailed the ritual symbolism, but this could be examined as an example of the efficacy of symbols. We need not bother with the actual effect (if any) of Chinese medicine, because it was not used during the session. More pertinent is the group support given the patient by the assistants, other clients, and his family. Like virtually all folk healing activities, this was a public event. Not only the supportive response of people in the shrine but also their presence when the patient spoke about his problems may have reinforced whatever catharsis occurred and the persuasive aspects of the care. The danger here (and in studies of healing in general) is that we have recourse to so many possible explanations.

Instead of these, let us bring to bear the theoretical framework advanced above: the social reality of clinical care, and its peculiar cultural construction in this society and in this shrine. Like the great majority of patients with depression in Chinese culture, this patient did not admit to being depressed. Rather he presented physical complaints, some of which were biological concomitants of his primary affective disorder. His concern was with these and with the business failure he had suffered. Not only is it unlikely that he had ever expressed his depressed affect before, it is also unlikely that his family had ever confronted him with what was such an obvious but psychoculturally dangerous problem. To have done so would have caused great embarassment, made the patient (the family head) lose face, and gone against basic cultural rules governing the communication of emotion. Indeed, had this patient seen a Chinese-style or Western-style doctor he almost certainly would have received the culturally appropriate label of neurasthenia, even if they secretly diagnosed and treated his depression, so that he could occupy a socially legitimate medical sick role rather than a highly stigmatized psychiatric sick role.

With this in mind, we can appreciate that here is an instance in which the healer provided the patient with an explanation, socially endorsed by the shrine, that allowed him to recognize his problem for what it was, and at the same time provided an appropriate cultural model that could be used to treat him. The fact that the patient used the word "depressed" to refer to himself is of great significance. The god told him he was depressed, and what is more, gave him a supernaturally meaningful explanation; one that the patient could understand and to which he would know how to react. The god also sanctioned the business reverses in the most culturally appropriate way, by blaming them on bad fate. And the *tâng-ki* provided treatment for the hungry ghost, the bad fate, and even for the physical complaints, which he discounted and reassured the patient he need not worry about, but which he nonetheless treated with the prescription for Chinese medicine. The therapist's explanations were sanctioned both by their sacred source and by the social ethos of the shrine, where explanations such as bad fate and hungry ghosts are more real than biological phenomena. Each explanation was linked to a treatment, and the more treatment given the better, but the therapist cannot simply diagnose and not treat, or place responsibility for treatment on the patient alone.

It is important to see these explanations as anchored in this shrine's particular clinical reality. There was really nothing exceptional about the therapist's use of these ideas—they are basic concepts in the cognitive system of sacred folk healing in Taiwan, and are also part of widespread popular beliefs. (I grant, of course, that the *tâng-ki's* skill came in communicating all of this in a clinically effective way to the patient.) Therefore, they are explanations that convey personal and social meaning to the patient, his family, and the other people in the shrine. Whereas the label "depression" could not be used by the patient or his family, it could be used by the god. It is unlikely that the patient would have accepted this diagnosis as readily elsewhere, and many patients attending the Psychiatry Outpatient Clinic at National Taiwan University Hospital do not accept this label when it is applied by a psychiatrist. Nor could a psychiatrist sensitive to these issues have given the same explanation in the clinic and gotten away with it. Not even the *tâng-ki* can have the same impact outside the appropriate setting. (I was told that on several occasions shamans were invited onto psychiatric wards to treat patients, but did not have a beneficial effect.) When these explanations are lifted out of the social reality they are embedded in, they seem trite and flimsy because they have lost their meaning and their reality. They don't amount to much in an academic seminar room. For the power of the explanation is precisely that social reality, the culturally constructed clinical world, which functions as the "real world" for shaman and patient. In this sense, it is the clinical reality, not the clinician, which is effective. Here, in an instance much more striking than what usually happens in even a *tâng-ki*'s shrine, the explanation itself is therapeutic.

Several weeks later the same *tâng-ki* treated the following case: an obese, elderly female who had returned again and again to his clinic for a multiplicity of seemingly endless and usually vague and different physical complaints. I diagnosed this lady as suffering from hysteria. She also had been using the services of a number of Chinese-style and Western-style doctors. In the U.S., such "chronic functional" patients are the bane of medical clinics. They do not do well in psychotherapy, since it is the somatic complaints not psychological issues they wish to talk about. In Taiwan, such patients are part of an enormous group of cases of somatization which may account for as much as 50 percent of all general medical practice.

This patient had spent twenty minutes telling everyone in the shrine about her complaints, and remarking that the Chinese medicines the *tâng-ki* gave her had been of no help. She clearly was delighted (just as patients with chronic functional complaints are in medical clinics in the U.S.) at demonstrating that nothing could help her problems, and that there was no end to the physical problems she could report. Before the séance began, the *tâng-ki* was clearly irritated, and I found myself responding in much the same way:

Client: "I wish to ask about my illness."

Tâng-ki: "You are so fat who will believe you have illness. You want to eat, you want everything to go smoothly and be easy."

Client: "I feel discomfort."

Tâng-ki: "This year is very unlucky for you. Mind your own business, don't mind others. Don't quarrel with others. Recently, you get angry with people too easily. Do you know this?" (The *tâng-ki* had heard the woman criticize her husband and children for various things, and also gossip about her family problems before the séance.)

Client: "I didn't know. I am thinner than before." (The client begins to relate a long list of symptoms, but the *tâng-ki* breaks in and prevents her from going on by singing loudly.)

Tâng-ki: "To be thinner is better for you."

Client: "Do I have pain in my abdomen?"

(A sacred folk practitioner in Chinese culture should be able to tell the client his symptoms because of the god's reputed ability to see them, just as the popular ideology holds that a Chinese-style doctor can tell symptoms from the pulse alone. This patient is challenging the *tâng-ki*.)

Tâng-ki: "Not only pain in the abdomen. You have many other symptoms. I won't tell you. I will prescribe medicine for you. I won't tell you about your other symptoms so that you don't worry so much about your illnesses."

Client: "I had physical pain yesterday and could not walk. . ."

Tâng-ki: "I know! I know! Even now you feel like you don't want to walk."

Client: "Do I have pain in the stomach? I have taken so much medicine for my stomach problems."

Tâng-ki: "Finished! Finished! You shouldn't take stomach medicine because your symptoms will go to other places from now on."

(The patient had been acting in her usual fashion, listing one problem and about to go on from there, but she was taken aback by the *tâng-ki*'s remark: she seemed embarrassed and she laughed. The *tâng-ki* sang out the prescription, indicating that the session had ended.)

This example illustrates several features. First, it suggests that this group of patients seems to elicit the same annoyance from clinicians worldwide. Second, to understand the *tâng-ki*'s response here, it must be seen in its clinical context. Though annoyed by her behavior the *tâng-ki* recognizes that this troublesome patient has come with problems for him to treat, and I think he even saw that complaining too much about symptoms (hypochondriasis) was part of her illness. He responded by giving her a prescription. Not to have done so would have been to have acted "unprofessionally." It would not have been expected of the god. Third, within the limits of his skills he managed this case with considerable psychological insight. Many other *tâng-ki*s and Western-style and Chinese-style doctors would have performed much worse under these difficult circumstances. Again he is aided by the socially constructed reality within which he operates: the god can get away with calling the patient fat, criticizing her faults, and even implying strongly at the end that she would purposefully defeat the treatment, because he is the god. Not many other situations in Taiwan would legitimize such behavior. If a physician said these things the patient might have been outraged. Furthermore, several times the *tâng-ki* skillfully manipulated his audience to laugh at the patient; at the very end this seemed to help the patient laugh at herself. In fact, when this session ended, the patient bantered lightly with other clients and assistants, even criticizing herself for her tendency to worry about her health so much. I doubt this session had any lasting effect, but I also doubt that this patient will present herself again in this shrine in her habitual style, though she might do so elsewhere. Since modern psychiatry has very little to offer such a patient, I do not feel I have the right to criticize the *tâng-ki* for not treating her psychopathology and chronic abuse of the sick role. In this case, Chinese culture, by sanctioning so readily all physical illness sick roles, works against treatment of this particular disorder.

While praising the positive side of this special form of clinical reality, we should also face up to its negative aspects. The *tâng-ki* is working under some difficult restrictions. He is not given time to obtain a full history, and the popular ideology argues that he should be able to divine the symptoms. These are all-too-real handicaps. If he were operating in a small village where he knew his clients well, perhaps it would not matter so much. But in many cases he is unable to obtain all the facts he requires to make the most effective use of the psychocultural explanations available to him. He lacks a method which enables him to respond consistently in each case. Lacking follow-ups he has no clear notion of what works and what doesn't work. And he lacks adequate technological interventions. Perhaps his most difficult problem, however, also relates to the social reality of the shrine. He employs, as we have seen, explanatory models not just from the sacred folk tradition but from secular folk traditions, popular cultural beliefs, and at times even Chinese and Western medicine. He runs into trouble if his clients do not understand certain of these models. When he employs them he is transplanting them to an alien context. For the clients in his shrine the supernatural explanatory models are stronger and more real than are the others. Yet at times the *tâng-ki* would like to make more use of the others and less use of the supernatural model. He has justified this to me by saying "that is what the patient (his word) needs." When he deals with sick people, this *tâng-ki*, along with the other *tâng-ki*s I have studied, focuses in on *illness* as the central problem, and tries to bring to bear whatever he thinks will have an effect.[3] I have caught him, and other shamans, in seeming contradictions, making use of ambiguities, illogicalities, and even ideas which are blatantly false from his own standpoint. This is not surprising to me. As a clinician I have done some of this myself when I thought it indicated. It is part of the explanatory patchwork that is sometimes effective, at other times ineffective. But in the shaman's practice it is not brought under the self-critical scrutiny that should be practiced (but usually is not) in scientifically based clinical care.

For example, on two occasions in the same afternoon I observed the same *tâng-ki* consult with ladies complaining that their husbands were causing them problems. In the first case, a thirty-five year old mother of two complained that her husband had girl friends, wasted money on gambling, and was infrequently at home. She had responded with anger, and when he returned she would scream at him and they would then fight. The *tâng-ki* inquired if she and her children were supported by her husband, and learned that indeed he supported them quite well. He then reminded her that this was important. He told her her husband had terrible fate this year, but it would change next year. She had to be patient. She should not scold him since his behavior was beyond his control, and he was not responsible for it. After learning that she had a uterine coil for contraceptive purposes, he (the god) told her to have it removed and in fact to have another child. I thought this was a remarkable example of making good clinical use of his cultural sensitivities, which led the *tâng-ki* to encourage intimacy (which made a good deal of psychosocial sense in this case) in a culturally sanctioned manner, and in so doing, to act in the client's best interests, while espousing, as is typical of shamans, a culturally conservative viewpoint (strengthening family bonds). My delight turned to disappointment in the second case, however, which reveals some of the limitations of shamanistic healing. In that case, a forty-five year old Taiwanese mother of eight, looking pale, fatigued, and chronically ill, complained that her husband (a mainlander who had retired from the army) refused to work but would not let her stop her taxing work selling vegetables in order to follow her physician's orders and get plenty of rest. This client was as shocked as I was by the *tâng-ki*'s advice that she too should remove her uterine coil and have more children. When we visited her at home, we found her living in terrible poverty with a tremendous workload: caring for young children; acting as the bread winner for the family; suffering a lazy husband who made it clear he had no intention of working and who himself entirely consumed his pension payments; and in the midst of this trying to keep her diabetes under control. She had been further upset by the *tâng-ki*'s advice which seemed to her (as it did to me) unhelpful and frankly dangerous. I have seen other *tâng-ki*s have more ruinous effects, but not often. The social reality which is the great strength of this form of care also is its great weakness, and in a number of ways makes it unlikely that this type of care (at least as it is now practiced) can be readily integrated into a modern health care system. This incompatability includes the fact that *tâng-ki*s often categorically state that their gods cannot be told what to do and not do by Western-style doctors, and is substantiated by their evident disinterest in learning modern medical or psychiatric concepts and practices. My prediction is that *tâng-ki*s will not become Taiwan's barefoot doctors just as they apparently have not filled this or other modern medical roles in the People's Republic of China.

There is a very well-known, and previously studied (Wang 1971), *tâng-ki*'s shrine near National Taiwan University where a resourceful *tâng-ki* has developed a cult with almost 100 followers. These followers attend each night's séance and sleep in the shrine. About half of the cult members exhibit trance behavior regularly. Of these, about five or six are females who themselves are able to heal while possessed by their gods, and would be considered *tâng-ki*s in other settings. These women, as well as many of the other female cult members, are middle-aged or elderly mothers who leave their families each night to pray, trance, and sleep in this shrine. The *tâng-ki* encourages this behavior by telling many cult members that if they do not come nightly to the shrine their tutelary gods will become angry and the symptoms that brought them to the shrine in the first place will return. A research assistant and I were able to interview and perform mental status exams on ten of these women. We found that most of them had remarkably similar life histories: born and raised in poor farm villages or market towns; early marriage with subsequent migration to Taipei; relatively impoverished circumstances requiring them to work as maids, laundresses, and laborers in what they now refer to as "the sea of bitterness" (*k'u-hai*); family problems involving marital discord and/or strife with in-laws; and histories of chronic non-specific physical complaints as well as conversion reactions, dissociation states, and eruptions of hysterical behavior. Several women had suffered short-lived psychoses without sequelae, perhaps best regarded as hysterical psychoses. Several others had histories of sexual promiscuity. In behavior, most of the cult women I interviewed were dramatic and quite egocentric, and unusually emotional, impulsive, and coquettish for women in Chinese culture. Some of these labels were applied to them by family members, many of whom were unhappy with their membership in the cult and especially with the fact that they slept overnight in the shrine. To my mind, these women combined hysterical personalities with somatization and hypochondriasis quite suggestive of the clinical syndrome hysteria. For them the role of cult member was preferable to the chronic sick roles they had occupied; and indeed none were still seeing doctors or going to hospitals and clinics. In place of the sick role, these women can be seen "performing" nightly at the tâng-ki's shrine, where they trance and heal clients. Their trance behavior involves a great deal of physical exertion. They jump around, sing, act out the characteristics of the gods who possess them, and at times tremble and shake violently. At other times, their activities take on clearly sexualized forms. Perhaps most impressive of all is the release of strong affect while entranced, otherwise so unusual in Taiwanese society.

This cult structures and participates in a form of social reality which has been adaptive for some of its members who previously were ill. In this instance it is the social world they have created that has provided socially legitimated roles for their behavior—behavior which had previously been labeled deviant both by themselves and others. Whether we call this healing or not, it represents very impressive psychosocial change, with loss of symptoms, improvement of family problems, and seemingly more adaptive and personally satisfying social roles.

Tâng-kis differ in a number of ways: some spend more time communicating with clients, others spend more time performing elaborate ritual activities; some have many clients and earn much money, others are poor and have few clients; some are charismatic, others are unimpressive; some have cults or specialize, others do not. But almost all the ones I observed were skilled at responding quickly to intra- and inter-personal crises. A final example from another tâng-ki's shrine will demonstrate this.

Well before the séance begins, while clients are still assembling and the tâng-ki is sitting smoking unobtrusively in a corner, a handsome woman in her early 40's rushes into the shrine. She is extremely distraught; she paces back and forth. Occasionally, she sobs. At first, her speech is very rapid and incoherent. From the moment she enters all eyes focus on her. At last, with angry curses she begins a lengthy monologue. A thief has broken into the secret place where her money is kept, and has taken most of her money and gold. All the doors of the house were locked. She suspects the thief is someone they know very well. The client breaks into sobs and wails. Other clients begin to talk with her softly. They try to comfort and console her, but she seems to be uncontrollable. While this is going on, the tâng-ki quickly enters his trance. Before he enters the trance he says loud enough for her to hear: "The thief has no guilt." Other people tell her the thief has no conscience. Someone says: "Why did you put it all in one place?" The assistant tells her: "Don't be too sad in the loss of your money. It must have some meaning."

Although many others were ahead of her, the *tâng-ki*'s assistant calls her as the second case. The *tâng-ki* begins to speak, but the client questions him repeatedly, sometimes angrily. Finally, the *tâng-ki*'s voice and bearing become much more authoritarian. He commands her to silence. Then he tells her: "It is not the gold and money that matter. This is a very bad year for your fortune."

Client: "I know the god knows who did it. I know I won't get the money and gold back. But the thief also took something from my ancestors that I want to get back."

Tâng-ki: "Forget the money and gold. You must lose it. If you didn't lose it, then something else very bad would happen to you. The things are gone . . . you will not get them. They are lost. But more important is your fate this year. You must do something about that. I will help you." The *tâng-ki* goes on to tell her that it is a person close to her who is the thief, and that he stole the things after unlocking the door and then locking it again.

Client: "Is the thief a relative or a neighbor?"

The *tâng-ki* at first did not respond, then he told her the thief would receive a great punishment. The session ended when the *tâng-ki* performed a ritual to treat her bad fate. Altogether the *tâng-ki* spent hardly more than ten minutes with this client. That is more than twice the time he spends with most cases, however, and there were more than twenty other clients waiting. Other clients and his assistant helped translate and interpret. He sent the god's soldiers (mythical figures) to search for her money; he gave her many charms. The *tâng-ki*'s assistant refused to receive any money from her even for the incense she had burned.

This is not a case of illness, yet it represents a universal clinical task. The clinician must respond quickly to crises. His knowledge, his sources of power, the clinical relationship he establishes with patients, the social context in which he practices, all are used to cope with such immediate stress threatening the patient and his family. Illness and other personal and social crises are "dis-orders" which undermine personal and social order. They threaten the social reality of daily living. Clinical reality imposes order on those chaotic events. In exigent cases such as this last one, just as in diseases which cannot be cured, the construction (or re-ordering) of cultural meanings may be all that therapy (and efficacy) consists of. Here the *tâng-ki* applies one of the most powerful Chinese cultural interpretations in his conceptual armory: the idea of fate. This idea is widely diffused in Chinese culture, and its application is not limited to the *tâng-ki*'s shrine. But by its ritual application in that setting the concept acquires greater meaning than when employed in the family context. At the same time, by crystallizing one of the most profound sources of explanatory power in Taiwanese popular culture around the problem, something can be done to cope with this difficult psychosocial stress. Again, this is only one of several different coping strategies used to manage this crisis. The client also received considerable social support, including sanction to reveal her anguish. After the session several people in the shrine offered her practical advice about what to do next. In Taiwan one hears people say that bad fate and bad health need to be "patched" (Gould-Martin discusses this in Chapter 3). This is an apposite metaphor to apply to clinical work. Something tears (body, mind, family bonds) and must be patched; the patch itself (the intervention of sacred and/or secular healing) is a local cultural and social artifact, the meanings and techniques at hand; the act of patching (treating, relieving suffering, coping with crises) is more important than the composition of the patch; and the social construction of clinical reality is the thread that fixes the patch to the fabric (lesion, person, family, etc.). This is a view of clinical reality I found myself sharing with most practitioners I studied. Now let us turn to another traditional type of patchwork.

Practitioner-Patient Interactions 2:
Ch'ien Interpreters

In most temples of any size in Taiwan, there are *ch'ien* or fortune papers. These contain one's personal or family fortune, usually expressed by fragments of archaic poetry as vague and obscure classical allusions. Often the *ch'ien* paper is divided into separate sections, or there are different *ch'ien* papers, covering the major questions people ask about: health, business, marriage, children, and the like. The system of using *ch'ien* begins with a person praying to the temple's god(s) and then throwing divining blocks until they fall in such a way as to indicate that the god has agreed to let the individual ask about his fate. Since each person must first select a bamboo stick with a number on it before casting the divining blocks, he uses that number to obtain a fortune paper with the same number. For most people these *ch'ien* papers are virtually uninterpretable. Therefore, they turn to specialists, generally old men with some connection to the temple, who sit in a prominent booth in the temple and interpret the *ch'ien*. These men sometimes make use of books which contain the *ch'ien* along with commentaries on them.

Ch'ien interpreters are only one type of diviner; in Chinese culture there are many other specialists who interpret fate. We saw shamans do this. They often make use of the eight characters associated with a person's year, month, day, and hour of birth in order to divine his fate. Fortune-tellers also calculate a person's fate by this technique and others based on the Chinese classic, *I Ching* (Book of Changes). Astrologers, physiognomists, and geomancers all read fate from different sources. As we have already seen, fate (literally heaven's fate, *t'ien-ming*) is one of the most powerful explanatory models employed by folk specialists and in the popular culture generally.

But, as we shall soon see, the interpretation of fate is considerably more than a categorical and arbitrary answer. As Aberle (1966) has noted for divination generally, what makes diviners and their explanations powerful is that they predict from essentially unknowable and uncontrollable sources, often quite trivial, which give an almost random answer for problems that themselves are essentially unknowable and uncontrollable, but usually quite important. Efficacy is derived from the application of cultural belief systems which order reality through ritualized activities (e.g., fortune-telling, divination, chĭen interpretation), dependent on trivial and arbitrary techniques (e.g., casting divination blocks, blindly selecting a numbered bamboo stick), by symbolically linking personal and family problems to highly ordered natural events (e.g., the movements of the stars) and the systems for interpreting them that are socially legitimated as powerful sources of prediction and control. The symbolic efficacy of chĭen interpretation, then, is dependent on providing cultural order (Young 1977). But its efficacy also is a function of several other things: the "performative efficacy" resulting from the ritualized activities being carried out appropriately (Tambiah 1973); and more importantly, the instrumental efficacy resulting from psychosocial interventions in the context of the chĭen interpreter-client relationship. In Taiwan, the reading of the fortune only begins with the announcement of good or bad fate. From that point on it is best described as a transaction between explanatory models giving rise to culturally sanctioned psychotherapy or supportive care (see Tseng, Chapter 16).

Although the interpretation is supposed to come from an objective reading of the chĭen paper, this obviously does not happen in most cases I have observed. Furthermore, most chĭen interpreters readily admit that they do not transmit a reading of fate that is utterly bad. They will either lessen the impact of the reading of the fate by a careful choice of words and the use of understatement, or they will ask the client to go back and choose another chĭen paper, telling him that he has not followed the rules correctly for asking about his fate. A few chĭen interpreters admit openly that based on their own sense of the person and his problem, they will reinterpret the chĭen, sometimes changing a bad fortune into a not so bad or even slightly good one. Even if a bad fortune is transmitted, and in fact many are, it will be reinterpreted in terms of the client's particular situation. When really bad readings are given, almost simultaneously the client is shown how he can respond by having his fortune treated (made better) by a shaman or a priest or ritual expert. One group of chĭen interpreters ask the client for his age and date of birth before revealing the fortune. They use these to determine his fortune by another method, then select for the client either the better reading or the one they feel better suited to his problems. When expressed, however, the fortune is read as if it came directly from the chĭen paper, which confers on it the god's sanction. One chĭen interpreter finally admitted to us that he frequently payed no attention to the chĭen paper whatsoever, but interpreted solely on the basis of what he felt would do the client most good. Chĭen interpreters most often give culturally conservative advice, and, as we shall see, advice based on both long experience with similar problems and astute psychosocial assessments of the situation. Although the body of information they work with is limited, they break the cultural rules governing interpretation, which theoretically prohibit taking biographical and situational information into account, by asking about the client's personal and family history and trying to get him to reveal more about the problem. They are not supposed to give practical advice or information, but do that anyhow. Since the reading is quite public, other clients and onlookers are encouraged to add additional commentary, advice, support, etc. Some *chien* interpreters told me they keep in their mind a schema of the most common problems people of different ages, sex, social and educational backgrounds are concerned about, so that they know from the onset what is likely to be troubling their client and what might be most helpful for him/her to hear. Although women still predominate, *chien* interpreters see middle-class as well as lower-class clients, and men of all ages as well. Consultations average only two or three minutes each, though some take five minutes or more.

Below are *chien* consultations from several different interpreters. I think they speak for themselves. Compare the clinical reality pictured in these cases with that structured in Chinese-style and Western-style doctor-patient relationships in the following sections. Here again we see explanatory models used to "patch" problems in which the chief concern is not the beauty and consistency of the explanatory models, but their utility in providing meaningful psychosocial interpretations of difficult situations. They are powerfully sanctioned coping strategies. As we have already seen, illogicalities, contradictions, and even frank dissimulation may be part of these explanations, if that is deemed necessary for treating a particular case. This is an example of practical clinical reasoning which aims at being convincing and relevant in order to resolve a concrete human problem, as opposed to abstract theoretical explanations meant to accurately articulate a body of knowledge. Chinese culture, like other cultures, involves both of these, but the former has more to do with what actually happens in clinical care than does the latter (which is frequently elicited by the anthropologist or clinician from the practitioner outside the context of acute care).

*   *   *

Chien interpreter: "What is the problem?"
Client (a lower-middle-class woman about 35 years of age): "Marriage. The man has a concubine."
Chien interpreter: "Don't marry him. The *chien* says not to marry."
Client: "I'm already married to him. Should I separate?"
Chien interpreter: "Do you have children?"
Client: "Yes."
Chien interpreter: "Does he give you money?"
Client: "Yes, he gives me at least half the money."
Chien interpreter: "Then don't separate from him. It is not good to separate."

(This culturally conservative advice appears to be the opposite of what is written on the *chien*, but seemed to make sense in this case. And after the client left, people standing around the interpreter as well as my research assistants approved his remarks.)

Ch'ien interpreter: "What is your question?"

Client (attractive, healthy-looking girl in late teens appearing anxious and worried): "Health."

Ch'ien interpreter: "Is the person you ask about young or old?"

Client: "Young."

Ch'ien interpreter: "There is an illness. It is not serious. She will recover quickly."

Client: "She has stomach upset."

Ch'ien interpreter: "How does she treat it?"

Client: "She uses patent medicine."

Ch'ien interpreter: "If it is not serious then she should watch her diet. Also worrying too much can make this worse. She should worry less. Does she vomit?"

Client: "No."

Ch'ien interpreter: "She should not use patent medicine but go to a doctor (Western-style) for a checkup, and take X-rays."

Client: "She always uses patent medicine rather than going to doctors."

Ch'ien interpreter: "Patent medicines are not good. She should go to a doctor to make sure it is not serious and to get a full check-up. Is this person married yet or not?"

Client: "Not yet married."

Ch'ien interpreter: "Then she should take care of this now before she gets married. When she gets married she will be busy and there will be no time to go to the doctor, and she will need all of her strength."

(At the end of this interview several things happened: they both switched from the third person and directly referred to the client herself as the person involved. The *ch'ien* interpreter told a joke and the client laughed, she was noticeably less anxious and troubled than at the start of the interview. She left smiling. She seemed relieved. Since medical care is relatively expensive in Taiwan, people avoid going to doctors, and deciding to go to a doctor is often a large decision. Here the client had that decision made for her.)

*   *   *

Client (a middle aged female asking about her daughter's fate for marrying. In this society this is a complex and divisive question, since parents still try to arrange marriages for their children and claim that marriage occurs between families, not individuals; but children increasingly demand to arrange their own marriages or hold "veto power" over their parents' selections. In turn, parents usually have to agree to the choices their children make.)

Ch'ien interpreter: "Does your daughter have a boyfriend yet?"

Client: "Yes. A friend introduced this man to her."

Ch'ien interpreter: "Does your daughter agree with him or not? If she agrees, then you come back to ask again."

Client: "My daughter won't say anything. She has no opinion about it."

Ch'ien interpreter: "You can make a decision only after your daughter has agreed. This *ch'ien* says . . . 'not suitable', maybe that's the reason why your daughter does not give her opinion. You can tell her that the god here said 'not right yet'. What's your opinion?"
(The client did not answer but went off smiling as if she appreciated this interpretation.)

*   *   *

Clients (Several relatives have come to ask about the fate of health of another family member. They look concerned.)
Ch'ien interpreter (looking at the *ch'ien*): "It is not good. What do you specifically want to ask about?"
Clients: "This relative is a man with liver disease. Our family would like to send him to Japan to cure this liver disease. We wish to ask if it is good to send him to Japan?"
Ch'ien interpreter: "It's fine to send him to Japan. To change doctors if the patient is not improving is good for the patient." (This interpretation actually runs counter to the *ch'ien* which should have been interpreted as *no* in this case. The *ch'ien* interpreter, however, obtained the same impression my research assistant obtained that the family was looking for a positive answer to sanction their desire to send this family member to Japan.)

*   *   *

Although I have been generally impressed with the positive effects of *ch'ien* interpretation, there are of course negative effects as well. Especially in regard to health care problems, we see that *ch'ien* interpreters do not have enough information about the case to work with, possess limited knowledge of modern health care, and tend to refer patients either for sacred healing rituals or for Chinese-style medicines. Indeed, one commonly finds the name and address of a specific Chinese pharmacy listed at the bottom of the *ch'ien* paper. (The pharmacy's owner probably donated money to the temple or donated the *ch'ien* paper itself.) For example, in one case, a mother asked what she should do about the chronic tonsilitis of her 20 year old daughter and was told her daughter's fate was bad and that she also was suffering from "fright" and needed a ceremony performed to "call back the soul" and make her fate better. In fact, that girl had a chronic illness (probably chronic hepatitis) and the tonsilitis represented an intercurrent infection. This interpretation delayed appropriate treatment. Nor is the *ch'ien* interpreter educated to make appropriate triage decisions when he deals with diseases. In another case, a pregnant woman went to a *ch'ien* interpreter with symptoms suggestive of hypertension and perhaps early toxemia. The *ch'ien* interpreter referred her to a Chinese pharmacy, saying that Western medicines were dangerous to take in pregnancy. While that is certainly true, some Western medicines are effective in maintaining pregnancies and treating some of its more serious problems, including the one she was suffering from. Moreover, Chinese medicines can produce abortion and other dangerous effects in pregnancy (though these are rare), but this is not recognized in the popular culture's system of beliefs. Fortunately, most patients go to several different kinds of practitioners (including Western-style doctors) in succession or simultaneously. The patient himself then can select what is technically effective and what is meaningful from different sources, but this is not always easy to do. Clients also commonly go to more than one *chien* interpreter with the same question in order to obtain the answer they desire. That allows them to choose the advice which seems to them most pertinent to their case, and at the same time enables them to receive cultural sanctioning for that advice.

Practitioner-Patient Interactions 3:
Chinese-style Doctors

In this section of the paper and the next, I simply wish to describe observations made in the offices of Chinese-style and Western-style practitioners in Taipei. This is not the place to detail the stories of Chinese medicine and modern scientific (Western) medicine in Chinese culture (see Kleinman 1976 and Kleinman et al 1976). Since I had the opportunity of working out my own clinical formulations for certain cases side by side with Chinese-style physicians, and then comparing my evaluations with their evaluations, I shall try to outline several of these comparative exercises to reveal more about differences in the cultural construction of clinical reality.

Comparing Chinese medicine with Western medicine, we can say that the theories are greatly divergent, the diagnostic systems unalike, the treatments quite distinct, and the social reality of clinical practice considerably different. Most of our attention will be devoted to examining these differences. Before we do so, it is important to underline one universal characteristic. As a clinician, I found that many, though by no means all, of the approximately twenty-five Chinese-style doctors whom I studied took a "clinical" approach to their patients that I could readily understand and feel comfortable with. Although the Chinese medical concepts they employed frequently were remote from my own orientation, when a sick person came before us, I discovered that that abstract medical theory was translated into a practical clinical approach which, though still considerably different from my own clinical perspective, paralleled the translation I made of medical scientific theory into actual clinical strategies. That is, we both made use of clinical concepts which were transforms of theoretical concepts; and we both approached *illness*[3] as an orienting problem which focused our quite different systems of knowledge and action and which forced us to search for immediate solutions and to attend to the exigent human problems created by sickness. These mutually shared aspects of clinical practice were undeniable, and were as impressive to some of the Chinese-style doctors as they were to me.

The differences were also clear. If trance and charms symbolize the social reality of *tâng-ki*s' clinical practice, and if *chien* paper and the negotiated interpretation of fate symbolize *chien* interpreters' work, then taking the pulse and especially writing out the prescription are the core symbols of the clinical reality of Chinese medicine. That social reality is not constructed in a temple, of course, but in a doctor's office, often one which is part of a Chinese pharmacy. But it is not what we think of in the West by the term doctor's office. There is virtually no equipment in this office, unless the Chinese-style practitioner uses acupuncture or bone setting techniques, which most Chinese-style doctors in Taiwan do not use. There is a desk, and on the desk a small cushion, usually old and dirty, where the patient places his hand and wrist. Often the desk is out in the open across from the counter of the Chinese pharmacy in which it is located, so that consultations are public occurrences, just as in the practice of *tâng-ki*s and *chien* interpreters. Thus patients tell their tales of illness and receive treatment in front of other patients and their families. Though this is somewhat strange to Westerners, it is part of the "clinical set" patients in Chinese societies bring to doctors' offices. It plays an important role in what is said and what is suppressed. And it reflects certain basic cultural differences in the definition of bodily complaints and treatment as private or public concerns.

The offices and pharmacies of Chinese-style practitioners open directly into the street, just as do most Chinese businesses and temples, their fronts completely open without door or wall. A few private Western-style practitioners' office do the same, but most houses of Western medicine are closed to the busy commercial streets. They are walled off, and are both more remote and more formal. Similarly, although their popular image is that of a Confucian scholar, most Chinese-style practitioners in Taipei are members of the lower middle class. They practice more like local businessmen and shop-keepers than do their Western-style medical colleagues, who, as middle-class and often upper-middle-class professionals, live in a different social world from that of most of their patients. Though Chinese-style doctors usually do not maintain this wide social distance from their patients, they do cultivate a distance between the knowledge they hold and that held by their patients. The ancient medical classics and the medical books passed down in the family containing "secret prescriptions" which stand behind the desks of Chinese-style physicians make this point. Their medical knowledge is special, and access to it is strictly limited.

Most Chinese-style practitioners I interviewed believed their patients knew very little about Chinese medicine. As a result, unless a patient asks, they rarely explain about cause, pathophysiology or course of illness. They may not even name the illness. What they do is to give patients detailed prescriptions. For most patients coming to Chinese-style doctors that is all that matters. The prescription is what gets them the mixtures of Chinese medicinal agents, mostly herbs, which they view as the source of efficacy *and* meaning in Chinese medical practice. Chinese patients pay *only* for treatment. Whether the doctor spends one hour or one minute with them, it is the access to medicines that they pay for, nothing else. (This view is carried over into all other forms of practice— the *tâng-ki* is payed for his treatment—herbal and ritual—not for his explanations; the Western-style doctor is payed for his antibiotics and sedatives, not for his physical examination, history, or tests. Since talking with patients is *not* considered treatment, the psychotherapist (and this is one reascn there are hardly any in Taipei) does not get payed for listening and talking for 50 minutes but for prescribing tranquilizers, etc.)

In a typical case a patient (people of all socio-economic classes, levels of education, and both sexes go to Chinese-style doctors) walks in and sits down at the doctor's desk. He rolls up his sleeve and places first one arm and then the other on the doctor's small cushion. He may give a complaint, but frequently doesn't. He may say something about the effect of his treatment if he is returning for a follow-up visit. Since the Chinese-style doctor spends several minutes taking the pulse at each wrist, they sit in silence while the patient looks around at the calligraphy mounted on the walls which represent testimonials of satisfied patients and moral exhortations from the Confucian classics. At the same time, the physician is examining the patient's face—making an assessment of color, odor, type of hair; looking at the eyes and perhaps also the tongue.

The doctor then asks questions. For a Westerner this is the strangest part of Chinese medical practice and the Chinese-style doctor-patient interaction, because these questions seem so bizarre and often seem to have nothing to do with history taking. In Chinese culture, the popular medical ideology holds that the skills of a clinician are demonstrated by his ability to ascertain what is wrong from the pulse and perhaps from a few short questions. The fewer the questions the better. A great doctor need ask nothing. Thus, for a clinician the pressure is on from the outset to make as rapid a diagnosis as possible and to do so with the smallest amount of information he can get away with. For obvious reasons, however, experienced clinicians do nothing to discourage patients from talking about their problems, and try to obtain the crucial aspects of the history through a small number of questions which cover the chief problems they associate with each age group, sex, and life-style.

The questions Chinese-style doctors ask seem strange to a Western-style doctor, as we shall soon demonstrate, because they make sense in the framework of Chinese medical theory, not modern scientific medicine. Similarly, the behavior of Chinese-style practitioners and their transactions with patients make sense in the context of the clinical reality sanctioned in Chinese medical practice. Yet there are substantial similarities with Western-style practice, which in Taiwan is obviously also affected by Chinese cultural factors. For example, both types of doctors relate to their patients in terms of the Confucian father-son, teacher-student paradigm which determines so many relationships in Chinese culture. Thus, both Chinese-style and Western-style doctor-patient interactions are strictly authoritarian. But Chinese-style doctors tend to communicate more with patients and often demonstrate more personal concern for their patients' problems (see Chapter 3 by Gould-Martin and Chapter 5 by Ahern above). Also, both Chinese-style and Western-style doctors go to lengths to announce their medical genealogies in order to conform to the popular Chinese belief that medicine is a hereditary profession in which secret knowledge and special healing powers are transmitted along medical kinship lines.

When Chinese-style doctors explain things to patients they transform traditional concepts into modern forms. They usually do not use the classical ideas of *ch'i, yin/yang*, or *wu-hsing* (Five Elements), but rather use other words from Chinese medicine which can be applied in a modern idiom, frequently an idiom from Western-style medicine, which they believe their patients better understand at present. Thus, *huo*, fire, is used in the sense of inflammation, not in its classical Chinese medical sense, where it denotes a type of energy, *huo-ch'i*. Instead of talking about a state of imbalance between the interrelated *functions* of the internal organs, a central idea in Chinese medicine and one Chinese-style doctors often use amongst themselves in formulating a clinical problem, they talk to their patients about "liver fire" or "stomach fire" or "brain fire" in the modern scientific sense of specific organ pathology, an idea foreign to Chinese medical thinking. They do this not only because they feel this is what their patients can understand, but also because they themselves have begun to combine their concepts with those from modern scientific medicine.

Chinese-style doctors tend not to be confused by complaints of diabetes, asthma, tuberculosis, post-surgical complications, and the like, although these problems are not part of classical Chinese medical theory. They have developed practical translations from Western medical terminology to Chinese medical terminology, and vice versa. However, since they are not systematically schooled in medical science and since translations tend to be haphazard, misconceptions and miscommunications abound.

Neurasthenia, *shen-ching shuai-jo*, is an example of this process of medical assimilation and syncretism. It was picked up by Chinese-style doctors in the 1920's and 1930's, ironically just when it was being discarded by Western medical science, and made to fit neatly with Chinese medical theory. It is still used to signify a syndrome with multiple manifestations characterized by psychological problems such as anxiety and depression along with a range of non-specific physical complaints. Because Chinese medicine views all disorders as essentially somatic, even though they may have social or environmental determinants, neurasthenia is regarded by Chinese-style doctors (and by their patients) as a physical disorder. This diagnostic category, then, fulfills an important social function, for it legitimizes minor mental illness, psychophysiological disorders, and interpersonal problems with a medical sick role. Interestingly, it is still used by Western-style practitioners in the same way, because their patients frequently express their complaints via this popular cultural category.

On the other hand, there is much in Chinese medicine that patients don't understand, and Chinese-style practitioners appreciate this. For example, one of the most important concepts in Chinese medicine is *ch'i* (vital breath).In a survey of several hundred patients and family members in Taipei I found 90% had no idea what this term meant. As in our own society, one finds that patients possess packages of information which are strange combinations of traditional and modern ideas about illness. Chinese-style doctors seem to be much more sensitive to this problem than

Western-sytle practitioners. Yet most Chinese doctors whom I observed rejected popular and folk medical notions, such as ghosts, geomancy, bad fate and astrological beliefs. These they regarded as superstitions. While Chinese-style practitioners sometimes disparage these ideas, they tend on the whole to be less intolerant of them than Western-style doctors. Patients recognize this, and are more likely to tell Chinese-style doctors their real beliefs, though they will not reveal these ideas to them nearly as readily as they will to sacred folk practitioners.

Chinese-style doctors also possess their own unusual packages of knowledge, packages that combine modern scientific ideas with Chinese medical notions and certain folk ideas with Chinese medical concepts, and which contain different versions of Chinese medical theory. Since most Chinese-style practitioners have studied under a relative or some other "master", have read one or two medical classics, but not others, and have followed one particular school of orally transmitted clinical knowledge, their conceptual systems frequently differ considerably. For example, acupuncturists follow the ideas in the *Huang-ti nei-ching* (Yellow Emperor's Classic of Internal Medicine), while herbalists tend to follow the ideas in the *Shang-han lun* (Treatise on Cold Disorders), in which the concept of the *wu-hsing* (Five Elements), so central to the *Nei-ching*, is not used at all. But here I am going well beyond the narrow focus of this paper. I merely wish to stress that Chinese-style doctors vary considerably. Besides different knowledge bases, some are more theoretical and others much more practical (indeed, I have worked with a few who hardly payed any attention to theory at all); some use many Western concepts, others hardly any; and some are skilled professional clinicians, while others are not nearly so experienced or adept.

One of the most skilled was Dr. Lim, a sixty year old Taiwanese Chinese-style doctor who reminded me of certain experienced, skilled, kind, and quite pragmatic modern medical doctors (usually internists in family practice) whom I have encountered (not all that frequently) in our own society. Let us sit in while Dr. Lim treats several cases. Realize as we watch Dr. Lim that he keeps full records of his cases; that he believes "most patients who come to Chinese-style doctors nowadays come with minor illnesses or chronic illness"; that he feels, as do most people in Taiwan, that Chinese medicines work slower than Western medicines but unlike Western medicines produce no side effects and eventually cure the "underlying disease", not just the symptoms; and that he knows that many patients will not return and that they consider themselves, not him, primarily responsible for their care.

*   *   *

Patient (a middle-aged woman with a hoarse voice who has recently had an operation on her nose by a Western-style practitioner. She has been to see Dr. Lim before but he cannot locate her chart): "I still have a problem with my nose. I took Western medicine and it caused epigastric discomfort."

Dr. Lim (who is feeling her pulse during this interchange): "How long ago did you have your operation?"

Patient: "Three months ago. I still have treatment. One nostril is all right, the other is not good."

Dr. Lim: "Since you know which side is bad you can buy a type of Japanese medicine which you can put on locally with cotton. You can treat yourself and take medicines. That will get you better. You have inflammation of the tissues of your nose. (Here he used the Western medical terminology.) You treat yourself and take the medicine and the inflammation will get better. The tissue itself will shrink."

Patient: "Now I'm still taking the Western medicine for the inflammation."

Dr. Lim: "If your stomach cannot tolerate the Western medicine then only take the Chinese medicine. Take with it 5 parts of the white section of large onions, and eat hot (he means temperature, not symbolic hotness) food not cold food. Do you yourself boil the medicine or does someone else?"

Patient: "Me."

Dr. Lim: "When boiling the medicine breathe in the steam. If it is too hot then stop for awhile then breathe it again. If you do this the tissue in your nose will gradually shrink. It takes about two months to cure sinusitis with difficulty breathing."

Patient: "I still have some discharge from my nose."

Dr. Lim: "Do you go to an ENT doctor (he means Western medical specialist) to have your nose washed?"

Patient: "Yes. I have gone."

Dr. Lim: "After having the nose washed you can treat yourself."

Patient: "I always go back to have my nose washed. Still it feels uncomfortable in the nose."

Dr. Lim: "You can treat yourself after that. Maybe the ENT doctor didn't cut all the tissue."

Patient: "The operation took two hours. The doctor showed me the tissue. The operation was on both sides."

Dr. Lim: "If he cut out the tissue completely then there should be no more problem. Was part of the surgery done in the throat?"

Patient: "Yes. Why am I still hoarse? What is the medicine for?" (Dr. Lim has begun writing out the prescription.)

Dr. Lim: "Medicine is for letting breath get through the blocked nose. From the time of the operation until now have you had tonic with wine?"

Patient: "No."

Dr. Lim: "If not it is all right, I was afraid you had taken tonic."

Patient: "Since the inflammation of the nose is not cured, I cannot have tonic."

Dr. Lim: "Take this prescription for one week. Then the nose will get better."

In this case I think anyone familiar with general medical problems can follow Dr. Lim and feel that what he does is fairly similar to what a

Western-style doctor might do, although certain of his questions and recommendations relate only to Chinese medical beliefs. Most of the time Dr. Lim spends less than one minute talking to patients (including asking questions). Thus, this case is atypical. Moreover in other cases, Dr. Lim's conceptual model is quite different from that of modern medical science, and so his questions and his entire approach become much more difficult to follow and may be at variance with modern medical diagnostic evaluation.

*　　*　　*

Patient (a tall, thin, chronically ill-appearing middle-aged man): "I have great difficulty swallowing sputum."

Dr. Lim (who is looking into the patient's throat): "You have a white spot on your throat. How about the medicine I gave you last time?" (patient did not answer.)

Dr. Lim: "Indigestion?"

Patient: "Ah?" (He indicated he could not hear Dr. Lim's question because of the loudness of the pharmacy's TV which was showing the funeral procession for Chiang Kai-shek.)

Dr. Lim: "Pain?"

Patient: "I can't digest. Also have a little difficulty breathing."

Dr. Lim: "How about urine?"

Patient: "At beginning clear, now white. Stool is too soft."

Dr. Lim: "Kidney is weak. Stomach is not well."

Patient: "I had some fever before."

Dr. Lim: "Your kidney has some fire. Do you do heavy labor?"

Patient: "I drive a bicycle truck." (This is a very strenuous activity.)

Dr. Lim: "Some pressure is on the lower part of your body."

Patient: "I am not strong enough to use my feet to peddle. That causes my stool to be soft too."

Dr. Lim: "Dream much?"

Patient: "At first no dreams. When dawn comes, I will dream. Medicine could be somewhat stronger!"

Dr. Lim: "Pass gas?"

Patient: "No gas. Have an ache in the side of my neck."

Dr. Lim: "How about nausea?"

Patient: (I could not hear his reply.)

Dr. Lim: "Bad taste in mouth?"

Patient: "I still have a bad taste. Difficulty swallowing. Can these symptoms be treated altogether?"

Dr. Lim: "No! Step by step." (Dr. Lim begins to palpate the patient's abdomen.) "Feel any pain?"

Patient: "Not pain but can feel something uncomfortable. Powdered medicine doesn't work so well. Medicine I took before made my urine white."

Dr. Lim: "I suggest three days medication this time." (He wrote out a new prescription.)

I did not follow Dr. Lim's reasoning in this case. The questions and their order made no sense to me. Afterwards when we went over it again he described it in terms of traditional Chinese medical concepts which linked it to a particular prescription but did not explain it as a disease or single syndrome. Nor could I decide what was wrong, since I had not been able to elicit the information necessary to make a differential diagnosis and could not do a physical examination or laboratory tests. But my impression was that I would want to determine if a chronic disease was present as well as define more clearly the white spot in the throat, which I perceived as an acute local problem (pharyngitis) responsible for the difficulty swallowing and perhaps also for the difficulty breathing and the fever. I could not convince Dr. Lim of the importance of doing this just as he could not convince me of the validity of his approach. Here is a basic conflict in conceptual models. It points up the values built into the social reality of clinical practice, because not only did I not understand Dr. Lim's approach, but I felt strongly he was wrong and was giving this patient poor care.

In another case, a middle-aged lady complained of stiffness in the neck and headache. Dr. Lim spent only five minutes with this patient, and during that time asked his usual questions to evaluate the reputed functions of the five interrelated organs comprising the *wu–tsang*'s internal functional system. I could not relate his concerns to my own. I was wondering if the case was one involving an acute viral illness, early signs of a neurological disorder, the sequelae of hypertension, or somatization because of anxiety neurosis, depression, or hysteria. Nor could I determine what was wrong (using my own conceptual framework) based on the information he had gathered (using his conceptual framework). I felt that not only did I have to ask an entirely different set of questions, but that my evaluation would be valueless without a physical examination.

In most cases Dr. Lim and I were in general agreement on the problem (arthritis, low back pain, measles, hepatitis, etc.). But we were not in agreement about what was to be done. This kind of disagreement is fundamental unless the observer shares the expectations and beliefs of the culturally constructed world of clinical practice. Dr. Lim would have had the same disagreements had he watched me practice. But this is not completely fair. Dr. Lim has a niece who is an internist in the U.S. and whose training and skills he deeply respects. Frequently he told me that scientific medical reasoning was more accurate and inclusive than his own conceptual approach. Most Chinese-style doctors I met felt this way. Thus, in the confrontation of Chinese and Western medicine, it is the Chinese-style cognitive framework which appears less adequate (for certain problems) than the Western scientific orientation, and which is undergoing most change: it is attempting to build in elements from Western medical science—but does not do so systematically. This is a view shared by Chinese-style and Western-style doctors and patients also.

Other Chinese doctors I studied labeled diseases with names that meant a specific entity to themselves and their patients, but held no meaning in modern medical terms: *yin-yang* imbalance, summer fever, cold (symbolically cold) disorders. These labels led to very specific remedies. They structured the experience of illness and the course of care for the patient as well as for the physician. Western-style practitioners could neither diagnose nor treat these problems in the terms that are understood by patients and Chinese-style doctors. Much of the social reality of Chinese medical practice is a shared (even if only superficially shared) framework for assessing symptoms, categorizing them, and applying treatment, which patient, family, and doctor use. This is usually not the case in Western medical practice in Taiwan.

Nonetheless, many patients complain that Chinese-style doctors don't explain enough to them, take too little time, sometimes use medical labels they can't understand, and show insufficient "caring" interest in them. These same complaints are also applied to Western-style doctors, but with stronger criticism. Dr. Lim clearly demonstrates to patients his professional competence, his concern for them as sick people whom he wishes to help, and his ability to give them medicinal agents which are sometimes empirically effective. But he often can be faulted for not explaining much to his patients. From a psychiatric standpoint, he and many of his colleagues do very little psychologically oriented practice, although they do give general support. Indeed, Dr. Lim doesn't consider psychological disorders "real" illnesses. He has a somato-psychic viewpoint, one in which physical problems can produce psychological problems but not vice versa. He has recently begun, however, as have several other Chinese-style doctors I know, to see psychological stress as a potential cause of certain physical illnesses. Patients do not expect him to talk to them about their personal and social problems, and he does not do this. Why then do so many patients come to him and his fellow Chinese-style doctors with primary psychological problems and somatization, just as they go to Western-style doctors with these problems? They do not get from these professional doctors the kind of sensitive psycho-cultural responses that *tâng-ki*s and *chien* interpreters give them. Nor do they seem to expect that. Instead, they go to doctors to get herbs or injections for their reputed efficacy in treating symptoms, and also to obtain legitimation for a medical sick role. Patients realize that for care which is personally and socially meaningful this is no more the right clinical reality than is Western-style medical practice, and therefore they go to *tâng-ki*s and *chien* interpreters for another kind of clinical reality. They go to Chinese-style and Western-style doctors, when they want more potent technical interventions than they can get in the social context of folk medical care. As we have seen, they often do both together: an example of a split in the traditional functions of clinical care which has usually included in the same setting (and practitioner) both technical remedies and social and personal meaning for the experience of illness (see Kleinman 1974).

In closing this section, I will sketch other *styles* of practice in Chinese medicine. Some Chinese-style doctors go out of their way to cultivate traditional appearances: long finger nails; scholars' gowns; their own calligraphy and paintings on the walls of their offices; discourses on medical theory to patients; formal etiquette and language; and so forth.

Others, especially acupuncturists, go to great lengths to appear like Western-style doctors: they wear white laboratory coats; they use blood pressure devices and other modern medical equipment; they take symptom histories along modern medical lines; they send patients off for X-rays, blood tests, and urinalyses. In one case I am familiar with, a father who is a Chinese-style practitioner runs a large clinic which employs his two sons, who are Western-style doctors, well-trained in treating liver and kidney disease. The father sees all the patients first. He has nurses who perform urinalyses and blood tests. If patients have demonstrated abnormalities they are sent to his sons for Western-style treatment, and if they have no demonstrated pathology they are treated with Chinese medicine. These different versions of practice point to an aspect of health care in urban Taiwan that I have not discussed—the marked competition by a huge number of practitioners for a limited supply of patients who can afford to pay. The styles described have obvious appeal to different patients in that pool.

One Chinese-style practitioner I studied in detail, Dr. Ao, managed to combine Chinese and Western ideas and practices in a syncretic clinical approach that seemed quite effective and which reminds one of the success Chinese culture has always shown in developing syncretic systems. Dr. Ao is a 55 year-old man who owns a large Chinese pharmacy and specializes in the treatment of women's and children's diseases. He has read modern medical textbooks on obstetrics and gynecology and pediatrics. He knows all about modern contraceptives and their side effects. He knows about the anatomical and physiological changes of pregnancy and menopause. He knows a great deal about early child development, and spends time advising young mothers how to care for children. He uses both Western and Chinese medical concepts, and makes frequent referrals to modern hospitals and laboratories. He does not claim to possess herbs that can cure cancer, something that many Chinese-style doctors claim. He recognizes the limitations of his treatment, something most Chinese-style doctors do not recognize. He diagnoses and frequently treats both hysteria and depression, which makes him much more psychologically sophisticated than most Chinese-style and Western-style doctors in Taiwan. He has created a clinic atmosphere that seems to combine the best of both systems—he is virtually the only Chinese-style doctor I know who has successfully done this. He has done this because he is a clever man who wanted to practice the best clinical medicine he could and because these changes have led to a truly enormous clinical practice that has made him very wealthy. (He has visited the U.S. three times, including visits to several major university medical centers.) He is the exception which proves the rule: the clinical reality structured in the clinics of most Chinese doctors is quite different from the world of Western-style medicine and from the sophisticated syncretism practiced by Dr. Ao. It too, however, is a professional view of clinical reality, and as such is further from the patient's perspective on clinical reality than is most folk medical practice.

Practitioner-Patient Interactions 4:
Western-style Doctors

Chinese patients in Taiwan believe Chinese medicines contain the power of the indigenous Chinese medical tradition. Those who know herbs and other medicinal agents do not bother to go to a Chinese-style practitioner but self-administer them. Similarly, in the popular cultural view, injections are the crystallization of all that is powerful in Western medicine. These two therapeutic agents symbolize the distinctive clinical realities of Chinese-style and Western-style practice. In the popular ideology, which we recorded in our family-based interviews, Chinese medicines are seen as cumbersome and crude in form, difficult to prepare, slow to work, but delicate and without danger in their actions which result eventually in a "radical" or complete cure. On the other hand, Western intramuscular and intravenous injections are viewed as streamlined, ultra-modern, and quickly and easily administered. They are believed to be extremely powerful with dangerous side effects, but are said to work immediately to cure symptoms or not to work at all. These are deeply ingrained beliefs, and they help determine the social realities of clinical practice.

In the popular view (a view clinicians are sensitive to and admit being unable to resist), going to a Western-style doctor, no matter what the problem, should eventuate in symptom improvement after two or three visits (over not more than two or three days) or something is wrong—with the doctor and his treatment. People, even educated people, describe Western medicine as "the magic bullet." And in Taiwan it is practiced in line with this metaphor.

In fact, the administration of antibiotics (the original and perhaps only magic bullets) was the *technological* intervention that had the largest impact on the practice of medical care in Taiwan, as in many other developing nations. (Nutritional, social, and economic changes, of course, had a far greater impact on public health and health care in Taiwan as in most of the world (Kleinman et al. 1976), but this is not mentioned by lay people or practicing doctors.) Along with intravenous hydration, antibiotics had a significant impact on treating the chief killers of infants and children, the pneumonia-diarrhea complex of diseases (though social changes clearly were essential here as well). Antibiotics also were dramatically effective in adult infections which previously had been deadly. But this metaphor has been carried over to all aspects of medical care in Taiwan, including many areas where it is absolutely the wrong image, such as in the management of chronic diseases, in the treatment of the diseases of the elderly, and in the care of mental illness.

This is the popular perspective, and it is a compelling social reality, especially for doctors in private practice. As unusual as it may sound, of several hundreds of cases I have observed in the offices of Western-style practitioners fewer than 25 percent failed to receive injections of one sort or another. There is a strong financial motive here. In Taiwan, as we have already noted, practitioners *only* get paid for treatment. Most doctors (Chinese-style and Western-style) provide their own medicines—sold in small pharmacies on their premises. If a practitioner gives the patient a prescription, he does not get paid, the pharmacy where it is filled is paid. If a practitioner gives the patient medicine to take orally, he does get paid, but less than if he gives the patient an injection. Furthermore, to give an injection is to give the patient the message that you are giving him the best treatment you possess. Consequently, almost all medicinal agents that can be given by injections are so administered. That includes medicines—vitamins, mild sedatives, antipyretics, antiinflammatory agents, medicines used in the long-term management of chronic illnesses like hypertension, etc.—for which there is no good clinical reason for parenteral administration, and for which there are good reasons *against* it: since it may increase the incidence of dangerous side-effects, and can add complications like iatrogenic infection. (Indeed, epidemiologists are now investigating this as a possible source of the extremely high incidence of hepatitis in Taiwan.)

Many Western-style doctors I interviewed told me this was a dangerous practice, quite unnecessary, but one they could not relinquish given the "realities" of clinical care in Taiwan. That is, they feared not being able to earn sufficient money from their practices and the possible loss of patients. Since referral by satisfied patients is how most people in Taiwan get to doctors, it is not surprising that doctors fear that going against such expectations will ruin them. There is some preliminary evidence from my work that the few doctors studied who do not follow this ideology have not been seriously affected by their deviant clinical practice. But doctors clearly are part of this social reality, and are responding to its ideology and the fears that ideology generates.

The results of this ideology can be horrendous. Almost every case of hepatitis (no matter how mild) that I saw in the offices of private practicing Western-style doctors was receiving intravenous saline or dextrose in water. These treatments are absolutely unnecessary in the vast majority of such cases; and worse yet, they might help spread hepatitis to other patients, nurses, and the practitioners themselves. Much the same is done with run-of-the-mill cases of enteritis, again for poor clinical reasons. E.C.T. is the supposedly magic bullet in psychiatry, and is administered excessively and in situations where it is of doubtful value.

Probably owing to this practice, over the past decade or so penicillin reactions increased greatly, including some deaths from penicillin allergy. In some of these cases the only reason penicillin was even given was because the patient had fever, and bacterial infection was a possible, though not very likely, cause. Medical-legal litigation followed swiftly on the heels of these deaths. Awards have been relatively high, and this is terrifying to Western-style doctors since there is no malpractice insurance and some doctors have had to go into bankruptcy to pay off claims. Even where suits have not been filed, families have taken the traditional Chinese approach of bringing the corpse in its coffin into the practitioner's office until the claims are met. This has had a disasterous effect in the last few years. Private physicians now fear treating any case who might die. They turn down cases of pneumonia for treatment, and many other kinds of acute medical problems. Managing chronic illness has come to mean being prepared to "dump" the patient into a hospital before the patient dies. Moreover, recourse is now made hardly at all (outside hosptials) to penicillin, which has become a fearsome symbol to physicians (though it remains an excellent drug if properly used), but instead to a vast array of "new" antibiotics—many of them with severe side-effects but less immediate than those of pencillin. The fear of suits and the large numbers of suits have brought the private practice of major surgery virtually to a halt. E.N.T. has overnight become a medical subspecialty, since its surgically-trained practitioners fear performing surgery. This has put an enormous burden on government and military hospitals, especially the National Taiwan University Hospital, which are carrying most of the load of major surgery and the care of the acutely or dangerously ill. Here is an example then of the clinical reality of Western-style medical practice working against the best interests of patients and doctors, and also against good medical care.

But there is much more to culturally constructed Western-style clinical reality in Taiwan than this. Of several hundred patients my research assistants and I have studied in private medical practice in Taipei, most get to see the doctor for 2 or 3 minutes. During that time there is barely time to express fully the chief symptoms. Virtually nothing is explained to the patient, unless he or she asks. This varies by education and social class. Upper middle-class patients and patients who are professionals or students get explanations; laborers and semi-literate or illiterate housewives get none. When explanations are given they are very limited and expressed in terms that are either too general or too abstract for patients to make much sense of. Even more than Chinese-style doctors, Western-style doctors regard patients as essentially ignorant. As others have shown (see Ahern, Chapter 5, Gale, Chapter 19, and Gould-Martin, Chapter 3 above), if you ask a question in the doctor-patient interview, you most likely will be ignored or given an inadequate answer. Patients realize this and do not ask questions. Over a two-day period in observing ten hours of doctor-patient interactions involving five Western doctors and about fifty patients, I clocked an average of less than one minute spent explaining to patients, and one-fourth of these patients heard no explanations at all. What was explained was on the order of "you need several shots, that will make you better." Three-fourths of the patients I interviewed afterwards were unsatisfied with the care they received because they were told so little, and almost all of these admitted that they had definite questions they wanted to ask in order to obtain specific information about their illnesses and treatments, but they didn't ask these because they felt intimidated by the doctors.

What we have said so far holds principally for private medical practice, but practice in government and military hospitals is not much different. It holds less, but still to some extent, for practice in the local university hospital, where many excellent physicians are faced by a stupendous work load. Patients in Taiwan see the National Taiwan University Hospital as the court of last resort, and large numbers of patients attend its clinics, even though many come from areas in Taiwan that are far away. For example, two interns, two residents and one senior psychiatrist see four to twelve new cases, and usually more than fifty, and on some days more than a hundred, return cases each morning four days per week. These include "problem" cases referred for careful evaluation. In such a setting only the most severe and immediate problems can be effectively managed, and there is essentially no time to talk with the patient about personal, social, and less immediate or severe problems, or to do more than a cursory psychiatric evaluation. This is a great handicap for modern psychiatric care, and it is not surprising that less severe cases choose to go instead to traditional practitioners for care. Because there is virtually no psychotherapy, the disenfranchised patient is one who is better educated and more modern, since he is often unwilling to see a *tâng-ki* or *chien* interpreter. I have seen dozens of cases of masked depression, for example, who were excellent candidates for short-term psychotherapy, but for whom none was available. Many of these were college graduates who refused to consider my suggestion that they go to a local temple or a particular *tâng-ki*, because they had rejected folk beliefs and no longer believed in these traditional forms of care.

At the same time, in medical clinics as many as 50 percent of all cases may be suffering from primary psychological or social problems with secondary somatic symptomatology. There is no possibility that these cases can get the psychological treatment they require in those clinics because the clinical reality systematically enforces the medical sick role and makes no provision for psychological treatment. This also works against the use of effective biological agents for mental illness, as in cases of masked depression —a large segment of this patient group—who frequently would respond to anti-depressant therapy, but who go un-diagnosed.

This clinical reality has a very interesting effect on how patients evaluate Western-style medical care. I compared several groups of patients with respect to their evaluations of care: twenty-five patients in the clinics of private Western-style doctors; twenty-five patients in the general medical clinic at the local university hospital; twenty-five psychiatric outpatients at the same institution; and fifteen patients seen by *tâng-ki*s, including twelve seen consecutively by one *tâng-ki*. All were interviewed at home with the same questionnaire and by the same interviewers. Patient satis-faction for all of the Western-style groups ran between 30 and 35 percent. Patient satisfaction for the shamans' group was greater than 80 percent. (I also am investigating a Chinese-style practitioners' sample, but do not yet have the results.) This is a very complex problem for analysis of the factors involved, but, crudely put, most patients in the Western-style group complained of lack of sufficient time and explanations. Most patients in the shamans' group stressed the importance of meaningful explanations. I reported these findings at the local university hospital, where they were received with polite laughter as demonstrating the obvious. "Obviously if we had more time, we would explain more," I was told. This is not in fact the case: it is the clinical reality (the expectations and culturally shaped behavior of clinicians and patients) which leads to this undesirable situation. I observed Western-style doctors on many occasions with much time and only one or two patients. They still behaved as if there were no time and as if they were overwhelmed with patients, spending less than

5 minutes with their patients in spite of ample time available for much longer consultation. Similarly, the patients involved did not demand different behavior from their doctors under these very different circumstances. Analysis of early findings gives me the distinct impression that under the same circumstances Chinese-style doctors do spend more time talking with patients. If real, this may reflect the fact that in cultural beliefs and social distance they are closer to patients than are Western-style physicians.

These findings need to be balanced against other facts before conclusions are drawn about health care in Taiwan. Notwithstanding all these clinical care problems, the standard of care and the availability of care in Taiwan is clearly higher than in most Southeast Asian countries. Many of the problems described are relatively minor when compared with the fact that in Chinese society before 1949 there was virtually no modern medical care outside of the large cities. Furthermore, the quality of care has in fact improved as physicians have received better clinical training. The unfortunate loss of 1,500 doctors from Taiwan via emigration to the U.S. has had an unquestionable influence on these problems. Finally, some of the problems raised above are not limited by any means to Taiwan, but are found in other Asian and developing countries, and in the U.S. as well. For example, the failure to provide adequate and meaningful explanations in clinical care seems to be almost universal in modern medical practice throughout the world. In research with Dr. Thomas Hackett at the Massachusetts General Hospital, I found this to be a large problem about which physicians tended to be insensitive, in spite of the concern with which it was viewed by their patients. Our findings, yet to be published, suggest that this problem had a significant effect on the care these patients received. The question is inescapable then: could it be that (as our Taiwan and U.S. findings seem to suggest) modern physicians are socialized into a clinical reality which has certain systematically negative effects on the human aspects of care?

The cognitive structures of professional, folk, and popular care differ significantly. When patients and doctors talk, they are translating between different languages of medicine. Those languages are rooted in social worlds which to the actors represent "truth," "reality," and even positive moral values. In Taiwan I found Western-style practitioners who could not understand how their patients could believe in ghosts or gods, even though their own mothers and wives believed in them. These practitioners could not carry on dialogues with their patients about illness, since their patients told me they would not tell them their real beliefs because they would be "laughed at." Just as patients do not understand classical Chinese medical theory, they often do not understand scientific medical concepts, or they combine popular beliefs with scientific ideas. I interviewed families who remain largely ignorant of the germ theory of illness, even though this theory is actively and widely propagated in Taiwanese society. Moreover, many informants told me they would never allow their children to have measles vaccinations since measles involved the release of poison which came out from inside the body only when the rash appeared. To suffer measles meant to let the poison out and never to suffer from it again. To be vaccinated, they believed, was to have the poison suppressed. They feared this might cause major problems when children grew older since the measles poison would remain in their bodies.

By not eliciting patient views, doctors lose the opportunity to educate patients and to educate themselves. But to elicit such views means stepping outside the social reality of modern medicine, and this many physicians (in Taiwan and the U.S.) seem unable to do. This is an indicator of the enormous impact clinical reality holds for the practitioner. In Taiwan, strange as it may seem, it is difficult to talk to psychiatrists and physicians about the impact of Chinese cultural factors on illness and care. Not that they disbelieve this impact, but it is not as interesting to them as the biological perspective they have been socialized with in the course of their medical training. This is a disheartening experience. Again and again I pointed out to psychiatry residents and interns how Chinese culture influenced the behavior of their patients in clearly demonstrable and clinically important ways. And again and again, I learned that more "real" to them than this direct clinical experience was what they read about psychiatric problems from American textbooks. For example, when cases of schizophrenia were presented in which possession states occurred, residents were much more interested in learning about the World Health Organization concepts of what schizophrenia was than trying to figure out why schizophrenia in Taiwan, though able to be diagnosed by Western standards, still differed in presentation from schizophrenia in the West. The psychiatry and internal medicine practiced in Taipei is based entirely on models developed in the U.S. and England, as if the patients and the cultures were the same. Why has there been so little attention given to masked depressions and somatization in Taiwan when clearly they are such enormous problems? Because they are not major problems in the psychiatric frameworks developed in the West. The same is true of the small amounts of attention given to hysterical psychoses and culture-bound disorders. It has been estimated that by the year 1980 close to one out of every four people in the world will be Chinese and more than three-fourths of the world's population will be non-Western. Yet it is likely that psychiatry in those populations will be based then, as now, on psychiatric concepts developed almost entirely in research and treatment with Western populations. This is a product of the cultural bias built into the clinical reality created by modern scientific medicine, and it is as powerful an influence amongst modern medical doctors in Taiwan as amongst their colleagues in the U.S.

Several examples are worth mentioning briefly before the close of this section to illustrate how Chinese culture provides its own peculiar influence on clinical reality in the Western medical sector. Most Western-style doctors I interviewed could not believe that any of their patients failed to comply with the medical regimen. They pointed out that Chinese patients would never spend money on medicine and then not use it. But preliminary analysis of our findings gives the impression, as in the West, that large numbers of patients fail to comply with doctors' orders, perhaps as many as 50 percent of patients we have studied. Chinese cultural values also place the chief responsibility for patient care on the family rather than the practitioner or State; this was affirmed in our family-based study, but much more dramatically illustrated by a tragic case. In a tour of private mental hospitals, I came across a pretty, single twenty year old girl with an acute manic psychosis (her first episode), sitting and crying on her cot in the midst of a squalid room in which were five other women, all suffering from chronic psychoses and lack of socialization and behaving in various autistic ways, several chained to their beds. They had been in the hospital (and in that very room) for more than ten years each. They had developed the social breakdown syndrome, and that was this girl's fate as well, as she saw only too clearly. She was not receiving the proper antipsychotic medications. (How could she when the hospital received the equivilent of one U.S. dollar each day from the Taipei City government to cover all the costs of her hospitalization.) Nonetheless her psychosis was mild, and in the U.S. she would have been treated as an outpatient. Since her family had rejected her, however, and since she therefore had no place to go, she had to remain in this hospital indefinitely; perhaps for life I was told. I was shocked by this case and expressed my dismay to the public health officials who were with me, all of whom seemed incredulous that I could not understand the appropriateness of this disposition. Over and over again they said, "But her family has rejected her . . . it is her family's responsibility . . . if her family will not care for her then there is nothing we can do." This is a tragic instance of the dominant role the family still plays (for ill as well as good) in Taiwan's health care systems, even in the public health domain.

After one gets to know Western-style practitioners, and even medical scientists, one learns some interesting things about their cultural beliefs. Although in their clinics and laboratories they operate with the explanatory models of medical science, at home they make use of a range of explanatory models some of which come from Chinese popular culture or the folk healing traditions. I know mental health professionals who, after professional hours, visit *tâng-ki*s to ask the gods if their diagnoses are correct and to divine the prognosis of difficult cases. I have met nurses, who, under the stress of repeated illnesses in their families, have called upon geomancers to see if geomantic forces were producing this family misfortune. Similarly, there are medical people who hesitate to undergo surgery or any potentially dangerous medical treatment in the lunar month when hungry ghosts are believed to leave the underworld and raise havoc amonst the living—a reputedly very dangerous time. Some first-rate laboratory scientists return to their homes where they maintain the traditional ancestral worship and report strong beliefs about the influence of ancestral spirits on their lives and those of their relatives. Psychiatrists report corroborating support for the contemporary genetic view of major mental diseases from the popular Buddhist views, taught to them by their grandparents and parents, that mental illnesses are inherited or passed on in the same families because of sins members of those families committed in previous lives. And then, of course, Western-style doctors and medical scientists in Taiwan, like their colleagues the world over, are capable of trotting out explanatory models in other fields that are strange combinations of ideas from science, folk religion, and the higher-order, classical Chinese tradition. We see this so commonly amongst ourselves that we take it for granted—but from the perspective advanced in this chapter should we? Are we not fumbling here with a huge problem that touches upon a question that makes us all uncomfortable: namely, the rational structures by which we live, and their relation to our scientific orientations, on the one hand, and our cultural beliefs on the other. What makes this a valid question for this paper is that in the clinical encounter these popular cultural rationalities interact with clinical rationality which itself is only partially scientific, and in part is built out of these same popular rational structures. The study of this issue in Chinese culture is especially germane to the situation in our own society. Chinese culture is a heterogeneous culture where modernization has produced a large array of explanatory models of illness and treatment which are loose integrations of professional, popular, folk and classical beliefs. The cultural construction of clinical reality in Taiwan is the result of these combinations. In turn, the Taiwan example challenges us to look carefully at clinical reality in our own society, an even more heterogeneous one, where plural-life worlds have important, if still poorly understood, influences on practitioner-patient communication and other aspects of health care. Here we are left with a tangle of terribly difficult questions, such as how to "rationalize" health care so that scientific rationality is only one of several alternate rational components in a broader framework, and how to compare the cognitive structures of scientific, clinical, and ethnomedical traditions. While not answering these questions, this chapter argues that they are essential and that their solution rests on an appreciation of the cultural construction of clinical reality.

Implications

Had I additional space I would describe a case I studied in Taiwan which I was able to view in a Roshomon-like multiperspective based on the ways this case was "seen" by different professional and folk practitioners. I would stress not the differing content of each perspective, but the strength by which the perspectives compelled the loyalty and action of these practitioners, none of whom was able to step outside his own culturally constructed clinical world. I could do exactly the same for cases I have studied in a similar way in Boston. It is this compelling "truth" or "realness" of clinical realities which expresses this chapter's chief implications. Recently, a Navajo speaker at the Harvard Medical School talked about indigenous Navajo medicine, yet never was able to recreate this alien clinical reality in the midst of the dominant scientific clinical reality at the Harvard Medical School. Conversely, in the tâng-ki's shrine, in the Chinese-style doctor's office, and perhaps most importantly, in the homes of Chinese families, that scientifically constructed clinical reality is no longer the only way of looking at clinical problems; it loses its dominant grip on the minds of its audience, which has changed from an audience socialized into it to one outside of it. Cross-cultural studies of medicine and psychiatry, and anthropological and sociological perspectives on health care, are powerful and of considerable value precisely because they force us to step outside the culture-bound clinical reality constructed by the social and cultural context we are in, including ·that of modern scientific medicine.

The implications this argument holds for teaching are easy to visualize. This view is a corrective to the dangerous scientistic perspective imparted to many medical students and house staff. It is a way of introducing social science into their thoughts and work so that it can have an impact on clinical care. It is a way of getting them to move beyond this culture-bound professional medical perspective and to integrate into their viewpoint the visions of clinical reality held by patients and families. That change holds important implications for clinical care. It suggests a way of humanizing care by opening it up to the personal and social realities of illness and treatment. It suggests that the perspective of the clinician, perhaps unlike that of most biomedical scientists, must hold together quite different conceptions of reality—biological, psychosocial, and cultural. And, of course, it demands that we work out mechanisms and strategies by which this anthropological concept (and closely related ones) can be systematically and rigorously taught and applied to clinical care, so that, for example, clinicians can be taught to negotiate between their own and patient views of clinical reality.

Lastly, there are important implications for research. I have tried to spell these out in programmatic terms elsewhere (see Kleinman 1973c and 1976b and c). I am presently analyzing data from a comparative study, attempting to quantify the cognitive and communicative dimensions of clinical realities and their impact on measurable health care outcomes. This chapter should underline the need for comparative studies of the culturally constructed realities of clinical care. Such studies must bring together anthropological and clinical approaches in cross-cultural field work. That such a comparative clinical venture is required, regardless of the evident limitations of this chapter, is certain, even if the actual form it will take remains uncertain.

NOTES

1. This subject is treated in somewhat more detail in Kleinman (1973a and b, 1976b). My approach is based on the now classical statement by Peter Berger and Thomas Luckman (*Social Construction of Reality*. New York: Doubleday, 1967), which itself is based on the seminal work of Alfred Schutz (for example, see *On Phenomenology and Social Relations*. Chicago: University of Chicago Press, 1970). Another statement of this position is found in: Burkart Holzner: *Reality Construction in Society*. Cambridge, Mass.: Schenkman, 1968. Translation of the concept of social reality to the medical field is principally the result of writings by Eliot Freidson (see *Profession of Medicine: A Study of the Sociology of Applied Knowledge*. New York: Dodd Mead, 1970.) See also Joan Emerson: Behavior in private places: Sustaining definitions of reality in gynecological examinations. In: H.P. Dreitzel, ed.: *Recent Sociology, No. 2*. New York: Macmillan, 1970. In the history of medicine, certain of the writings of Michel Foucault come close to being historical studies of clinical reality: *see Madness and Civilization* (New York: Mentor, 1965) and *The Birth of the Clinic* (New York: Pantheon, 1973). Anthropological studies in the medical field frequently make use of this perspective, though most tend to focus on definitions of illness or limit their analyses to symbolic healing systems. The patient-practitioner transaction has not yet become a major focus for such studies, but clearly it should.
2. For general statistics see *China Yearbook, 1974* (Taipei: China Publishing Co.); and for general medical statistics see *Republic of China, Health Statistics 1972-1973* (National Health Administration, Republic of China). See Baker and Perlman (1967) for a detailed study of health manpower. For medical statistics concerning Taipei see *Public Health in Taipei, 1973* (Taipei City Health Department). All health statistics for the 3 districts of Taipei City studied come from the Taipei City Health Department.
3. Medical anthropological and sociological studies suggest that *illness* and *disease* aspects of sickness be distinguished. By illness is meant the perception, cognizing, valuation, and panoply of psychosocial and cultural reactions to sickness by the patient and his family. That is, illness means the personal and social problems created by sickness. Disease, on the other hand, refers to the biological maladaptations and malfunctionings involved in sickness. Primary concern for illness is shared by most of the clinicians described in this paper, and is a universal characteristic of clinical reality, though it is weakest amongst professional practitioners, especially Western-style doctors, who often are primarily oriented toward disease. (See Eisenberg 1976).

REFERENCES

ABERLE, D.
1966   Religio-magical phenomena and power, prediction and control. *Southwestern Journal of Anthropology 22*: 221-230.

AHERN, E.M.
1976a Sacred and secular medicine in a Taiwan village: A study of cosmological disorder. In Kleinman et al below. (Chapter 2 above).

1976b Chinese style and Western style doctors in northern Taiwan. In Kleinman et al below. (Chapter 5 above).

BAKER, T.D. and M. PERLMAN
1967   *Health Manpower in a Developing Economy: Taiwan, a Case Study in Planning.* Baltimore: the Johns Hopkins University Press.

CROIZIER, R.C.
1968   *Traditional Medicine in Modern China.* Cambridge, Mass.: Harvard University Press.

EISENBERG, L.
1976   Conceptual models of physical and mental disorders. In Ciba Foundation Symposiums #44: *Research and Medical Practice.* Amsterdam: Associated Scientific Publishers.

GALE, J.
1976   Patient and practitioner attitudes toward traditional and Western medicine in a contemporary Chinese setting. In Kleinman et al below. (Chapter 14 above).

GALLIN, B.
1966   *Hsin Hsing, Taiwan: A Chinese Village in Change.* Berkeley: University of California Press.

GOULD-MARTIN, K.
1976   Medical systems in a Taiwan village: *Ong-ia-kong*, the plague god as modern physician. In Kleinman et al below (Chapter 3 above).

HSU, J.
1976   Counseling in the Chinese temple: psychological study of divination by "chien" drawing. In W. Lebra, ed.: *Culture and Mental Health in Asia and the Pacific*, Volume 4. Honolulu: University of Hawaii Press.

JORDAN, D.
1972   *Gods, Ghosts, and Ancestors: The Folk Religion of a Taiwanese Village.* Berkeley: University of California Press.

KLEINMAN, A.
1973a Toward the comparative study of medical systems. *Science, Medicine and Man 1:* 55-65.

1973b Medicine's symbolic reality. *Inquiry 16:* 206-213.

1973c Some issues for a comparative study of medical healing. *International Journal of Social Psychiatry 19:* 159-165.

1974 Cognitive structures of traditional medical systems: Ordering, explaining, and interpreting the human experience of illness. *Ethnomedicine 3:* 27-49.

1975 The symbolic context of Chinese medicine. *American Journal of Chinese Medicine 3* (1): 1-25.

1976a Medical and psychiatric anthropology and the study of traditional medicine in modern Chinese culture. *Journal of the Institute of Ethnology, Academica Sinica* 39: 107-123.

1976b Social, cultural and historical themes in the study of medicine and psychiatry in Chinese societies: Problems and prospects for the comparative study of medical systems. In Kleinman et al below. (Chapter 20 below).

1976c The use of "explanatory models" as a conceptual frame for comparative cross-cultural research on illness experiences and the basic tasks of clinical care: Appendix in Kleinman et al below.

KLEINMAN, A. et al, eds.
1975 *Medicine in Chinese Cultures: Comparative Studies of Health Care in Chinese and Other Societies.* Washington: D.C.: U.S. Government Printing Office for Fogarty International Center, National Institutes of Health.

LI, Y.Y.
1976 Shamanism in Taiwan: An anthropological inquiry. In Lebra *op. cit.*

LIU, C.W.
1974 *Essays on Chinese Folk Beliefs and Folk Cults.* Taipei: Institute of Ethnology, Academica Sinica, Monograph No. 22. (In Chinese).

1975 Shamanism in Taiwan. *Ethnos in Asia 3:* 56-67. (In Japanese).

PORKERT, M.
1974 *The Theoretical Foundations of Chinese Medicine.* Cambridge, Mass.: M.I.T. Press.

TAMBIAH, S.J.
  1973   Form and meaning of magical acts. In R. Horton and R. Finnegan eds.,: *Modes of Thought*. London: Faber.

TSENG, W.S.
  1972   Psychiatric study of Shamanism in Taiwan. *Archives of General Psychiatry 26*: 561-65.

WANG, C.M.
  1971   *A Folk Doctor and his Cult on Keelung Street in Taipei*. B.A. Thesis, Dept. of Anthropology, National Taiwan University. (In Chinese).

YOUNG, A.
  1977   Order, analogy, and efficacy in Ethiopian medical divination. *Culture, Medicine and Psychiatry 1*: 183-200

CHAPTER 18

THE RELEVANCE FOR DEVELOPING COUNTRIES OF THE CHINESE EXPERIENCE IN THE HEALTH FIELD

JOHN KAREFA-SMART

World War II was almost immediately followed by an era during which most of the colonial territories and dependencies in Africa and in Asia achieved political independence and became responsible for the economic and social welfare of their citizens. As far as health care was concerned, the only models that were readily available were the systems of health care in Europe, North America and in the Soviet Union. Experience has since then shown that these models were not easily adaptable to the conditions in the new countries, mainly because they were devised and developed for economically advanced and industrialized societies while, for the most part, the newer countries were unindustrialized and unable to command the technologies on which the models were based.

More recently, however, when normal relationships became possible between the PRC and the Western World and opportunities for visits to China increased, more attention has been given by public health leaders all over the world, including those in the "developing countries." This paper tries to examine the question as to whether or not the Chinese experience in the delivery of health care has any advantages over the other models for the developing countries.

It is generally accepted that the following are the conditions which all developing countries have in common, in dealing with the health problems of their citizens:

First: poverty. A characteristic of most developing countries with the exception of those blessed with huge reserves of petroleum, is a very low gross national product and a correspondingly low true per capita income per individual. Under such conditions of poverty, the standard of life is at a subsistence level and there are no savings with which to pay for any improvements in some of the basic requirements of health.

Second: in most developing countries where upward of 70 percent of the population live in rural areas which are generally poorer than the urban areas, a disproportionally higher concentration of the already inadequate available health services are to be found in the urban areas. This results in very slow progress in reducing the major causes of illness and death among the majority of the population.

Third: and as a corollary of the poor distribution of health facilities, there is generally a paucity in the number of trained professional as well as auxiliary health personnel, and these are also concentrated in urban areas where they are not available to the majority in the rural areas.

Fourth: a high prevalence of infections, communicable and parasitic diseases is a general characteristic of developing countries, and as is to be expected, general mortality rates are much higher than in the industrially developed countries and the age-specific mortality rates of infants and pre-school-aged children and of women in their childbearing years are also much higher.

Fifth: because of the combination of poverty, or poorly-developed agriculture and processing technology, and of low levels of health education, particularly of nutrition, the nutritional status is generally low in developing countries, and the incidence of malnutrition and particularly of protein-caloric deficiency is generally high.

Last: again for reasons nearly all of which are related in one way or another with poverty, developing countries are generally unable to deal very efficiently with problems of environmental sanitation—especially those related to the disposal of wastes, the control of insects and other carriers of disease and the provision of adequate quantities of safe drinking water.

Reports brought back by visitors have indicated that China has dealt with most of the conditions described above with varying degrees of success but adequately enough to present a picture of health conditions much better than those in the developing countries. It is reported, among other things, that poverty seems to have been abolished. Every citizen, whether in the urban or in the rural areas, is said to be adequately housed and clothed and has access to sufficient food. In addition each citizen is reported to have an equal access to educational opportunities with the consequent elimination of mass illiteracy.

It is also reported that effective health education is widespread and that everywhere the visitor encounters evidence of public participation in programs directed at public-health problems. It is said, for instance, that effective fly and rodent control has been made possible by the complete cooperation of every citizen in the specific campaign against these carriers of disease.

Similarly it is reported that participation in the making of health policies and in decision-making on most programs is extended to all. The members of a commune are said to make all the major decisions about health services that they require and that they receive general guidance about standards, and financial supplements, from regional and national authorities. An interesting and important example is the choice by the commune of which of its members are to be trained as commune or "barefoot" doctors, and so on.

It is also reported that the health services available to the rural areas do not differ in quality or quantity from those available to the cities—with the exception, of course, of regional and specialized treatment facilities.

Although medical schools where Western medicine is taught have been continued and even enlarged, it is also reported that all the old schools of indigenous Chinese medicine have been revived, new ones built, and all encouraged to pursue a serious study of Chinese systems of medicine. Practitioners of both systems are urged to cooperate, and opportunities are provided for continuing education at all levels.

Perhaps the most important observation is that during the years when not much contact was maintained with the outside world, health measures and services were developed entirely within the available resources, and relevant solutions were applied on the basis of local motivation and policies. Foreign solutions were not only not possible but were even discouraged.

The reported Chinese success, as has been stated above, raises questions about how much of it can be emulated by other countries which face the problems which seem to have been overcome in China. It would appear that, while it would be just as unwise to try to "copy" the health-care systems of China, as it has proved ineffective to copy those of the Western World, the developing countries can learn some important lessons from China.

First, it is clear that the basic changes which led to the abolition of poverty and which led to equal distribution of opportunity and facilities in urban and rural areas are based on a firm ideological commitment. Change was not brought about by chance, and once the decision to change had been made, economic and social structures had to be adapted to the new ideology, and health policy was only an application of the values of the new ideology. The lesson for developing countries might be that they will not be able to get rid of poverty as a hindering factor until a serious ideological commitment is made to establish equality for all.

A second important lesson might be not to look on foreign models as necessarily more desirable and always to be copied. A serious effort to find indigenous solutions might not only prove to be less costly but might also result in more acceptable programs and services.

Finally, the mere existence of a model such as China which offers an alternative source of inspiration is in itself important to the developing countries. Often it is the absence of suitable alternatives that leads to an uncritical adoption of the only available model. Now that Chinese health authorities, in keeping with their international obligations as a member-state of the World Health Organization, will report more fully on vital statistics, epidemiological situations, training facilities, and on their national health programs, and will participate in the provision of health advisors and consultants as part of the advisory services of WHO, the developing countries and the rest of the world will gradually get a fuller understanding of the successes and of the remaining problems of the Chinese health system, and be able to extract what is relevant and adaptable to their own problems. Equally helpful will be the increasing opportunities for a full exchange of visits, and a full exchange of ideas at the national and the international professional meetings and conferences.

CHAPTER 19

HEALTH CARE IN THE PEOPLE'S REPUBLIC OF CHINA: IMPLICATIONS FOR THE UNITED STATES

H. Jack Geiger

Great social experiments, like new species which have adapted precisely to a particular ecological niche, are rarely if ever directly transplantable from one society (or environment) to another. Even mere technologies can run into trouble (as anthropologists and engineers alike have learned to their sorrow) as they spread across national and social borders; and if they do prove functional, in the narrowest technical sense, they can still have unanticipated—and dreadful—secondary social consequences.

When technological change is intimately and deliberately interrelated with social, political and economic change, as in the health-care system elaborated over the past 24 years by the PRC, the limits of direct transplantability are narrowed even more drastically. There is a story—possibly apocryphal—of the Cuban health planner who was asked by an old friend from the United States how we might apply some of the lessons learned in the Cuban health experience of the last decade. "Well, the first thing you do," the Cuban responded, "is make a revolution."

I mention these considerations at the outset to underscore my view that there is no way to talk sensibly about any direct and immediate translation of the Chinese health-care delivery system to the U.S. If we accept that premise, we still have a wide range of positions for comparative analysis. At one extreme is the position that, because of profound political, social, demographic and developmental differences which I will mention subsequently, there are *no* implications for the U.S. in the Chinese health-care experience. At the other extreme is the view that there are multiple implications—none of which can be realized until and unless the U.S. has undergone a comparable political transformation. My own position in this discussion is somewhere between these two, though at a point closer to the latter. While understanding that the Chinese health-care experience of the past quarter century represents a response by the PRC to a particular set of environmental, demographic, epidemiologic and developmental problems—a response, furthermore, heavily shaped by political and social commitments—I believe we can review that experience for evidence of goals, techniques, strategies (*general principles* of response, if you will), and then as a series of questions. Do these principles, or goals, or strategies, have any applicability to our own society, our own health and health-care delivery problems? If so, to which segments of our society, and to which problems? Under what circumstances? And at what requirement of other, broader types

379

of change beyond the technical aspects of health-care delivery?

This last question is clearly political, just as choices of a health-care delivery system, and many of the causes of ill health itself, are political, and lie in the social order. To search for the "implications" of the Chinese experience for the U.S. may really be to ask any one of a series of political questions, depending on one's point of view: "What do we do in health care 'til the revolution comes?" or "What can we do in health care to further revolutionary change?" or "What can we do in health care if we believe that a revolution will never come?" or even "What can we do in health care to forestall general revolutionary or political change?"

No matter which question is chosen, in my view, any assessment of China's health care "implications" for the U.S. must begin in the same way. First, one must look at some of the profound differences between the two societies, and then at some similarities, with due attention to the problems of insufficient data and the difficulties of interpretation that may obscure the clear identification of both differences and similarities. Then one must try to extract some key variables or general principles in the Chinese experience that may over-arch the differences and difficulties. Finally, one may examine the ways, and the conditions under which, these principles might be applied in the United States. Only the explicitly political questions—whether these principles *should* be applied, in preference to other principles or strategies with different political connotations—will then remain.

Some Differences

In no rank order, the important differences between the PRC and the U.S. include differences in the stage of development and industrialization; differences in demographic profile; differences in the nature of the major health problems confronted in the past quarter century; differences in the degree of uniformity or diversity in the society; differences in the interplay between "scientific" and "traditional" or folk beliefs about health and illness; and differences in political and economic systems. Each deserves brief mention here, though none requires extensive discussion for our purposes.

By most classic economic or socioeconomic indicators, China is a developing nation—a most unusual developing nation, to be sure, with a limited industrial base established before 1949, and with a long indigenous tradition of scientific and cultural development, but nevertheless a nation still very different from the highly industrialized, highly affluent Western nations exemplified by the U.S. Even after 24 years of rapid industrial development, China—in contrast to the U.S.—is a primarily rural and primarily agricultural society. Figures for gross national product per capita, kilowatt production, energy consumption, or output in such basic areas as steel production range from one-sixth to one-thirtysixth of U.S. levels. While industrialization is proceeding steadily, China is still a labor-intensive rather than capital-intensive society which has concentrated for much of the past decade on the development and stabilization of agricultural output to achieve self-sufficiency, and which has moved only more recently to the stage of rapid growth in industrial productivity. The major and apparently successful effort has been to provide the agricultural and industrial floor necessary to meet basic needs for food, housing, clothing, transportation, control of the environment, and a variety of human services such as health care and education.

Next, even if we rely on the relatively crude estimates now available from China, there are the major demographic differences—in sheer magnitude of population, in age distributions, and in population densities in both rural and urban areas.

Third, there are profound and major differences in the health problems the two nations have faced in the past 25 years. The development of China's health-care system was heavily influenced by the major tasks and priorities it confronted in the 1949–73 period: infectious and parasitic disease, malnutrition, and problems of control of the physical and biological environment. Only relatively recently, in considerable measure because of the successes in the struggle against poverty, malnutrition and infectious disease, have cancer and cardiovascular disorders become the major causes of death, as in the U.S. It is not yet clear what changes in the current patterns of health-care delivery and health planning will be required by these newer patterns of morbidity and mortality in China, nor that the system that has dealt so successfully with infectious disease will be optimally effective in the immediate future.

The next differences, which I have lumped under a general heading of "uniformity versus diversity," are a bit subtler. First, it should be recognized that it is a very different task to *construct* a health-care delivery system (or at least the "transnational scientific" components of a health-care delivery system) from a near-zero base of prior experience with such health care on the part of 90 percent of the population, as compared to *changing* a highly-developed, highly-sophisticated health-care system (in our own case) with which many people have had prior experience, for which there is sophisticated demand, and which represents many vested interests. Second, the health-care delivery system in the PRC in the past several decades had to address highly uniform, albeit overwhelming, needs and problems. It may be, in such instances, easier to act and to design a system to match the needs, to have greater social coherence between the health-care delivery system and the social and biological needs, than in the American situation of a widely varied society, a great deal of socio-economic and micro-environmental diversity, and a great deal of diversity in the distribution of health problems. As a corollary, it may be easier to win wide acceptance of new health services and related social services when the programs are of direct and obvious relevance to major life problems and uniform community needs, as was the case in China, than it is when the "fit" between new services and diverse and varying problems is not as readily apparent.

A great deal has been written concerning the integration of "scientific" and "traditional" forms of medical belief and practice. As we all know, there is a vast literature in the U.S. on traditional or folk beliefs held by minority and ethnic groups, and on variations by social class and region in beliefs and attitudes toward the health-care system, conceptual formulations of illness and treatment, and so on. Nevertheless, I would argue that our primary folk-culture with regard to medicine and health care is a magical belief—that is, a non-rational faith—in the efficacy of scientific technology and pharmacology, a popular belief which is shared and engendered by the practitioners of the system. This belief, reflected in our language in such terms as "miracle drug," acts powerfully in several ways to influence the future development of our health-care system. On the one hand, it tends uncritically to support technological solutions—millions of dollars invested in coronary bypass surgery without evidence of efficacy, as a recent example, or pyramiding investments in intensive coronary care units. On the other hand, it promotes a conceptual resistance to the recognition of relationships between life-style and illness, or between the social environment and illness, and it may be argued that it inhibits the development of individual responsibility with regard to health care. These contrast sharply with the probable consequences of Chinese folk beliefs, and in particular with the political emphasis on individual responsibility for health care and on the importance of social and community factors—a model still held from the massive efforts to clean the environment in defense against infectious and parasitic disease.

Finally, and most importantly, no implications can be considered without recognition of the profound differences between the political and economic systems of the two nations. The overall difference between a health-care service operated and controlled by the State as a social utility, on the one hand, and an imperfectly regulated, imperfectly distributed "free enterprise" health-care system preferentially serving the wealthier and healthier segments of the population, on the other, cannot be overstated. The most significant differences in terms of health care may center on China's ability absolutely to control the payment, location and mobility of professional personnel, and on the fact that the Chinese health-care system seems to be socially rather than professionally dominated. China's ability to control population movement in general, and to assure stability, or at least planned change, in population distribution, in contrast to the high-mobility, rapidly-shifting U.S. population, is also a major difference affecting the planning and delivery of health services.

Some Similarities

While these specific differences are obvious and significant, they should not, in my view, be permitted to obscure some striking, though more general, similarities. Both China and the U.S., in their approach to health-care problems, try hard to be pragmatic and to emphasize pragmatic efficacy—what is necessary? what will work?—even over questions of ideology. An example is China's development in rural areas of a Cooperative Medical Service System that relies heavily on local participation in funding, a locally varying version of national health insurance including some co-payment, and a variety of controls on utilization.

Second: both societies make strong commitments to the principle of self-reliance, and both—though in very different political frameworks—emphasize local control and development of programs and local variation in their implementation. To a degree that is surprising in a socialist state, for example, the implementation of the new, shortened 3-year medical school curriculum appears to vary substantially from one medical school to another, and schools seem to have substantial latitude, as in the U.S., to adapt their educational programs to meet local or regional needs.

Third: both nations make at least rhetorical commitments to the importance of having a vision of what life should be like on personal, community and national levels, and to the translation of that vision into some kind of coherent national health policy. This commitment seems to me to lie somewhere between the issues of political form, on the one hand, and pragmatic efficacy, on the other. It is a statement that certain human services including health care are essential components in the quality of life, and therefore require significant national investment of resources and effort. Among both developing and industrialized nations, there are many in which this commitment does not have the importance attributed to it in China or the U.S.

Some Difficulties

Even such broad and general statements of differences and similarities must be tentative, and when we attempt to move to a level of greater specificity, a number of difficulties—the difficulties besetting short-term American visitors to China reflecting on health-care implications for the U.S.—become clearer. First among these is the lack of specific Chinese data as a basis for comparisons. We do not yet have reliable or detailed demographic data from China. We do not have epidemiologic data. We lack detailed information on utilization of health services, both ambulatory and in-patient, by defined Chinese populations. We know very little about the quantitative distribution of services obtained from professionals (in the Western sense) and paraprofessionals. On another level, we have almost no data on costs or on health-care budgets, local, regional or national. We have only sketchy information on decision-making structures and processes in health care, or on budgeting and policy-making procedures. And we have only crude data on health manpower and its distribution.

The lack of data is compounded by the problem of bias. Like other American visitors of widely varying political persuasions, I have had to struggle against the tendency to see selectively in China those things I expected to see. Even more distressing is the realization, which I am sure others have experienced as well, that many of the lessons China taught me were lessons whose truth was apparent to me before I left these shores. A related danger for the American visitor is the tendency to assume or construct false analogues to his own experience; this might be called the "Take Me To Your D.H.E.W." syndrome. It is easy to overlook that "similar" governmental structures in China may not be similar to their apparent American counterparts, or that they may have different functions, or that both structure and function themselves may be defined differently.

Some Key Variables

Given these differences and difficulties, is there a useful way to approach the question of implications of the Chinese experience for health care in the U.S.? One can, of course, list a variety of China's approaches and policies that we might consider for ourselves, and suggest strategies for their adaptation to our circumstances. I will do that shortly. But neither the specific substantive list nor the strategic agenda, in my view, would have much social meaning unless we first recognize some fundamental and broad aspects of the Chinese health-care effort that distinguish it sharply from the U.S. experience. I believe there are three such variables:

(1) *The socialization of health goals*

By this is meant the belief, in China, that good health has a social purpose, that it is important to be healthy (or to have health care) not merely because it feels better to the individual, or is better for one's family, but because good health is better for the community and is, indeed, one of the social purposes of the nation—what is expressed by the rhetorical phrase "forward together" as applied to health. This sense of community, social and national purpose about individual health derives from Chinese political beliefs about the relationships between the individual and the society, but it seemed to me to be real and immediate. It contrasts sharply with the American tendency, equally politically derived, to consider health essentially as an individual or family concern, rooting its justification in the quality of individual life and the fulfillment of individual rather than social purpose.

(2) *The sense of coherence between the health-care delivery system and the rest of the social order*

In part, I believe, this derives in China from the relative uniformity of the health problems faced during the last several decades; in part from the "public health" nature of those problems—infectious disease, malnutrition and the like—and their obvious relationship to housing, food and environmental control; and in part from the fact that a health-care system was being constructed simultaneously with other elements of a new society. It is, of course, enhanced by the socialization of health goals. It differs from the American tendency to deal with the health-care system and with "health policy" much more categorically, as an essentially technological system unrelated to policies, programs or systems in other fields.

(3) *The adoption of multi-causal approaches to health care*

By this elliptical phrase is meant the inclusion of social and environmental factors as concerns of a health-care system, rather than its definition as a technical, highly specialized and essentially non-socialized enterprise. This is not an "either/or" question in China or the U.S.— we do not have to make a choice either of social approaches to the causation of illness or the provision of medical care or of medical technology, equipment and skills, because it takes both—but as a matter of balance. In the U.S., all three variables, but especially the last, lead to commodity-consumer relationships with the health-care system: the patient becomes the purchaser of a technical commodity, has an adversary relationship in which he tries to get from the system the technical services (there is little social dimension) he thinks he needs, and tries with even less success to get caring as well as curing from the system. The system itself is not viewed as being under patient or consumer control, nor (except in the most general sense) of having coherent social purpose.

Some Implications

What, then, are some of the principles, or goals, or methods that we might consider for ourselves on the basis of the Chinese experience? The list is astonishingly similar to an agenda that many American health workers have been urging for years. That, in turn, is not surprising, both because of the problems of bias and value choice I have already mentioned and because the significance of the Chinese experience, to many, is the demonstration that this agenda can be, has been, carried out with at least partial success on a vast scale, although in circumstances that differ substantially from ours. The list includes:

(1) As a goal, the creation of universally available health care, at a single standard of quality, without barriers of cost, distance or fragmentation.

(2) Emphasis on populations at highest risk and need, with the differential provision of more resources for such populations.

(3) Decentralization of health services to the local level, with emphasis on local institutions responsive to defined communities and populations.

(4) Regionalization of health resources, in a system in which patients move up to increasingly higher levels and more specialized sources of care as they need them, *and* in which, at the same time, highly specialized professionals move down the chain to work for significant periods of time giving service and providing training and supervision in local units and outlying areas.

(5) Community participation and control—that is, accountability of the health-care system to its users, rather than professional dominance and autonomy. To maintain quality, in the technical sense, this requires the separation of expertise and elitism.

(6) The fusion of preventive and curative medicine, of "public health" and clinical medicine, and of "social concerns"—housing, transportation, nutrition, the environment, incomes policy, working conditions, education—with health-care delivery.

(7) Changes in the recruitment pool, and the recruitment process, for health-work training, to make the opportunity available to (and ultimately, to make the health work force reflective of) all segments of the population.

(8) The wide use of paraprofessional health workers. As corollaries, the substitution of performance criteria for credentialism, and the creation of opportunities for on-the-job training and upward mobility in health careers.

(9) The integration of "folk" and "scientific" beliefs and resources in a health-care system.

(10) The socialization of health and health care—the recognition that health has social as well as individual purposes, and the definition of health-care services as a social utility, a central responsibility of the society.

In neither the U.S. nor the PRC, of course, has this agenda been fully achieved, though the limited information available to American visitors suggests that China is closer to its achievement in many respects and is moving more explicitly toward these goals. Furtherance of this agenda in the U.S.—that is, adaptation of these implications of the Chinese effort to our very different circumstances—implies four major areas of change in this country:

(1) Institutional, organizational and locational change in the health-care delivery system;

(2) Change in the recruitment, organization and utilization of health manpower;

(3) Change in the professional educational system; and

(4) Change in two aspects of the relationship between the health-care system and the rest of the social order: in the coherence between the delivery system and other social policies, and in the accountability of the system to, and its control by, consumers of health care.

Some Strategies

If adaptation of some of China's approaches to our circumstances is to be deliberate, it must also be selective. Just as the health-care approaches of the PRC may have greatest relevance for developing nations, so—within the U.S.—they may be most immediately applicable in those areas and among those populations which, because of impoverishment and discrimination, have developing-nation characteristics: dangerous environments, high birth rates, high death rates, high infant, neonatal and maternal mortality rates, high rates of infection and malnutrition, low mobility, low income, low education and low employment. Rural blacks in the south, rural Chicanos in the southwest, and rural whites in Appalachia are the obvious examples. To a lesser extent, inner-city areas and the populations of urban-ghetto blacks, Puerto Ricans, Chicanos and Asian-Americans may be useful strategic sites for selective inplementation of these new approaches.

It is in these populations that the needs are most overwhelming and clear-cut. Given the obviousness and interrelatedness of the causal problems, it is easiest, at least in the rural areas, to strive for coherence between a health-care delivery system and the major social needs. It is equally important that these areas often lack any existing health care and human service resources, let alone the multiplicity of organized agencies that exist in cities, each with its own existing turf to defend and each likely to resist the integration of various kinds of approaches and services into a single coherent agency or package.

For other reasons as well, it is easier in impoverished rural areas to attempt to create new kinds of health-care organizations. There are in many such areas intact community structures and community institutions, and a powerful sense of community. As in China in the period of early revolution, the pressures of sheer survival have led people to help each other, to form and strengthen groups, and to recognize that they suffer systematically—that is, as members of a class, or a race, or both—rather than by individual mischance. It is on these existing community networks and structures (of which the clearest but not the only example is the black church) that new health-care institutions may be developed.

The likelihood of building and funding such new institutions, capable of adapting some of the Chinese approaches, will be increased by the advent of national health insurance *if* the latter is flexible enough to permit more than the mere purchase of technical health service as a commodity from existing providers in the existing system. Through community organization efforts, the health-care funding provided each individual or family must come in a form that permits its pooling to build new local institutions and services, and there must in addition be both standards and capital support for such institutions—whether they are called health centers, or health maintenance organizations, or group practices; and their mandates must be broad enough to include not only traditional medical services but also, at the least, environmental and nutritional services.

If the national health insurance funding and the organizational flexibility are such as to permit interested health workers and local impoverished rural or urban populations to create such new health-care institutions, it is hoped—again as an adaptation of the Chinese models— that such institutions would be used consciously as levers for broader social change. It remains a source of surprise to me that we have done so little in this country to make such broader social use of health-care programs and institutions. They are particularly useful for this purpose because they have salience to the population served—they are not abstractions, they begin by meeting real and evident needs—and because they have sanction from the larger society. Simply and directly put, it is possible to do more in the direction of social change if it is done under the umbrella of health needs and health services.

This is not mere surmise. In one program in a black, rural, deeply impoverished area of Mississippi, for example, it was possible, under special and flexible federal funding, for interested health workers to join with the population to create a new local health center to serve some 18,000 people. The health center program included all of the traditional clinical health services. But it also included a major environmental health unit which dug safe wells, built sanitary privies, rehabilitated plantation-shack housing and in some instances designed and obtained the funding for new small-town sewer systems and water supplies. It provided nutrition services, legal services, day care, youth guidance services, home economics and home management services, and an area-wide public bus transportation network.

Equally or more important, the health center's community organization section, building on existing networks and institutions in the 10 communities in this service area, was able to help organize thousands of residents into 10 local health associations, which merged to form a non-profit health council and community development association which ultimately assumed control of the health center. From this there stemmed the development of a savings and loan association, plans for cooperative low-cost housing, and the organization of more than a thousand families into a new economic unit—a farm cooperative whose 5,000 impoverished member-owners developed, worked and ultimately owned a 600-acre farm devoted to the production of badly-needed food as well as cash crops such as cotton and soybeans.

The community organization was not, as it might have been in the Chinese model, called the Revolutionary Committee—but the results of this effort ranged far beyond change in health status. Among the consequences are an extremely high level of black voter registration, the election of more than 50 blacks to public office, the survival of the farm cooperative without federal subsidy, an appreciable rise in income level for the black population of the area, and the admission of more than 70 blacks from the area—many after paraprofessional training and employment at the health center—to college, nursing school, law school, social work school, environmental engineering programs or medical school. These accomplishments, in the long run, may have a substantially greater impact on the health of the population than the traditional health services.

To repeat such adaptations of the Chinese approach in the U.S. on any significant scale—even in carefully selected rural and some urban areas—will require changes in professional training and education, change in the recruitment pattern for health workers, change in the locus of training from the tertiary-care hospital to the community institution and ambulatory facility. It will require health workers, particularly those with professional status, who have quite a different view of their relationship with, and accountability to, the community they serve. To some extent, it will require the recognition both by health workers and the community that health and health care are social rather than merely technical concerns.

It has been noted frequently in the literature that the definition of health care services as a "rational scientific activity" rather than as a social activity tends to serve the interests of its constructors and practitioners, rather than the interests of its consumers. Yet consideration of any organized effort to change this brings us, at the close, to the central barrier to adaptation of Chinese health-care approaches in our own society: the enormous difference in the basic social ethic, there and here.

We live in a society in which the highest good is defined as individual freedom, individual advancement, individual fulfillment and the protection of individual freedom from the power of the society and the State. In the People's Republic of China there is a very different social ethic in which individual freedom and fulfillment, while by no means neglected, are seen as less important than the social good, the advancement of the community and the development of the nation, or as achievable only through collective improvement of the social order. The question is whether we can find some middle ground, maintaining individual freedom while restoring that sense of community and society that will give social concerns, the needs of all of us as compared to any one of us, equal priority. The answer to that question will probably have more to do with the implications we find in other social orders, our ability to adapt them, and the health delivery system we evolve here, than any technical problems of health or health care.

SECTION III
THEORY AND METHODS

CHAPTER 20

THE COMPARATIVE ANTHROPOLOGICAL
STUDY OF MEDICAL SYSTEMS IN SOCIETY

PETER KUNSTADTER

These comments are made under the assumption that the comparative study of medical systems is not a discipline unto itself, but allows us to address questions of more general interest to medical and social sciences. Fred Dunn (1975) has suggested we look specifically at the patterns of interaction between social and medical scientists doing collaborative studies related to practical problems of improving people's health. He has reminded us that one of the difficulties in this interdisciplinary enterprise is that we enter with different goals. If we recognize this explicitly from the outset, we should not be dissatisfied when the anthropologists do not turn out to be brain surgeons and the doctors do not become professional ethnographers.

It is the job of the anthropologists to develop a comparative science of human behavior, and to look at both the sociocultural and the biomedical aspects of the continuing interaction between man and his complex environment. Thus I will refer to both the biological and the cultural realms in what follows, but from the perspective of an anthropologist.

Medical Systems as Cultural Universals

In all human societies from which we have data, some more or less formal, conscious, organized behavior is directed at the avoidance and cure of illness, and at the promotion of health. "Illness" generally seems to imply interference with normal functions, and health seems generally to be considered as a state in which normal functions are possible, but there has been virtually no systematic attempt to discover the content or range of these concepts cross-culturally. Universally applicable definitions of health and illness have yet to be worked out empirically.

The problem of definition is not trivial in as much as we have good evidence of the interaction of culture and illness, and thus feel that illness is in some important senses culturally defined (e.g., in the patterned interpretation of symptoms by participants in any cultural system), and even culturally created (e.g., by behavior patterns which have known associations with risks of illness, such as smoking in our culture, or hunting lions in Africa). We also know there is a biological component of at least some illnesses which we feel is universal, not subject to cultural re-interpretation (e.g., the relationship between smallpox disease and smallpox virus conforms to Koch's postulates in New Delhi, just as well as in New York).

It is a mistake, but an understandable one, to confine our concern as anthropologists to formal, conscious, purposive behavior. It is undoubtedly true that there are aspects of behavior which may not be recognized or intended as such by the participants, but which nevertheless affect the health of the members of the society.[1] Sociocultural anthropologists whose work is contained in this book, not surprisingly, have stressed the cultural analysis of the first kind of behavior (consciously directed at health and illness) and have been concerned with it as a symbolic system, rather than the much more difficult job of examining the biomedical, epidemiological and ecological health consequences of all patterned human behavior, regardless of the intentions and understanding of the participants. The intrinsic difficulty of this task, the fact that it cuts across disciplines involving different theories, methods, techniques and purposes explains why anthropologists have tended to stick to analyses of cultural aspects of medical systems, rather than looking at sick people per se.

This suggests a large field remains for collaboration between medical and social scientists in describing the health systems (holistically conceived), and how they function ecologically, epidemiologically or biomedically. If, as Kleinman asserts (Chapter 21) following Alland (1970), Dubos (1965) and others, the medical system is to be viewed as having biologically adaptive functions (presumably for the individual, the population, and the species) this perspective must be pursued systematically. Comparative studies of medical systems must consider the parallel evolution of man as a social and cultural being and the evolution of man's diseases (Fenner 1971, Kunstadter 1972: 315–326).

Medical Systems and Cognitive Systems

The symbolic-cultural analysis of medical systems as cognitive systems is obviously well under way, but where can it lead us? For example, what difference does it make if there are parallels between cosmology and beliefs about the body and healing, or if there are incongruities between these thought systems? Do people really try to organize their thoughts and their behavior consistently, and what difference does it make if they do not or cannot? Who actually does the organizing, just the literati, or people in general? We have several suggestions from the papers in this book, but are left with many unanswered questions about what I take to be basic aspects of the way people think. These are common questions in anthropology and other social sciences. Comparative studies of medical systems are an excellent place to look for answers because we have found both theoretical (cognitive) and practical (behavioral) components in the systems we have examined in this book, and we have identified more or less clearly the scientific, scholarly, popular and folk levels of theory and practice. Further exploration is required to define these levels, and exactly who believes in them, and who acts under what circumstances in accord (or discord) with them.

One job of anthropologists is to classify behavior and look for common features in the welter of cultural differences. We are no longer content to classify "primitive medicine" in terms of the disease causes such as "spirit intrusion" or "soul loss," etc. as mere culture traits (Clements 1932), and several of the papers in this book attempt to look at the thought processes involved in responses to illness. A thought process which seems to underlie Burmese, Chinese and Thai responses to some illnesses may be outlined in the following paradigm:

(1) There is no necessary relationship between symptom and underlying cause.

(2) It is essential to know the cause in order to select the proper treatment.

(3) The correctness or incorrectness of the diagnosis of the underlying cause will be shown in the response of the patient. Alleviation of the symptoms indicates the correct diagnosis was made (cf. Ahern: Chapter 5; Kunstadter: Chapter 9 ; and Spiro: Chapter 10; all in this volume).[2]

Given the variability in the course of most illnesses, all causes which might be proposed will, from time to time, be given some support, but no cause will be correct all the time. Perhaps this thought process itself is the basis of the existence or persistence of plural, parallel causal schemes in the medical systems described in this book.[3] The paradigm outlined above suggests that the ability to control (or to appear to control, by relief of symptoms) is equated with the ability to name and thus understand (i.e., to "know" the correct cause). This is a "labeling theory" discussed by Ahern, citing Levi-Strauss, not quite the same use of the term "labeling theory" in which ascribing a name to a condition determines the social reaction to that condition (e.g., alcoholism or drug abuse may be "labeled" either a disease, and thus subject to medical treatment, or a crime, and thus subject to police and judicial treatment). If either argument is correct, it suggests that the comparative study of cognitive processes associated with medical systems is one important source for the study of causal thinking as applied to instrumental tasks. Similar thought patterns should be sought in other areas, for example agriculture or hunting, in which people have accumulated practical knowledge, but in which they have imperfect control. As both Kleinman (Chapter 21) and Mendelsohn (Chapter 22) imply, we should look at the ways in which the technical practical knowlege and the thought and reasoning patterns are combined.

Professor Spiro (Chapter 10) has suggested that the "rationality" we have reported repeatedly in Chinese, Indian, Burman and Thai medical systems is a "primitive way of thinking." This suggests that medical systems in their historical and cultural settings are important places to look for the emergence of scientific thinking. A similar theme is foreshadowed in Kleinman's discussion (Chapter 21) of the dichotomy between "traditional" and "modern scientific" medical systems, and Mendelsohn's discussion (Chapter 22) of the emergence of scientific medicine in the West. The discussion needs to be pursued further for both practical and theoretical reasons. Except in rare instances, we do not know the extent to which medical *practice* (as distinct from medical *research* and public health) is "scientific" even in the West, and in fact we need to examine in detail the context in which the term "scientific medicine" can be properly used. If science is the attempt to use specified methods to arrive at verifiable generalizations, perhaps it can be argued that medicine as practiced in the West is more properly described as an art (application of techniques to *particular cases*), whereas the medical system of the PRC, as exemplified in the venereal disease control program (Worth 1975:481-483) is one of perhaps the world's largest-scale (though perhaps imperfect) integrated uses of scientific medicine (application to individuals and *populations* of decisions arrived at on the basis of probabilities, with results tested according to defined rules).

Ahern and Porkert on the one hand, and myself seem to be on different sides of the question of cognitive dissonance (as represented by multiple and perhaps inconsistent medical theories), as a determinant of behavior, including acceptance or rejection of "Western" or "modern scientific" medicine, and as productive of stability and instability in thought or action. I believe it is a mistake to rely, as an explanatory hypothesis, on the tendency of humans to bring their thought and behavior patterns into strict consonance or orthodoxy. Surely some people try to do this (often the literati in some societies) but clearly not all people do so. All the systems described in this book include explicit or implicit examples of multiple subsystems, and perhaps it is time we consider heterodoxy as normal, and orthodoxy or homogeneity as unusual and abnormal. The comparative study of medical systems in societies is, in fact, an ideal locus for the study of the roles of orthodoxy and reform movements and the literati who create them, versus the cultural pluralism which seems characteristic of all large-scale societies and many, perhaps all, small-scale ones. Beyond the empirical observation that multiple systems of medical thought and action co-exist, we can note that medical systems of thought and action always deal with uncertainty of outcome in an atmosphere of emotional tension. Perhaps we can go beyond Malinowski, magic, and game theory here to hypothesize that plural systems of thought and action will co-exist wherever such uncertainty and tension exist. In order to test such an hypothesis, and in order to understand the structures and function of medical institutions, our comparative study of medical institutions must consider comparisons with other (non-medical) institutions, as well as searching for cross-cultural regularities in medical institutions themselves.

One task of anthropologists since the days of Tylor (1899) has been to explain the perpetuation of cognitive systems and their associated behavior, even when they seem to be "outmoded" (survivals). How does the existence of alternative intrepretations or courses of action influence the evaluation and perpetuation of the cognitive system and its associated patterns of behavior? Obeyesekere (Chapter 12) has suggested that traditional cosmologies provide a clue to the future of any society's medical system, since they represent very widely and deeply held patterns of thought. Thus, he implies, they will tend to persist at least in some contexts, with regard to some categories of behavior, even in the presence of objective proof that other theories explain more and other techniques derived from these theories work· better than those related to the traditional cosmology. This theory of cultural inertia deserves to be examined in further detail in the context of medical system changes.

Jack Dull (1975) from the perspective of Chinese history, has raised a number of points with immediate relevance for comparative anthropological studies of medicine in society. He correctly reminds us that texts (which may represent ideals of medical practice) do not necessarily indicate how medicine was actually practiced, or how the practitioners of medicine were organized. The anthropological contributions in this book might likewise be criticized for failure to consider the textual statements and the classical origins of many of the contemporary patterns. Dull also suggests that the question of medical pluralism, at least in China, is evidently quite ancient, and for the anthropologist this should raise the question of how different traditions are maintained, side-by-side, for many centuries.

Some commentators who have written on current conditions in the People's Republic of China have referred to "miraculous" transformations of Chinese thought patterns and associated health behavior. Even if we reject the idea of miracles, and point to the systematic application of well-understood principles of decision-making and action in the PRC, the rapid changes there are apparent. Assuming radical changes have taken place in thought patterns, what does this imply about the basic flexibility of human thought patterns or the conditions under which they may change rapidly? Clearly the recent history of the PRC is a test case in which we may attempt to resolve the difference in implications of theories of cultural inertia versus extreme cultural plasticity. In a broader context, one may wonder about the implications of the rapid changes in the PRC for the persistence of Chinese *culture* versus Chinese ethnic or national identity. Aside from political differences, what are the limits of cultural change beyond which ethnic identity (in this case "Chineseness") will be lost?

Health Systems and Human Ecology

The analysis of health and illness as a part of human ecology has not progressed very far. By this I mean to suggest we need to adopt a view which emphasizes the understanding that medical technology, medical social organization, beliefs about medicine, and the biological environment are parts of the epidemiological ecosystem which determine the distribution of disease in a population.

We have tended to separate the beliefs, behavior, technology and environment, and study them with separate disciplines and toward different goals. The basic orientation of this book and the conference from which the chapters came was to try to look at these dimensions simultaneously. However, other than Dunn's remarks (1975), already referred to, there has been little attempt to put this idea into practice. Perhaps Worth's paper (1975) is the clearest example of an explicit statement to the effect that a people's health is a function not only of available medical techniques, but also of the way in which the society is organized. This seems an obvious enough statement when put as baldly as this, but we still need detailed documentation of how the process of social transformation affects epidemiological transformation. There are important clues in Worth's paper, as well as in Taeuber's (1975) that one of the basic variables is the differential role of various segments in the society. The example which both of them use is the role of women, and they seem to have documented quite well the association between improved role of women and lowered female mortality. The changes in mortality apparently were associated with decline in deliberate female infanticide and the general favoring of male babies, as well as a general increase in the perceived social value of women. In turn this may have been associated with disease control programs directly affecting specific causes of morbidity and mortality (e.g., venereal disease).

We anthropologists have been happy enough to psychologize and assert "parabiological" functions for social institutions (curative or socially protective "functions" of traditional practices) but we have not put these to the test of a well designed biosocial study. Surely the type of collaborative study suggested by Fred Dunn (1975) is badly needed. For example, what are the physiologically measurable effects on patients of isolating curing from all other aspects of life and belief versus an integrated set of roles and processes of patient and healer? Do we really know if this makes any difference in curing people? Social-psychological explanations of the persistence of traditional curing patterns are not necessarily adequate as biological explanations of what they do for the patients, despite the common feeling that Kleinman (Chapter 21) is correct when he says that the loss of caring for the patient as a social being has major effects on recovery of the patient under modern Western treatment.

Social Structure and the Epidemiology of Mortality and Fertility

Jack Dull (1975) pointed to one extremely important aspect of Taeuber's essay. Irene Taeuber (1975) presented some convincing evidence of demographic consistency suggesting there has been some consistent pattern of *behavior* determining the vital rates throughout China despite major environmental differences and widespread political disruptions from the late Ch'ing up to about 1950.

If we are interested in the interaction of epidemiology and social structure we must examine in greater detail persistent behavioral patterns which influence vital rates (e.g., Davis and Blake 1956). They have obvious implications for understanding and controlling growth of human populations, and thus lead directly to what has become defined as a public health activity.

If we are to investigate such matters I think we need anthropological-demographic studies of people in communities, as contrasted with studies of statistical samples of population aggregates. This is directly parallel to what Kleinman (Chapter 21) has urged in the study of the operation of medical systems at the local level. We need to know the patterns of demographic fluctuation and persistence over time. A cross-sectional study of a statistical sample of a large diverse population is not going to answer these sorts of questions which Taeuber and others have raised concerning the interaction between social changes and changes in vital rates. How do people in societies without statistics perceive vital rates? How do people respond, through time, to perceived or perhaps imperceptible changes in birth or death rates and the balance between births and death? Much more work is needed on the relationship between subjective probability and behavior. We do not know what we mean when we are discussing "rationality" in this context, because we do not know what is in people's heads as regards their perceptions of birth and death rates, or their ideas about the connections between one of these rates and the other, nor between their balance and environmental crowding. How do people figure out what to do as regards reproduction in a world of uncertain and incompletely controlled mortality? How *can* they do this when they do not have access to statistics?

The question is one of more than academic interest, since it is alleged that fertility rates will not drop until and unless child mortality rates drop, that is, until the people see their own children will (probably) not die. But how can they recognize this? They have only a limited number of children—is that an adequate sample and do they have some sort of statistical operation going on in their brain which allows them to calculate rates and probabilities? Do they look at the experience of their village neighbors? Is that adequate when they are concerned with the survival of their own children? What are some of the relationships between perception and behavior as they affect the changes in birth and death rates implied in the demographic transition? Is this even a reasonable model of what has gone on in the PRC (and perhaps elsewhere), or have family goals and motivations been replaced or supplemented by goals and motives related to institutions beyond the scope of the family (commune, nation, occupational mobility, social insurance, etc.). What are the relationships between the demographic transition (produced by changes in mortality) and social institutions, for example, the family?

At a minimum we can predict changes in age composition within this basic institution, as a result of the rapid changes in birth and death rates. The Chinese population since 1950 has apparently undergone a simultaneous modification of both mortality and fertility patterns, and also family structure. For this reason I think the People's Republic is a very *poor* place to look at the interrelationships because so many things have changed simultaneously. We might do better analytically by picking some place where only one of these things has changed at a time. Clearly there must be important interactions between fertility, mortality and family composition changes on the one hand and "medicine," or "health," broadly conceived, because, for example, there is a strong and apparently largely biologically-determined relationship between age and parity of mother, birth interval, and successful outcome of pregnancy. Obviously we need comparative studies here if general principles are to be identified so we can learn from or even understand "the Chinese lesson."

Medicine, Nationalism, Colonialism and Social Change

Dull (1975) has called our attention to the common theme of medicine and politics in several studies. Pursuing the question further, we might ask what is the relationship between medicine, nationalism and colonialism? Several papers in this book and elsewhere (e.g., Brass 1972) have discussed "Western" medicine as an aspect of colonialism, and have implied that the "native" reaction to it was in part a function of the colonial situation. Medical systems have often been an important focus of "nationalism," revivalism or millenarianism, but specific comparisons between, for example Ghost Dance religion among American Indians, and traditional medicine in the colonial societies of Asia, have yet to be made. It would also be instructive in understanding the role of medical systems in society to make a comparative study to learn under what circumstances medical systems have been the focus of anti-colonial movements, and under what circumstances they have been unimportant.

Exclusive attention to a colonial historical model may cause neglect of the relationship of changes in medical systems to social change in general, either with respect to changes in the social organization of medicine, or in the conceptual basis for medicine. Medical systems have not been stable or homogeneous either in traditional or modern societies. We should not be so overwhelmed with the association between colonialism and Western medicine as to ignore the general question of interrelations between social change and medical system change. Access to modern medical care has been a powerful motive for social change in general, even under non-colonial circumstances (e.g., post World War II England). Regrettably, there have been relatively few studies of the associations between changes in the social organization of medicine, changes in the use of medical facilities, changes in the health of populations, and changes in belief systems concerning health or between these variables and broader aspects of social change.

Control of Knowledge and Control of Power

Medical systems are, in general, a good place to examine the hypothesis that knowledge is power, and the control of knowledge is control of power. Mendelsohn (Chapter 22) for example, has suggested comparative studies of the social effects of restricting versus freeing access to specialized knowledge. The "science ethic" is one of open publication, but the "professional ethic" is one of restricting the distribution of knowledge to qualified individuals. Are these really essential features of professionalization and science? What are the social effects of changing the balance between these two? Apparently one of the attempts of the government in the PRC has been to broaden the distribution of scientific knowledge ("mass line") and widen the participation in officially sanctioned curing activities while de-emphasizing some of the aspects of professionalism associated with medical practice in Western societies ("red versus expert").

Applications of Comparative Studies of Medical Systems

One of the motivations of Westerners for deliberately establishing contact between different medical systems, and one of the motivations for studying such contact, has been the desire to "do good," i.e., lower mortality through providing health care. Croizier (1975) raised the question of how much foreigners can aid in other countries, even if they desire to do good. Although it is clear from the examples in this book that Westerners can introduce innovations in medical systems in foreign countries, the caution needs to be kept in mind. What is perceived as good by the donor may not be viewed as good by the recipient, may be disruptive of the local system, may fail to supply all the functions provided by the original system even if it is manifestly effective for some specific purposes. Worse than that, it may be impossibly expensive in terms of local resources, and it may not even have much effect on general mortality rates (e.g., McDermott et al 1966).

Having announced these cautions, we can still be sure the attempts will continue to be made. This suggests there is a practical, humanitarian function to be fulfilled in comparative studies of medical systems. Clearly this will require specialized, sophisticated knowledge of both the operation of local medical systems and the science of modern medicine. The applicability of this kind of knowledge is not limited to exotic situations. Modern Western scientific medicine is not the only system available in Western societies. The nature and functions of the non-orthodox or unofficial systems have been largely ignored by participants in the orthodox system, or have been dismissed as superstition and quackery. Despite such condemnation, they persist and account for major portions of health expenditures, and they deserve attention just as much as spirit cults in Taiwan. Their interactions with the orthodox systems, mediated by the consumers, are just as important here as in the PRC in providing health care for the people. Beyond this we need more careful holistic assessments of the effects of all aspects of human behavior and social organization on health. We have accepted the "medical model" of health improvement almost without question, and it is time to consider as well a broader scope social model.

Needs for Better Definitions

The papers in this book range from specific studies of local communities to attempts at broad summary. With regard to the latter, it is often clearly necessary to speak more precisely as regards which medical system and which people are being referred to. The community-based studies clearly indicate there are many medical sub-systems which are incompletely integrated with one another, which may be subject to regional or dialect variations, as well as the variations resulting from recent political differences. In what sense is it even meaningful to speak of something as all-encompassing and abstract as "Chinese medicine"? One result of this book should be to emphasize the pluralistic nature of medical systems in any society, and to suggest that definitions of "the medical system" take pluralism into account.

Beyond the problems of defining the universe to which the descriptions and generalizations apply, Mendelsohn has raised another, and methodologically more difficult, question of definition in reminding us that "medical system" may be a cognitive category which is appropriate primarily to the social system in which it has risen. This is a common problem in the comparative study of any social institution such as religion, economics or politics. Perhaps it is easier to see in regard to medicine how incompletely *our* concept of medical treatment may fit the institutions of other societies, if we limit our concept to current orthodoxy. Contributors to this book evidently believe it is meaningful to speak of comparative studies of medical systems for reasons suggested earlier in this chapter, i.e., the universality of institutions purposefully directed at health, curing and the prevention of disease, and the functional importance of control of morbidity and mortality for the perpetuation of any society. I have suggested that the definition of medical system be broad enough to encompass both the symbolic aspects of medical systems and their biomedical, epidemiological and ecological features. A definition of this scope should facilitate collaboration between the disciplines.

Another area of definition which has emerged as a problem in this book is the multiplicity of terms applied to different medical systems within a given society. The display of terms in Table 1 suggests one of the sources of terminological proliferation is that we have been talking about a variety of things, using an inexplicit and unsystematic vocabulary. (The table is oversimplified in that it is not all inclusive, and does not indicate the multiple uses of several terms.) We do not yet know enough to write a theoretically-sound typology of medical systems. Rather than attempting to bring order to this chaotic situation by arbitrary fiat, I would suggest that in speaking of any particular medical system or sub-system, attention be given to all the dimensions suggested in the column headings of the table. For example, is it true that in any society one and only one system is viewed as orthodox, or to put the question another way, that there is official or formal recognition of the propriety of one system as contrasted with others? If so, the dimension of social approbation should be included in the definition or description of any medical system.

TABLE 1

ADJECTIVES ATTACHED TO MEDICAL SYSTEMS

Ethnic	"Religious"	Historical	Methodological (?)	Geographic
Chinese	Ayurvedic	Modern	Scientific	Western
Burmese	Taoist	Traditional	Supernatural	Cosmopolitan
Thai	Buddhist	Ancient	etc.	Asian
etc.	etc.	Contemporary		Local
		Historical		etc.
		Intrusive		
		etc.		

National		Social Segment	Social Approbation	Social Organization
PRC		Great tradition	Orthodox	Professional
Official		Little tradition	Heterodox	Non-professional
etc.		Popular	etc.	Para-professional
		Folk		etc.
		Literati		
		etc.		

Given the fact that most societies are not homogeneous, official sanction may not be given to a system which is associated primarily with some lowly subgroup in a given society. This suggests the importance of specifying the social subgroup(s) with which the subsystem is associated. Some subsystems have much wider applicability than others, and the degree of geographic spread may also be important in an adequate definition. In brief, we should specify to whom, by whom, when, where, under what circumstances, with what evaluation, with what method, under what form of organization, from what historical sources, the subsystem applies. At this stage, terminological simplicity ("traditional versus modern") is confusing and should be avoided.

NOTES

1. The importance of this point cannot be overstressed, because evidence is accumulating rapidly on the predominance of non-specific social factors in influencing general levels of mortality, e.g., general level of nutrition, availability of clean water etc., whether or not intended for "health" purposes (McDermott, Deuschle and Barnett 1972; Mata, 1977); Taeuber (1975) and Worth (1975)

2. I must confess to a certain uneasiness when using such abstract concepts as "necessary relationship," "underlying cause," etc., and the associated chains of inference from the sorts of observations I have made of how people behave, or what they tell me they believe. One of the issues we have not adequately handled in this book, or in the conference from which it came, is the technique for reaching such abstract conclusions from what is usually very concrete observational data.

3. Parallel or plural systems should be distinguished from multi-causal theories which may involve a belief either in the compounding of several factors (malnutrition *plus* exposure to a disease organism "causes" severe diarrhea) or the belief that several factors may result in roughly the same outcome (several different kinds of organisms "cause" diarrhea, but because they may be sensitive to different antibiotics it may be important to distinguish between them). The latter use of the term "multi-causal" is obviously closer to what we have been discussing in Chinese and other systems.

REFERENCES

ALLAND, A.
1970   Adaptation in Cultural Evolution: An Approach to Medical
       Anthropology. New York: Columbia University Press.

BRASS, P. R.
1972   The politics of Ayurvedic education: a case study of revivalism
       and modernization in India. Chapter 14 *in* Education and
       Politics in India: studies in organization, society, and policy,
       S. H. Rudolph and L. I. Rudolph, eds., pp. 342-371. Cam-
       bridge: Harvard University Press.

CLEMENTS, F. E.
1932   Primitive Concepts of Disease. University of California Publica-
       tions in American Archaeology and Ethnology 32:185–252.

CROIZIER, R.
1975   Medicine and modernization in China: an historical overview.
       Chapter 3 *in* Mcdicine in Chinese cultures: comparative studies
       of health care in Chinese and other societies, A. Kleinman,
       P. Kunstadter, E. R. Alexander, and J. L. Gale, eds. Washington,
       D.C.: Fogarty International Center, N.I.H., pp. 21-35.

DAVIS, K. and J. BLAKE
1956   Social structure and fertility: an analytical framework. Eco-
       nomic Development and Cultural Change 4:211–235.

DUBOS, R. J.
1965   Man Adapting. New Haven: Yale University Press.

DULL, J.
1975   Implications of Chinese history for comparative studies of
       medicine in society. Chapter 38 *in* Medicine in Chinese cul-
       tures: comparative studies of health care in Chinese and other
       societies, A. Kleinman, P. Kunstadter, E. R. Alexander, and
       J. L. Gale, eds. Washington, D.C.: Fogarty International Center,
       N.I.H., pp. 669-678.

DUNN, F. L.
1975   Implications for future medical research. Chapter 40 *in* Medicine
       in Chinese cultures: comparative studies of health care in Chinese
       and other societies, A. Kleinman, P. Kunstadter, E. R. Alex-
       ander, and J. L. Gale, eds. Washington, D.C.: Fogarty Inter-
       national Center, N.I.H., pp. 681-682.

FENNER, F.
1971   Infectious disease and social change. The Medical Journal of
       Australia 1971 1:1043 (May 15); 1099 (May 22).

KUNSTADTER, P.
1972 Demography, ecology, social structure and settlement patterns. Chapter 16 *in* The Structure of Human Populations, G. A. Harrison and A. J. Boyce, eds., pp. 313-351. Oxford: Clarendon Press.

McDERMOTT, W.
1966 Medical institutions and modification of disease patterns. American Journal of Psychiatry 22(12):1398–1406. June.

McDERMOTT, W., K. W. DEUSCHLE and C. R. BARNETT
1972 Health care experiment at Many Farms. Science 175(4017: 23–31. January 7.

MATA, L.
In press. The Children of Santa Maria Cauque. Washington, D.C.: Pan-American Health Organization.

PORKERT, M.
1975 The dilemma of present-day interpretations of Chinese medicine. Chapter 5 *in* Medicine in Chinese cultures: Comparative studies of health care in Chinese and other societies, A. Kleinman, P. Kunstadter, E. R. Alexander, and J. L. Gale, eds. Washington, D.C.: Fogarty International Center, N.I.H., pp. 61-75.

TAEUBER, I. B.
1975 Health, mortality, and population growth in the People's Republic of China. Chapter 29 *in* Medicine in Chinese cultures: comparative studies of health care in Chinese and other societies, A. Kleinman, P. Kunstadter, E. R. Alexander, and J. L. Gale, eds. Washington, D.C.: Fogarty International Center, N.I.H., pp. 443-476.

TYLOR, Sir E. B.
1899 Anthropology: An Introduction to the Study of Man and Civilization. New York: D. Appleton and Company.

WORTH, R. M.
1975 The impact of new health programs on disease control and illness patterns in China. Chapter 30 *in* Medicine in Chinese cultures: comparative studies of health care in Chinese and other societies, A. Kleinman, P. Kunstadter, E. R. Alexander, and J. L. Gale, eds. Washington, D.C.: Fogarty International Center, N.I.H., pp. 477-486.

CHAPTER 21

PROBLEMS AND PROSPECTS IN COMPARATIVE CROSS-CULTURAL MEDICAL AND PSYCHIATRIC STUDIES

ARTHUR KLEINMAN

Cross-Cultural Approaches to Medicine and Psychiatry: An Introduction

I begin by describing the relationship of medicine (here taken to mean health care generally, including psychiatry and public health) and culture.[1] Since it is not feasible to exhaustively review this very large subject here, I will briefly discuss its significance for this book's chief concerns by considering three major conceptual problems that tend to distort and diminish the value of studies in the culture and medicine field. The subject itself can be conceived to include all aspects of the interactions, correlations, and impacts between medical phenomena and their cultural environment. The conceptual difficulties are: (1) the tendency to describe cross-cultural medical phenomena via the overly simplistic, ambiguous, and often misleading dichotomy between traditional and modern forms of medicine; (2) the tendency to concentrate almost entirely upon social issues and thus to exclude from cross-cultural analyses individual behavior, especially its biological substrate and subjective dimension, and also the crucial interrelations between social and psychological processes; and (3) the failure to conceive of the enormous and confusing array of medical phenomena as organized into a *cultural system*.

Following that, I will outline a new conceptual framework for studying medicine as a social and cultural system. This framework, which is presently emerging from comparative medical studies, attempts to integrate seemingly disparate research materials and approaches in this very rapidly expanding but still quite poorly conceptualized field. This model will be related to other models that might be used to study this field and especially to the conceptual difficulties already mentioned, and then this new framework will be applied to medicine in Chinese culture, where it helps to reorganize what we know about that subject and to generate important questions for future research. This model should also aid in assimilating the very different kinds of presentations offered in this volume, since it tries (1) to link a comparative cross-cultural approach with the empirical field study of particular medical systems, such as those found in Chinese societies; and (2) to integrate a variety of social and behavioral science, public health, and medical field research perspectives. Finally, it raises future prospects and problems both for the study of medicine in Chinese and other Asian cultures and the general relationship of medicine and culture; these will be discussed at the close of the chapter with respect to their research, teaching, and practical implications.

(1)   The standard analytical dichotomy between *traditional* and *modern* medicine derives from the study of medicine in primitive and ancient societies. Early students in this field, including Rivers (1924), Sigerist (1951), and Clements (1932), made a fundamental distinction between primitive and modern medicine. They took the latter to mean contemporary medical scientific thought, technology, and professional practice, while the former they regarded as the remnant of an archaic precursor containing two entirely separate traditions: magical-religious and rational-empirical. The rational-empirical elements were assiduously culled from their cultural contexts and touted as embryonic forms of modern medicine, examples of the evolution of science. The magical-religious elements were held to be outside of the developmental line of modern medicine, contaminants from primitive religion, at best precursors of modern religion. Much subsequent research, and the theoretical reconstruction that has resulted, has of course shown these notions to be erroneous; but even the very insightful Sigerist gave in to this bias which not only characterizes early efforts in medical history and medical anthropology but also appears to represent one of the deep-seated convictions of the still largely ethnocentric modern medical profession.

This conceptual dichotomy also led to a division between ethnographic and historical approaches and materials which tore apart the total fabric of medicine's cultural context. Medical ethnography studied the primitive medicine of non-Western peoples; medical history applied itself to the background of modern scientific medicine in the West. The separation was almost total. Ancient medicine was often a disputed borderland between these different perspectives. Erwin Ackerknecht, for example, managed to make separate careers out of both, medical anthropologist in his early years and medical historian in his later years, but he made no attempt to bridge these two fields, which he apparently regarded as two entirely different medical domains (Walser and Koelbing 1971). The continuing implications of this dichotomy for cross-cultural studies of medicine are enormous, since no unifying framework has been elaborated for comparing medicine in its contemporary Western, historical, and non-Western contexts. Until quite recently, culture was studied as having significance for primitive, and, to a lesser degree, historical forms of medicine only. Modern medical science and medical care in fully modern societies were, for a long while, excluded from cross-cultural comparisons, and unfortunately still are even in some fairly recent studies (Read 1966).

This conceptual distinction is impossible to maintain. In part it results from confusing medicine's scientific with its health-care aspects, and also its professional structure with its fundamental social and cultural functions. It is also a scientistic prejudice that has been slow to dissolve despite much recent interest in studying the social context of science. The distinction blurs when ethnographers turn to folk and popular forms of medicine in modern societies (Harwood 1971, Nader and Maretzki 1973, Saunders 1954), or study the modernization and indigenization of medicine in developing societies and post-traditional states (Gould 1965, Leslie undated, Wolff 1965). Historians have further muddied the water by studying the historical development of folk medicine (Thomas 1971), the historical interactions between folk and modern medicine (Foucault 1965, Gussow and Tracy 1970), and the comparative history of Western and non-Western medical traditions (Temkin 1968). Medical sociology not only has demonstrated many basic similarities between "traditional" and "modern" medicine, but has made us realize that the latter is just as unstable a mixture of heterogeneous components as the former. Modern medicine includes within its orbit not merely professional medical institutions, and their cognitive and behavioral correlates, but also various folk medical traditions and the extremely important realm of popular medical beliefs and practices (Freidson 1970). In fact, owing to such work we now appreciate that the modern medical profession, with its social institutions, roles, and functions, is only one sector of the total local health enterprise. We are just coming to understand the other health sectors: folk medical systems and popular medical culture. We have hardly begun to examine their crucial interactions, which seem to be responsible for when patients are labeled sick, how sick persons regard their illnesses, when they seek health care, what kind of care they seek, how they utilize health care facilities, whether they comply with treatment programs, and how they evaluate the quality and success of treatment.

The simple dualistic model breaks down almost entirely when the major non-Western forms of medicine—Chinese and Ayurvedic medicine (Bowers 1973, Croizier 1970)—are studied.[2] For here we find forms of medical science that are neither Western nor modern, but rather different cultural systems of knowledge. They each contain a literate classical stream, preserved in ancient texts and interpreted by practitioners who may often be critical commentators and perhaps even investigators as well as healers, along with folk and popular traditions. Moreover, modern Western medicine has often been present in the societies containing these other major medical traditions for some time, so that it has become an aspect of the total indigenous tradition. Indeed, medicine from the West was introduced into such societies well prior to the development of the germ theory of disease and thus before it itself took on its modern scientific form. Ironically, then, the historical Western medical tradition, often accompanied by elements of Western folk medicine, joined modern medical science as part of these indigenous medical traditions. In such very complex and confusing settings, the notion of "traditional" medicine no longer conveys a uniform or precise meaning.

Because much field research is still conducted in small-scale, preliterate and modernizing societies, and because in such settings comparisons are often made between ethnomedicine and the advanced systems of professional medicine in the West, the conceptual division between traditional and modern medicine has been maintained and found to be useful. Moreover, medical sociology and anthropology, plus a range of public health and medical research disciplines from international medicine to transcultural psychiatry, have failed thus far to construct a generally accepted comparative model that takes into account the spectrum of medical forms designated by that simple polarity. No widely accepted alternative conceptual model has emerged, even though medicine in post-traditional and modern societies obviously is not at all well handled within the old framework. Perhaps this is merely a specific instance of the conceptual confusion surrounding cross-cultural studies of modernization generally (Berger et al 1973).

The unfortunate result of the implicit continuation of the traditional/modern schema in cross-cultural medical studies is a failure to make significant comparisons of the most fundamental aspects of health care. This is paralleled by an equally undesirable kind of disciplinary compartmentalization and fragmentation—until recently medical anthropology and medical sociology studied two entirely different types of societies. Strangely, this has been carried over into medical research: transcultural psychiatry joined anthropology in the field in "traditional" cultures, while social psychiatry and social medicine remained with sociology in modern settings. Disciplinary boundaries also affect the literature in the culture and medicine field, which is loculated in a surprisingly large number of disciplinary journals, creating very real barriers to communication and hindering interdisciplinary work.

As I shall attempt to demonstrate, China represents the limit case, in that the distinction between traditional and modern medicine neither does justice to the complex phenomena it attempts to organize nor provides a basis for future research. As a number of scholars whose are represented in this volume have already shown, local field studies in Sri Lanka, India, and Chinese societies (Obeyesekere 1976, Leslie 1969, Anderson and Anderson 1969) require that the investigator know something about the classical medical tradition and its historical development as well as about its multiple levels of interaction with modern professional, folk, and popular medical forms.[3] He must also try to explain these interrelations as they actually affect local health care. These requirements call for a much more sophisticated appreciation of local systems of medical care and their sociocultural determinants.

Given this obvious need for new theoretical directions and given the renaissance of interest in comparative cross-cultural studies of medicine and psychiatry, it is not surprising that we are witnessing many new comparative approaches take shape (Fabrega 1973, Kleinman 1973a, Leslie 1976, Litman and Robins 1971, Poynter 1969).[4] The book represents, in part, a response to that new comparative impulse.

I am not arguing for total abandonment of the inveterate conceptual dichotomy that I have been criticizing. Indeed, this would hardly seem possible simply owing to its widespread use and acceptance as a communicative device, as illustrated by the title of the conference (Comparative Study of Traditional and Modern Medicine in Chinese Societies). Rather I wish to see it refined into a much more inclusive and sophisticated model. Unfortunately, whereas early students in the culture and medicine field were strongly interested in theoretical issues, such as models for conceptualizing various aspects of medicine cross-culturally, and in universal principles and patterns that operate behind disparate healing beliefs and activities, the recent thrust of cross-cultural studies in medicine has not been very concerned with these issues. Not unlike medical science itself, which after all is the last science to elaborate a meta-scientific enquiry into its theoretical underpinnings, the culture and medicine field has made do with outmoded conceptual paradigms because it has refrained from rigorously examining its own theoretical structure (Kleinman 1973b). Such a poverty of theory has actively worked against the development of integrative comparative research, while perpetuating narrow discipline-bound research interests which fragment and distort the holistic quality of this subject. After discussing the two other conceptual difficulties which afflict research in this field, we present what is regarded as a new theoretical framework in cross-cultural medical research, a framework which bridges fragmented disciplinary interests, generates important issues for integrated multi-disciplinary research, and radically reorients our perspective on the traditional/modern dualistic model of health care.

(2)   If the first conceptual distortion could be traced to certain early anthropological and historical preoccupations, the second—the failure to treat the individual along with the social side of health beliefs and behaviors—can claim almost all of early social scientific work for its paradigm (Chombart de Lauwe 1966), excepting the symbolic interactionist tradition. This problem needs to be discussed both as conceptual and methodological distortion. In the medical sphere, one simply cannot divorce culture and person. In fact, some of the most interesting questions being asked today by epidemiologists, medical anthropologists, and psychiatrists have to do with correlations between these two realities (Hinkle 1961, Lazarus 1971, Lipowski 1969, Mechanic 1966, Nader and Maretzki 1973, Rahe et al 1964, Spradley and Phillips 1972, Teichner 1968, Wittkower and Dubrevil 1973).[5] Although we can study illness entirely in social terms, it is a truly impoverished notion of illness unless it reflects the subjective and physiological experiences of the sick person. Similarly, though health services research has tended to avoid individual interactions (i.e. doctor–patient and patient–family relations) in favor of structural and systems analyses of health care, it is precisely those individual interactions which are at the center of communicative and cognitive mechanisms and problems in health care. And yet the doctor–patient relationship, for example, remains almost unexplored (Waitzkin and Stoeckle 1972); nor are the fundamental activities of primary health care at all well understood. The healing process, of course, simply cannot be studied without relating the individual to his sociocultural milieu (Kleinman 1973c). Medical sociology has more recently grasped the

significance of this inherent tension between the individual and social sides of illness in its concepts of the sick role and illness behavior (Parsons 1953, Mechanic 1962, Twaddle 1974, Zola 1966). Medical research and teaching have institutionalized the same question in the field of psychosomatic research and in the resurgent interest being devoted to the relation of stress, adaptation, and illness (Lipowski 1968, Whybrow 1972). Psychiatry's unique contribution here has been to underline the importance of the "meaning" of illness on multiple levels: cultural, social, interpersonal, and personal (Lipowski 1968 and 1969).

Unfortunately, in the past most historical, anthropological, and social analyses of the cultural context of medicine have tended to disregard the cultural dialectic relating individual and social realities (Murphy 1971). They have relegated the individual to a very distant second place, far behind the predominant concern with social factors and at times completely divorced from them. I would stress that this was a mistake in theory and research which greatly reduced the impact of earlier social and behavioral scientific research in medicine. The result is that we still do not possess adequate cross-cultural phenomenological descriptions of illness experiences, though in the last few years we have begun to build a basis for such work (Fabrega 1972). Nor do we have a cross-cultural phenomenology of doctor–patient interchanges, or of other crucial relationships in the healing process. These are future prospects for comparative medical research.

The chief problem with social and behavioral science research that omits the individual side of health concerns is that it ignores a central question in cross-cultural studies of medicine: the relation of biological and psychological processes with culture. A highly relevant example of this problem is the study of therapeutic efficacy. Much recent research has demonstrated the importance of the individual meaning of illness for the course of illness and the therapeutic outcome; and especially for the evaluation of successful health care (Lipowski 1970). If the study of medicine and culture strips away particular persons and particular illnesses, removes the psychosocial and psychocultural linkages, then it makes cross-cultural studies in medicine and psychiatry largely irrelevant to major issues confronting health care.

(3) The third conceptual problem is the only one I shall attempt to offer a solution for, since it goes to the heart of our reconceptualization of this entire subject. Almost everything medical, of one sort or another and at one time or another, has been studied in relation to culture. A vast array of potentially significant medically-relevant phenomena face the student of cross-cultural medicine and psychiatry. One can focus on the cultural factors influencing illness, beginning with their effect upon illness causation and ending with their impact upon the expression and evaluation of illness. Much the same can be done for treatment. One can study medical classificatory systems, the enormous variety of healing rituals, different medical technologies, groups of patients, various kinds of healers, the institutional structures of medical care, health values, medical economics,

and on and on. Research can focus on different levels of health care from national systems to local communities; it can concern itself with external factors (political, economic, environmental, etc.) influencing health care or with its internal mechanics; and it can focus on organizational structures or social functions. The range of potential issues is very wide. It is discouraging to survey the literature and search for stable foci for comparative cross-cultural research that have been studied repeatedly and systematically. The culture and medicine field suffers from a lack of conceptual unification. Rarely has attention been devoted systematically to the total field of medical events. Lacking conceptual agreement as to what makes up a given medical context, it is not surprising that studies vary greatly and that comparative research has been very difficult to carry out. Nor has clinical or public health research provided an operational model of fundamental medical care functions that could be used for cross-cultural research.

This problem returns us to the question of methods. Here cross-cultural medical research partakes of the discipline-bound compartmentalization previously referred to. The very different methodologies of ethnography, ethnoscience, macro-sociological comparisons, systems analysis, transcultural psychiatry, epidemiology, health services research, social deviance research and labeling theory, historical research, and other research approaches have all been applied to different problems in the culture and medicine field. The participant-observer approach of most medical ethnographies and of medical and psychiatric field research, though producing perhaps the richest picture of medicine in different cultures, does not specify a systematic methodological approach to medical events which is reproducible and which can be directly propagated from one cultural setting to another—while the more rigorous and formal research approaches, such as ethnoscience and epidemiology, do not attempt to deal with a total field of medical events. The absence of well-formulated and accepted theoretical models has also contributed to the limited development of new research methods and strategies.

If this seems too harsh a judgment, it is not meant, in fact, to reflect what is taken to be a newly-emerging conceptual consensus in cross-cultural medical research which has important implications for research (Kleinman 1973a). This model, which I shall now describe, seems particularly given to comparative research and studies of medicine in complex cultural contexts such as Chinese societies.

Medicine as a Cultural System

Amongst the extensive and confusing panoply of medical phenomena found in any cultural context are certain fundamental structural features and activities which appear to be universal. To begin with, medicine always exists as a body of more or less systematically articulated beliefs and values concerning illness and responses to illness. This ideological and value system supports social institutions, relationships, roles and behaviors, and health care activities which taken together constitute a special segment of social reality—the *medical system*. The medical system, as it is defined here, represents a total cultural organization of medically-relevant experiences, an integrated system of social (and personal) perception, use, and evaluation. That is, medical systems are much more than particular kinds of medical facilities, practitioners, and practices. They are cognitive, affective, and behavioral environments in which illness and health care are culturally organized. Moreover, they are to be appreciated as such only on the local level, where they actually function.

Such systems are not coextensive with a particular professional healing tradition or social institution. Even where several different kinds of professional medical practice, and their institutional structures, coexist in a local setting, our model of the medical system is meant to include considerably more than their sum. In small-scale pre-literate societies, of course, where professionalization and compartmentalization may be entirely lacking and where no separate body of medical beliefs and practices may exist apart from the general cultural milieu, the medical system may be a completely homogeneous entity (although as Kunstadter demonstrates in this volume (Chapter 9) plural medical forms may exist even in these very traditional societies). Whereas in rapidly modernizing, post-traditional, and advanced modern societies, this social and cultural homogeneity is gone. Instead, it is replaced by separate and often quite different sectors of local health care systems—professional medical institutions; folk healing traditions; and popular medical culture. Each of these contains its own cognitive, behavioral, and evaluative patterns. Although other models of local medical systems might describe things somewhat differently, we shall employ this tripartite cultural organizational paradigm to help us understand medicine cross-culturally and especially in its Chinese context, where this paradigm will be more fully developed. (See Figure 1 below, Chapter 17 above, and Chapter 36 in Kleinman, et al, eds. 1976; pp. 604-622.)

Medical systems are perhaps best regarded as adaptive cultural responses to the stress of illness and its consequences (Alland 1970). They seem to have evolved in response to the social and personal stresses generated by illness. It is not surprising, then, that they often overlap with other cultural adaptive systems. In "traditional" cultures it is not always possible to separate medicine from the religious system, for example; and the latter can be thought of also as a cultural adaptive response, but to a much wider range of suffering and misfortune (Geertz 1965, Spiro 1967). We have only begun to examine medical systems from ecological and evolutionary perspectives in regard to their "internal" adaptive health care functions; the nature of the stresses they are responding to; and the "external" environmental, sociopolitical, economic, technological, and epidemiological factors that determine their patterns of response. For example, we can relate the efficacy of these systems' instrumental and symbolic responses to particular "internal" factors, such as the nature of the doctor–patient relationship and actual healing practices; and to "external" factors, including epidemiological maps of disease prevalence, rates of morbidity and mortality, and the like. Similarly, these responses can be correlated with level of technological development, sociopolitical organization, and other critical "external" factors. This would be an interesting framework for future cross-cultural comparisons of medical systems. Furthermore, few if any attempts have been made thus far to gauge the impact of medical systems on their sociocultural environments, which would seem to be another interesting direction for research.

Medical systems are virtually impossible to understand once they are removed from their cultural contexts. The cultural context does not merely tell us about the social and cultural environment within which a particular local system of medicine is situated, but also tells about the specific cognitive, behavioral, and institutional structure of that system, and the cultural constructional principles (values and symbolic meanings) underlying and determining that structure. Ideally, it should be possible to analyze medical systems in a way analogous to the study of another, but quite different, system of cultural meaning—language. We might even think of the basic cultural units of the medical system as "medemes" similar to morphemes and phonemes; and we could perhaps search for the structural rules which generate certain healing activities much as we look for the generative principles of particular languages. Indeed, though this interesting analogy is somewhat remote, detailed analyses of the symbolic context of medicine have in fact been carried out (Benveniste 1945, Lloyd 1964, Ingham 1970, Turner 1967, Yalman 1964). Such a linguistic model might also help us understand the system of rules governing decisions about illness and treatment and use of health-care facilities.

But rather than focus on structural factors, I shall examine certain basic adaptive functions which appear to hold for all medical systems. An appreciation of these fundamental health care operations allows us both to compare systems of medical care at the point of their most basic inner workings and to understand the total organization of health care activities at the local level. Ironically, we know less about this unique set of medical activities than we do about the biological basis of disease or the workings of the immunological system; yet these health care operations taken together define what medicine is chiefly about.

The basic functions of medical systems are principally concerned with ordering and controlling illness, and providing the experience of illness and its treatment with meaning. We might think of *five major functions* including: (1) the construction of hierarchies of health values; (2) the shaping of illness as a psychosocial experience; (3) the cognitive and communicative tasks of health care, such as labeling, classifying, and explaining; (4) healing (and preventive) activities per se, from empirical remedies and technological interventions to symbolic therapies; and (5) the medical management of therapeutic outcomes, including cure, chronic illness, and death.

With some necessary adjustments, we could describe almost any local system of medicine in terms of these fundamental health care functions: from that of the Subanum of Mindanao (Frake 1961) which lacks any separate professional medical structure; to that of contemporary communities in the U.S., where very different professional, folk, and popular medical institutions coexist and compete (Dreitzel 1971, Freidson 1970, Mechanic 1973); and on to the Chinese examples that we have examined (Kleinman Chapter 17). These functions are briefly elaborated so that they can be appreciated as a basis for understanding medicine in given cultural settings and for making cross-cultural comparisons. The first analytic task, however, is to reconstruct a *total* medical system. To do so, one must specify the cultural and historical context, as well as the ecological setting. Then one can use our paradigm of basic health care functions to describe the interior of the system. Again, it is essential to stress the system as a whole, the way these functions interconnect so as to unify diverse health-related activities and form a local medical ethos. That ethos defines what is health and what is illness. It provides illness with a cultural trajectory; and it gives a special form to health-care activities, from naming and explaining to treating and evaluating, which defines the particular healing ways of a given medical system.

By constructing cultural hierarchies of health values is meant that medical systems establish socially legitimated criteria for evaluating illness and treatment. These values influence all aspects of health care. Although we are accustomed to think of the impact of these values upon (1) the labeling of behavior as normal or deviant (Buckner 1971, Williams 1971), (2) the decision to seek out medical care (Zola 1972 and 1973), and (3) which kind of care is actually chosen (Freidson 1970, Kennedy 1973), the system of health values also strongly influences personal and social reactions to specific illnesses and symptoms, as well as the evaluation of therapeutic success (Fabrega 1972). Moreover, these values help determine needs, goals, and expectations throughout the medical system. But since health values are deeply embedded in a culture's universe of symbolic meanings and thus in its social reality, where they are internalized by the individual during the socialization process, it is in the cultural ethos itself, or in complex societies in the popular medical culture, that one finds these value hierarchies. They are not found in professional medical institutions, which of course contain their own value orientations. Here is one danger in failing to recognize that the medical system is considerably wider than the often very narrow confines of its professional institutions. Some of the most central values in health care have little to do with those institutions, but instead operate outside them in the general cultural milieu. For example, one can cite the popular concern with receiving explanations from physicians (well-documented in contemporary clinics in this country) which appears to be a major factor in the public's evaluation of health care as well as in compliance. This is a highly valued health-care function in the popular but *not* the professional sector of our health-care system. Furthermore, in complex societies, like the U.S. and China, several different hierarchies of health values may conflict on the local level. This may represent the conflicting interests of cultural subgroups, economic classes, religious groups, people of different educational background, etc. Conflicting and contradictory values, which may reflect the ideological pluralism of societies or differences and tensions amongst the separate sectors of medical systems, often raise major problems for health care, problems which are resolved neither by technological advances nor without taking into account the divergent interests of the professional, folk and popular sectors of medical systems.

In small-scale, pre-literate societies, as well as in many historical cultures, the fit between health values (needs, expectations, choices and evaluations) and healing (therapeutic approaches and outcomes) can often be very tight. And this congruity may be responsible in large measure for the social and personal evaluation of therapeutic success on a symbolic level, even when empirical evidence of efficacy is lacking (Kleinman 1973c). This would also seem to contribute, in part, to the placebo effect in modern systems of medical care (Shapiro 1959). By establishing a socially-sanctioned hierarchy of health values, a local medical system has initiated the healing process. When therapeutic efficacy for a given health problem is lacking, manipulation of health values and use of explanatory devices for providing meaning for the illness experience and the treatment intervention form the basis for whatever therapeutic success occurs. Obviously, this finding is not limited to "traditional" societies, nor to situations where empirically effective therapeutic interventions are absent. It can still play an important, if somewhat less powerful, role in pluralistic medical settings where alternative systems are available and even in certain parts of technologically-advanced health care systems. For example, in a study of the health value system on a psychiatric ward in a modern general hospital, I was able to show that these values significantly influenced the decision for discharge from hospital and the evaluation of therapeutic success by patients and staff.[6]

Closely related to the health value structure is the influence of culture on the experience of illness. For, though disease occurs as a biological and psychological phenomenon that may or may not have cultural determinants, illness is experienced as a personal and social reality. That is, illness is in large part a cultural construct (Nader and Maretzki 1973, Plog and Edgerton 1969). We learn how to perceive, attend to, value, express, and live illness. We learn socially legitimated ways of being ill, whether we call this the sick role, illness behavior, or the experience of illness (Siegler and Osmond 1973). Culture may significantly affect symptom formation, as well as psychophysiological processes in and reactions to illness (Schmale et al 1970, Zborowski 1952, Zola 1966). It also plays a role in disease causation (Katz 1971, Yap 1952). Moreover, stress seems to operate, at least on one level, through its cultural significance as a social and personal threat or loss (Spradley and Phillips

1972). But culture's greatest impact is on the meaning given to the illness experience. Such meaning holds great significance for the course and management of illness. Here we have an important interface between culture and biology. Sociocultural events, via processes of conditioning and early learning that are still not well understood, are able to affect physiology and behavior (Lipowski 1968, Werner and Kaplan 1967, Platonov 1959, Mauss 1950). This linkage is important not only for psychosomatic disorders but for all illnesses as well. All of which makes it clear that we must develop a much more sophisticated appreciation of illness as cultural experience and that this perspective is an appropriate direction for future comparative cross-cultural research.

Perhaps the core function of medical systems is their cognitive response to illness: that is, the ordering of illness via labeling, classifying, and explaining. Although these cognitive and communicative activities are universal, models and idioms vary greatly both cross-culturally and historically (Entralgo 1955, Horton 1967, Porkert 1974, Siegler and Osmond 1966). Moreover, they appear to be significantly different in the different social sectors of medical systems. Medical sociology has tended to stress the behavioral rather than the cognitive aspects of labeling (Rubington and Weinberg 1969). Most research on medical cognition has centered on classificatory systems in primitive societies. Both symbolic analyses (Rosaldo 1972, Turner 1967) and ethnoscientific studies (Berlin et al 1973) have demonstrated the extraordinary sophistication of even pre-literate medical classificatory schemes. Such studies attempt to reconstruct indigenous cognitive maps of how illness or treatment forms, such as medicinal herbs, are categorized. Very little work in this area has been done in modern societies, however.

What work has been done in modern societies, outside of a very few studies of clinical reasoning (Feinstein 1967, Lazare 1973, Ledley and Lusted 1959), has been limited to more general appraisals of medical knowledge, beliefs, and explanatory models in the popular sector of medical systems (Apple 1960, Freidson 1970, Mabry 1964, Samora et al 1962). Yet important work has been done on the explanatory structure of folk healing in modernizing societies (Fabrega 1973), and this may hold real significance for future research in complex modern societies (Engel 1973). Methodologies are now available to pursue cross-cultural studies of this and other aspects of medical cognition (Cancian 1971, Waitzkin and Stoeckle 1972).

Studies of cognitive and communicative processes would seem most relevant to the analysis of doctor–patient and family–patient relationships. In these contexts, one can study the transmission of information as well as the interactions that take place between quite different explanatory and evaluative models (Plaja et al 1968, Waitzkin and Stoeckle 1972). This aspect of the doctor–patient relationship seems particularly given to studies of the cognitive functions of and interrelationships between the different sectors of medical systems.

What we now know about this subject points up the tremendous importance of these cognitive activities for (1) organizing illness and healing activities as an integral part of social reality; and (2) providing them with meaning. As Mary Douglas and others have convincingly shown, illness and its consequences, especially chrönic disability, deformity, and death, are disordering events which provoke disruption and tension in the social nexus, the family, and the patient (Douglas 1970a, b, Turner 1969). On the cultural level, they threaten the most basic values, behavioral norms, and conceptions of order. The cultural response to illness is an attempt to order this threatening stressor within a well-articulated conceptual frame, to control its disruptive psychosocial effect on the sick person and his social network, and to make both it and its treatment personally and socially meaningful.

The explanatory functions of medical care represent a departure of modern scientific medicine from folk, popular, and non-Western forms of medical and psychiatric care. Horton has emphasized this disjunction between the explanatory systems of "traditional" medical systems, which are concerned with making the experience of illness culturally meaningful, and the explanatory systems of modern professional medicine, which are concerned with providing objective, scientific accounts of illness that are devoid of cultural meaning (Horton 1967). Thus, one of the most basic functions of health care seems no longer to be part of the modern profession of medicine. Rather, there is evidence that this crucial health-care function in modern medical systems has been left almost entirely to the folk and popular sectors. If so, then this represents one of the major problems resulting from the impact of modernization, and specifically scientific and technological development, on systems of medical care (Gallagher 1972, White et al 1972); and it tells of a fundamental change in medicine's historical and cross-cultural pattern. It may, in part, explain the resurgence of folk (including religious) healing forms and explanatory models in contemporary Western societies, along with some of the popular dissatisfaction with the "quality" and "success" of modern medical care. If true, it would also appear, on the one hand, to diminish the importance of traditional psychosocial and psychophysiological mechanisms in modern medical treatment; while, on the other hand, it represents the irrelevance of scientific explanations for social action outside of the narrow confines of the medical profession. The well-publicized efforts to integrate "traditional" and "modern" approaches to medical care in modernizing societies, such as the PRC, may, in part, constitute a response to the problems resulting from this radical change in medical practice.

Perhaps the ideal setting for studying medical cognitive activities is where very different medical traditions interact and where the professional, folk, and popular sectors of health care are both conspicuous and markedly different. The modernization process offers a rich context for such studies, while it also receives an interesting examination from this perspective. Scientific medicine is one of the vanguard forces of modernization at work challenging and undermining traditional cognitive models concerned with human suffering. And thus the study of the interaction between "modern" and "traditional" forms of medical cognition, especially in the context of doctor–patient relationships, is crucial for our understanding of the impact of modernization on human consciousness (Berger et al 1973). Comparative studies of medical beliefs and models of meaning should contribute to any future comparative cross-cultural study of systems of knowledge and ways of knowing. Furthermore, where different systems of medical knowledge interact, we have a "natural" comparative experiment in cognitive transfer and change, and the resulting problems in communication, which has tremendous importance for the teaching and practice of primary health care.

The richest cross-cultural findings in the culture and medicine field are directly concerned with healing activities (Kleinman 1973c). Although we have learned quite a lot about healing practices in different contemporary cultures (Frank 1961, Glick 1967, Kaplan and Johnson 1964, Kiev 1968, Leighton and Leighton 1941, Leighton et al 1968, Messing 1968, Nash 1967, Tambiah 1968) and historical settings (Entralgo 1970, Ellenberger 1970), rarely have these activities been looked at within the *total* context of the medical system and its other health care functions. This suggests a potentially vast subject that includes everything from healing rituals to modern psychotherapy, chemotherapy, and advanced surgical procedures. Under this heading we could also include the facilities and technologies of health services. One branch of these activities involves anticipatory and preventive practices. These too have been studied cross-culturally (Hughes 1963). For our present purposes, it is enough to point out that healing (i.e. psychosocial and/or physiological responses to treatment) is, in fact, going on at all levels of the medical system and in each of the health-care functions. It is also essential to recognize that healing practices are evaluated in terms of environing social and cultural factors, the system of health values, the particular cognitive and communicative models employed, and much else besides demonstrable empirical efficacy, important as this is when it actually occurs. Finally, from the perspective of healing activities we see that modern medicine has (1) failed to study adequately its most important and most universal function and, because of this, (2) allowed sociocultural models of medical events to be constructed which stress illness while de-emphasizing healing, thus distorting medicine for social scientists and physicians alike who work with these models (Whybrow 1972). It is argued that distorting medicine in this way has had deleterious effects for cross-cultural approaches to medicine and has contributed to many of our popular misconceptions about health care, including both devaluation and overvaluation of therapeutic practices and technologies. As with each of the other health care functions mentioned, healing practices readily lend themselves to comparative cross-cultural research.

As a last set of activities, medical systems operate on a series of potential outcomes, managing cure, chronic illness, permanent impairment, and death. The management of death demonstrates the extent to which medicine overlaps with religion and other cultural systems. Indeed, much of "traditional" medical practice is concerned with preparing for death and making the experience of dying meaningful (Cassell 1972, Fabian 1972, Racy 1969, Speigel 1964). In increasingly secularized modern societies, scientific medicine, for reasons previously mentioned, has run into great problems in this area, and at a time when it has been given ever greater control over aging and death (Morison 1973, Zola 1972). Here is a concrete instance of a medical-care function that is very poorly handled by modern systems of medicine. (At one time modern scientific medicine seemed to regard death as the ultimate defeat of health care.) And it is one that they could learn a great deal about from cross-cultural medical research. Nothing reveals more clearly the holistic structure of medical systems than recognition of their important roles both in structuring the illness experience and in managing dying. This subject is deservedly attracting much attention today from practitioners, health planners, and researchers, but its comparative dimensions have barely been explored (Artiss and Levine 1973, Parsons 1972, Weisman 1972).

From the standpoint of the health-care system, all attempts to understand illness and treatment can be thought of as *explanatory models.* Although they may differ considerably with regard to how much they can explain and the power of their explanations, scientific medical models of illness (see Englehardt 1974) and folk and popular beliefs (see Jahoda 1971; Snow 1974; Yap 1967) can be compared as explanatory models patterned by particular social and cultural determinants. Explanatory models can be objectively elicited as more or less formally structured coherent accounts of reality, though they may be and often are ambiguous and changing, and they may contain contradictions and various degrees of logical development (see Cancian 1971). As sociologists have shown (Freidson 1970; Twaddle 1974) the different sectors of health systems employ distinct explanatory models which may complement, compete with, or distort one another. See Figure 1 for a graphic representation of my conception of the interrelated sectors or subsystems of the health-care system and their explanatory models and other components. Interactions between such sectors, like interactions between "traditional" and "modern" medical systems in the same health-care system, involve transactions or negotiations between these different explanatory models. Similarly, health care involves exchanges between the holders or users of these models, who perceive, interpret, evaluate and respond to illness and treatment in terms of particular explanatory models. The doctor–patient relationship is an obvious setting for studying these exchanges. Patient–family, family–doctor, patient–folk practitioner, or patient–paraprofessional practitioner relationships are examples of other interactions between explanatory models in health care.

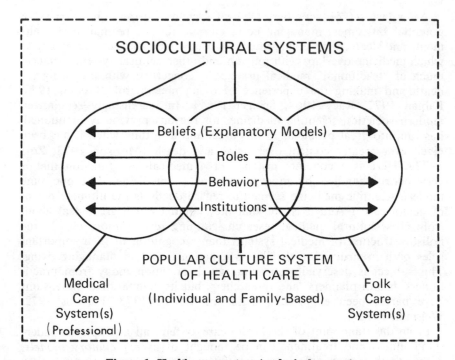

Figure 1. Health care system (ecological system).

This volume demonstrates how extremely rich are the interactions between different explanatory models in Chinese systems of health care (see the Chapters by Ahern (2), Gould-Martin (3), Tseng (16), Gale (14), and Topley (6)).

Compliance with medical advice and evaluations of the quality and success of medical care have been related to these cognitive and communicative interactions (Davis 1968; Haefner and Kirsch 1970; Stimson 1974). Medical modernization has also been studied from this perspective (Abramson et al 1961; Fabrega 1973). Explanatory models in our own society are studied in relation to how they reflect social class (Elder 1973) and ethnicity (Harwood 1971), but have *not* been studied to any extent thus far in terms of the beliefs and behaviors of the mainstream of American culture. Satisfaction with the quality and amount of explaining seems to have been a determinant of why patients in one recent study (Kane et al 1974) found chiropractors more helpful than physicians for the treatment of back pain. The studies mentioned above by Davis (1968), Haefner and Kirsch (1970), and Stimson (1974) demonstrate much the same thing. Other studies have documented that modern scientific physicians often perform poorly in explaining to patients (Ley and Spellman 1967; Reader et al 1957), while the chapters in this book by Ahern (5) and Gale (14) suggest that this is a clinical function especially well handled by folk practitioners (secular or sacred); though

Ahern (5) offers an observation that professional Chinese physicians may not do much better than Western physicians in this "traditional" clinical task. Recently, Lazare et al (1974) have shown that patient satisfaction with health care often reflects whether their explanatory models along with their general expectations have been elicited and responded to in the clinic.

In this volume, Tseng (Chapter 16) focuses on explanatory models as a fundamental factor in the efficacy of psychotherapy. Spiro (Chapter 10) also suggests that this is an important ingredient in folk psychotherapy in Burma. Hsu and Tseng (1972) have documented the difficulties surrounding inter-cultural psychotherapy in part owing to basic differences and conflicts in explanatory models; and Tseng (Chapter 16) describes these problems in the care of Chinese patients. I have had very similar experiences, but have also witnessed the tremendous impact of explanatory models on illness behavior and clinical care in our own culture. In Chapter 17, I present case illustrations of transactions between explanatory models. Those cases illustrate both the practical clinical and research significance of these explanatory model interactions in health care. I am presently analyzing data from a study in which an attempt was made to quantify differences between explanatory models functioning in actual health care encounters and relate these to various health care outcome measurements. Thus, this area would appear to offer clinically-relevant research opportunities.

Prospects and Problems in Comparative Medicine and Psychiatry: A Personal View

Throughout this chapter the writer has frequently pointed to issues that seem especially important for future work in the comparative cross-cultural medical field. We will now reconsider certain of these that touch upon theory, research, teaching, and practical health care concerns, and there will be suggested several steps that might be taken to advance this field.

To begin with, it is thought essential to encourage serious theoretical work which will better conceptualize medicine cross-culturally and which will attempt to unify the many different approaches and findings in this field. Concern with the theoretical issues is also important for defining key problems for research and establishing new methods for studying such problems. But perhaps just as significant a task for theoretical work are the implications of comparative research for our general understanding of medicine and psychiatry, since this viewpoint enables us to study universal features of health care and its most fundamental processes, along with the constraining forces of sociocultural patterns and change. Thus, comparative studies carry with them the possibility of a major critical approach to health-care activities, institutions, and policies, a unique opportunity to *rethink* medicine. The conceptual model presented in this paper is an attempt to reconceptualize medical and psychiatric care in cross-cultural perspective; it is not the writer's desire that it be simply accepted, but that it provoke other models as well as renewed interest in the basic conceptual problems that it tries to resolve. In this way, comparative medicine and psychiatry together can become a major source of theoretical development in the health sciences and perhaps in behavioral and social science also.

Elsewhere this writer has proposed that what are most needed in comparative studies are fully integrated and well-planned multi-disciplinary *research programs*. These should use the same theoretical formulations, research methods, and team of investigators to compare local medical systems both in different settings within the same culture and between distinctly different cultures (Kleinman 1973c). An example of this kind of research program, using the central focus of this book, would be comparative studies of local health-care systems in urban and rural Chinese communities and in similar kinds of communities in the U.S. Adding another Asian, or other non-Western, culture in a similar, or perhaps earlier, stage of modernization would make for an even more interesting comparison; while comparative field work on health care in different Chinese societies, such as Taiwan, Hongkong, Singapore, and in the U.S., would represent another important research strategy.

It is hoped that such a research program would include a team of investigators from several different disciplines (including perhaps medical anthropologist, medical sociologist, epidemiologist, and cross-cultural psychiatrist, or experts in social medicine and health services research) who would study simultaneously and in an organized way (1) the different sectors of health care and (2) the major adaptive functions of these systems. Indeed, this would seem to be the very best means for studying the complex types of multi-layered *interactions* between health-care components that have been stressed in this chapter.

Since this kind of research program would require a great deal of support and cooperation, including substantial funds and the capability of keeping a group of experts in the field for a considerable period of time, it may well prove infeasible in the era of scarcity that we have now entered. Although still believing that this is an ideal-type approach to comparative medical research that deserves to be tried, the writer will suggest a number of specific problems for comparative field research that lend themselves to either individual or small team efforts. Even if multidisciplinary collaborative projects are infeasible, the selective use of available experts and cross-disciplinary training of field workers, which in any event is greatly to be desired, could make for unusual contributions. For what we now need is certainly not simply more of what we already possess, but the new kinds of information and approaches mentioned above.

Issues worthy of comparative investigation are quite numerous, but a short listing might include:

(1) The systematic and holistic study of particular local health-care systems, emphasizing the interaction between their different sectors and the relation of health-care functions to those component parts.

(2) Focus on the cognitive and communicative aspects of doctor–patient and patient–family relationships, stressing comparisons of and interactions between explanatory models in popular, folk, clinical and scientific domains (see Chapter 17 above).

(3) Phenomenological descriptions and cross-cultural comparisons of the psychosocial and psychophysiological aspects of illness experiences, emphasizing the mechanisms by which culture molds behavior and biology. (This would seem to provide a frame for joining epidemiological, social science, and psychosomatic research approaches in actual field research settings.)

(4) The relationship between meaning (subjective and social) and efficacy in "traditional" and modern forms of health care, as well as the role of this relationship in determining how medical and psychiatric care are complied with and evaluated.

(5) Comparisons of these issues in a range of different societies, with special emphasis on the impact of sociocultural change and modernization.

(6) Comparisons of local medical systems as adaptive responses to specific stress factors in the physical and social environments, including particular diseases.

The writer has already shown that these issues are directly applicable to research in Chinese societies.[7] And already stressed are the unusual richness of and opportunities provided by the Chinese case for studying the interactional processes, especially conceptual transfer and transformation, between the different sectors of the medical system. Although, as has already been noted, it is very unlikely that research on local health-care systems of the type described in this paper will be conducted in the PRC itself, this research paradigm can still be used to organize what information is gathered about health care in that country.

Unfortunately, most research on medical and psychiatric problems in Chinese culture has neither involved medically-oriented nor medically-trained field workers; this is all too obvious from the kind of work that is being done. That research, though interesting for social scientific purposes generally, has *failed* to come to grips with (1) the basic internal features of health care in Chinese communities and (2) the interconnections between Chinese culture and the biological, psychophysiological, and psychosocial substrata of illness and healing. Thus, the writer would strongly encourage collaborative research ventures on studies relating to medicine and psychiatry in Chinese culture, and/or the use of medical personnel who possess the requisite social science and language training (or social scientists and sinologists with some kind of medical training). This book, and the conference from which it is derived, should demonstrate that such a category of scholars does in fact exist; and, more importantly, that cross-disciplinary training can greatly enhance the quality of research in this field and thus should be supported.

What next? Frankly, this writer sees this volume as a first step that needs to be followed by other specific steps if both the comparative approach to medicine and the study of medicine in Chinese culture are to become firm directions for research. Perhaps other conferences on comparative cross-cultural studies of medicine and psychiatry can be convened around (1) medicine in other cultural contexts; (2) conceptual models and methodological approaches; and (3) specific problems in illness and health care. Just as important, however, are local or regional seminars and workshops which bring together or, in the case of the participants here, maintain contact amongst scholars concerned with various aspects of this field. It also might be worthwhile to consider the possibility of a cross-disciplinary journal or the publication of future work in special issues or sections of existing journals.[8]   I see comparative medicine and psychiatry as a new branch of research and teaching, linking medical schools; schools of public health and departments in the social and behavioral sciences, that is in great need of new ideas, concrete plans, and active development.

Teaching and training are essential components of comparative cross-cultural approaches to medicine and psychiatry. They represent another important area for cross-disciplinary efforts. Undergraduate, graduate, medical, and public-health students are all appropriate for teaching; and I have had some very gratifying experiences teaching this approach not only to medical students and residents, but to undergraduates and graduate students. The opportunity exists here to structure an academic program with contributions from anthropology, sociology, area studies, medicine, psychiatry, and public health. The same holds for post-graduate training, where comparative cross-cultural studies are personally seen as a major future direction for advanced students of international health, medical and psychiatric anthropology, medical sociology, and related fields. Indeed, the comparative approach to medicine seems equally important as a unifying perspective for training as for research. And here also are its difficulties, since it can become an easy victim of inveterate disciplinary and inter-school barriers and rivalries.

Finally, we come to the practical implications of our subject for the delivery of health care in our own and other societies. The writer will expand on only one point, since this subject is covered rather fully in Chapters 18 and 19 of this volume. Both the comparative cross-cultural approach to health care and its specific application to the study of health care in Chinese societies lead us to new insights and new approaches which are not merely of heuristic value but can actually lead to reform. The point that the writer wishes to make is that these research interests center on some of the most basic "external" (sociocultural context) and "internal" (medical system and clinical tasks) issues in health care, issues which heretofore have been either ignored or considered only superficially. Yet these issues, such as conflicting values, dissimilar interests, and communicative barriers between popular and professional medical sectors, or the tendency of modernization to significantly alter fundamental health care functions, can be studied in depth from the perspectives advanced in this book, the results of which can then be applied either in the form of a critique or much more directly in making essential changes in the delivery of primary medical and psychiatric care. It is these basic tasks of health care—healing and the management of chronic illness, disability, and death—which we have so very much still to learn about and which we need to substantially improve (Snow 1973). The comparative interests here represented, if they center on the *primary* aspects of illness and care which are written of in this paper, can contribute both to our knowledge and praxis in medical and psychiatric care.

NOTES

1. The writer's approach to this subject is more fully presented in Kleinman (1973a). Other comparative approaches to the relationship of culture and medicine are found in works by: Fabrega (1973); Leslie (1976); Litman and Robins (1971); Poynter (1969); and Rosenberg (1969).

2. The writer does not include here another major system of non-Western medicine, Arabic medicine, because it developed in such close contact with and incorporated so many of the fundamental ideas and institutions of the classical Western medical tradition.

3. The general issue of the desirability for social scientific approaches to medicine and psychiatry to be historically-minded is discussed in Rosen (1973). This point has been made especially well for Chinese culture by Nathan Sivin (personal correspondence).

4. In May 1974 a workshop on "Conceptual Models for Studying Medicine in Different Social and Cultural Concepts" was held at Harvard University, organized by B. Rosenkrantz, A. Kleinman, and E. Mendelsohn, which considered different conceptual approaches in *comparative* social, historical and cross-cultural studies of medicine. An outcome of that workshop was the development of a fortnightly Harvard Faculty Seminar on "Cross-Cultural Studies of Illness, Doctor-Patient Interactions, and Clinical Care", October 1975-May 1976, under the sponsorship of Professors Eisenberg, Yalman, Pelzel, Mendelsohn, Good, and Kleinman. Papers delivered at the seminar by Harwood, Crapanzano, Zola, Leslie, Tambiah, Good, Eisenberg, Fabrega, Kapur, and others will be published in the journal *Culture, Medicine and Psychiatry* (see Note 8 below), and represent a substantial advance in medical anthropological and cross-cultural medical and psychiatric research.

   A general, if somewhat unsatisfactory, review of the comparative approach in social and cultural research is found in Etzioni and Dubow (1970).

5. Here we mean to draw attention to increasing recent research interest in stress and illness and psychosomatic and sociosomatic relationships. The development of research and teaching programs in biological anthropology, social biology, and psychosomatic medicine, as well as the long standing concerns of epidemiology, also attest to the cross-disciplinary interests in this crucial interface between the individual, his psychological and biological substrate, and his social and cultural environment.

6. These findings are part of unpublished results of an ethnographic study of the value structure of a psychiatric ward and its implications for the evaluation of therapeutic success, conducted by A. Kleinman at the Massachusetts General Hospital, 1972. (See A.

Kleinman: The Social and Cultural Context of Psychopathology and Psychiatric Care. In T. Manschreck and A. Kleinman, eds.: *Critical Rationality in Psychiatry*. Washington, D.C.: Hemisphere Publications, in press.)

7. Interested readers are referred to the larger paper from which this chapter has been extracted in A. Kleinman et al, eds.: *Medicine in Chinese Cultures*. Bethesda, Md.: Fogarty International Center, N.I.H., 1976; pp. 589-658. That paper contained a 20 page section on medicine in Chinese culture which applied the model developed in this paper to health care in Chinese societies.

8. Subsequently, a journal has been developed: *Culture, Medicine and Psychiatry*. This journal will cover 3 interrelated fields: (1) medical and psychiatric anthropology; (2) cross-cultural psychiatry; (3) related cross-societal clinical and epidemiological studies. Published by Reidel Publishers, the journal will appear quarterly from April 1977 in 100 page issues. It is edited by Arthur Kleinman, Department of Psychiatry, University of Washington School of Medicine, Seattle, Washington 98195.

REFERENCES

ABRAMSON, J., et al
  1961   What is wrong with me? A study of the views of African and Indian patients in a Durban Hospital. South African Medical Journal 35:690-694.

ADAIR, J. and K. DEUSCHLE
  1970   The People's Health: Medicine and Anthropology in a Navajo Community. New York: Appleton-Century Crofts.

ALLAND, A.
  1970   Adaptation in Cultural Evolution: An Approach to Medical Anthropology. New York: Columbia University Press.

APPLE, D.
  1960   How laymen define illness. Journal of Health and Human Behavior 1:219.

ARTISS, K. and A. LEVINE
  1973   Doctor–patient relation in severe illness. New England Journal of Medicine 288:1210.

BENVENISTE, E.
  1945   La doctrine medicale des Indo Européenes. Revue de l'Histoire des Religions 130:5.

BERGER, P., B. BERGER and H. KELLNER
  1973   The Homeless Mind: Modernization and Consciousness. New York: Random House.

BERLIN, B., D. BREEDLOVE and P. RAVEN
  1973   General principles of classification and nomenclature in folk biology. American Anthropologist 75:214.

BOWERS, J., ed.
  1973   Medicine in Chinese Society. New York: Josiah Macy, Jr. Foundation.

BUCKNER, H.
  1971   Deviance, Reality, and Change. New York: Random House.

CANCIAN, F.
  1971   New methods for describing what people think. Sociological Inquiry 41:85.

CASSELL, E.
  1972   Being and becoming dead. Social Research 39:528.

CHOMBART DE LAUWE, P.
  1966   The interaction of person and society. American Sociological Review 31:237.

CLEMENTS, F.
1932 Primitive concepts of disease. University of California Publications in American Archaeology and Ethnography 32:181.

CROIZIER, R.
1968 Traditional Medicine in Modern China. Cambridge: Harvard University Press.
1970 Medicine, modernization, and cultural crisis in China and India. Comparative Studies in Society and History 12:275.

DAVIS, M.
1968 Variations in patients' compliance with doctors' advice: An empirical analysis of patterns of communication. American Journal of Public Health 58:274-288.

DOUGLAS, M.
1970a Purity and Danger. Baltimore: Penguin Books.
1970b The healing rite. Man 5:302.

DREITZEL, H., ed.
1971 The Social Organization of Health. New York: Macmillan.

ELDER, R.
1973 Social class and lay explanations of the etiology of arthritis. Journal of Health and Social Behavior 14:28.

ELLENBERGER, H.
1970 The Discovery of the Unconscious. New York: Basic Books.

ENGEL, G.
1973 Personal theories of disease as determinants of patient–physician relationships. Psychosomatic Medicine 35:223.

ENGLEHARDT, H. T.
1974 Explanatory models in medicine: Facts, theories, and values, Texas Reports on Biology and Medicine 32:225-239.

ENTRALGO, P. L.
1955 Mind and Body, Psychosomatic Pathology: A Short History of the Evolution of Medical Thought. London: Harvill.
1970 The Therapy of the Word in Classical Antiquity. New Haven: Yale University Press.

ETZIONI, A. and F. DUBOW
1970 Comparative Perspectives: Theories and Methods. Boston: Little, Brown.

FABIAN, J.
1972 How others die—Reflections on the anthropology of death. Social Research 39:528–43.

FABREGA, H.
1972 The study of disease in relation to culture. Behavioral Science 17:183.
1973a An integrated theory of disease: Ladion-Mestizo views of disease in the Chiapas Highlands. Psychosomatic Medicine 35:223.
1973b Disease in relation to Human Behavior. Cambridge: M.I.T. Press.

FEINSTEIN, A.
1967 Clinical Judgement. Baltimore: Williams and Wilkins.

FOUCAULT, M.
1965 Madness and Civilization. New York: Mentor.

FRAKE, C.
1961 The diagnosis of disease among the Subanum of Mindanao. American Anthropologist 63:113.

FRANK, J.
1961 Persuasion and Healing: A Comparative Study of Psychotherapy. Baltimore: Johns Hopkins University Press.

FREIDSON, E.
1970 Profession of Medicine: A Study of the Sociology of Applied Knowledge. New York: Dodd and Mead.

GALLAGHER, E.
1972 The health experience in modern society. Social Science and Medicine 6:619.

GEERTZ, C.
1965 Religion as a cultural system. In Reader in Comparative Religion, W. Lessa and E. Vogt, eds. New York: Harper and Row.

GLICK, L.
1967 Medicine as an ethnographic category. Ethnology 6:31.

GOULD, H.
1965 Modern medicine and folk cognition in rural India. Human Organization 24:201.

GUSSOW, Z. and G. TRACY
1970 Stigma and the leprosy phenomenon: The social history of a disease in the nineteenth and twentieth centuries. Bulletin of the History of Medicine 44:425.

HAEFNER, I. and J. KIRSCH
1970 Motivational and behavioral effects of modifying health beliefs. Public Health Reports 85:478.

HARWOOD, A.
1971 The hot-cold theory of disease: Implications for treatment of Puerto-Rican patients. Journal of the American Medical Association 216:1153.

HINKLE, L.
1961 Ecological observations of the relation of physical illness, mental illness, and the social environment. Psychosomatic Medicine 23:289.

HORTON, R.
1967 African traditional thought and Western science. Africa 37: 150.

HSU, J. and W. H. TSENG
1972 Intercultural psychotherapy. Archives of General Psychiatry 27:700-705.

HUGHES, C.
1963 Public health in non-literate societies. In Man's Image in Medicine and Anthropology, I. Galdston, ed. New York: International Universities Press.

INGHAM, J.
1970 On Mexican folk medicine. American Anthropologist 72:76.

JAHODA, G.
1971 The Psychology of Superstition. Baltimore: Penguin Books.

KAGAN, A. and L. LEVI
1974 Health and environment—psychosocial stimuli: A review. Social Science and Medicine 8:225-241.

KANE, R. et al
1974 Manipulating the patient: A comparison of the effectiveness of physicians and chiropractic care. Lancet 1:1333.

KAPLAN, B. and D. JOHNSON
1964 The social meaning of Navajo psychopathology and psychotherapy. In Magic, Faith and Healing, A Kiev, ed. New York: Free Press.

KATZ, A.
1971 The social causes of diseases. In Dreitzel 1971.

KENNEDY, D.
1973 Perceptions of illness and healing. Social Science and Medicine 7:787.

KIEV, A.
1968 Curanderismo. New York: Free Press.

KLEINMAN, A.
1973a Toward the comparative study of medical systems: An integrated approach to the study of the relationship between medicine and culture. Science, Medicine, and Man 1:55.
1973b Medicine's symbolic reality: On a central problem in the philosophy of medicine. Inquiry 16:206.
1973c Some issues for a comparative study of medical healing. International Journal of Social Psychiatry 19:159–65.
1973d The background of public health in China. In Public Health in the People's Republic of China, M. Wegman, T. Lin, and E. Purcell, eds. New York: Josiah Macy, Jr. Foundation.
1974 Explanatory models in health-care relationships. In Health and the Family, Washington, D.C.: National Council for International Health, 1975; pp. 159-172.

LAZARE, A.
1973 Hidden conceptual models in clinical psychiatry. New England Journal of Medicine 288:345.

LAZARE, A. et al
1974 The customer approach to patienthood. Basic concepts. Archives of General Psychiatry 32:553-558, 1975.

LAZARUS, R.
1971 The concepts of stress and disease. In Society, Stress, and Disease, L. Levi, ed. London: Oxford University Press.

LEDLEY, R. and L. LUSTED
1959 Reasoning foundations of medical diagnosis. Science 130:9.

LEIGHTON, A. and D. LEIGHTON
1941 Elements of psychotherapy in Navajo religion. Psychiatry 4:515.

LEIGHTON, A. et al
1968 The therapeutic process in cross-cultural perspective. American Journal of Psychiatry 124:1171.

LESLIE, C.
1969 Modern India's ancient medicine. Transaction 46.
(Undated) The modernization of Asian medical systems. Mimeographed paper.

LESLIE, C., ed.
1976 Asian Medical Systems. Berkeley: University of California Press.

LEY, P. and M. SPELLMAN
1967 Communicating with the Patient. Liverpool: Staples Press.

LIPOWSKI, Z.
1968 Review of consultation psychiatry and psychosomatic medicine. III. Theoretical Issues. Psychosomatic Medicine 30:395.

1969   Psychosocial aspects of disease. Annals of Internal Medicine 71:1197.
1970   Physical illness, the individual and the coping process. Psychiatry in Medicine 1:91.

LITMAN, T. and L. ROBINS
1971   Comparative analysis of health care systems—a sociopolitical approach. Social Science and Medicine 5:573.

LLOYD, G.
1964   The hot and cold, the dry and wet in Greek philosophy. Journal of Hellenic Studies 84:92.

MABRY, J.
1964   Lay concepts of etiology. Journal of Chronic Diseases 17:371.

MAUSS, M.
1950   Les techniques du corps. In Sociologie et Anthropologie, M. Mauss, ed. Paris: Presses Universitaires de France.

MECHANIC, D.
1962   The concept of illness behavior. Journal of Chronic Diseases 15:189.
1966   Response factors in illness: The study of illness behavior. Social Psychiatry 1:11.
1972   Social psychological factors affecting the presentation of bodily complaints. New England Journal of Medicine 286:1132.
1973   Health and illness in technological societies. Hastings Center Studies 1:7.

MESSING, S.
1968   Interdigitation of mystical and physical healing in Ethiopia. Behavoral Science Notes 3:87.

MORISON, R.
1973   Dying. Scientific American 229:55.

MURPHY, R.
1971   The Dialectics of Social Life. New York: Basic Books.

NADER, L. and T. MARETZKI, eds.
1973   Cultural Illness and Health: Essays in Human Adaptation. Washington, D. C.: American Anthropological Association.

NASH, J.
1967   The logic of behavior: Curing in a Maya Indian town. Human Organization 26:132.

OBEYESEKERE, G.
1973   The impact of Ayurvedic medicine on culture and the individual in Ceylon. In Leslie, 1973, op. cit.

PARSONS, T.
1953   Illness and the role of the physician: A sociological perspective. In Personality in Nature, Society, and Culture, C. Kluckhohn and H. Murray, eds. New York: Knopf.

1972 The "gift of life" and its reciprocation. Social Research 39:367.

PLAJA, A., et al
1968 Communication between physicians and patients in outpatient clinics: Social and cultural factors. Milbank Memorial Fund Quarterly 46:161.

PLATONOV, K.
1959 The Word as a Physiological and Therapeutic Factor. Moscow: Foreign Languages Publications House.

PLOG, S. and R. EDGERTON, eds.
1969 Changing Perspectives in Mental Illness. New York: Holt, Rinehart and Winston.

PORKERT. M.
1974 The Theoretical Structure of Chinese Medicine. Cambridge: M.I.T. Press.

POYNTER, F., ed.
1969 Medicine and Culture. London: Wellcome Institute Publications.

RACY, J.
1969 Death in an Arab culture. Annals of the New York Academy of Science 164:871.

RAHE, R., et al
1964 Social stress and illness onset. Journal of Psychosomatic Research 8:35.

READ, M.
1966 Culture, Health and Disease. London: Tavistock.

READER, G. et al
1957 What patients expect from their doctors. Modern Hospital 89:88-94.

RIVERS, W.
1924 Medicine, Magic and Religion. New York: Harcourt and Brace.

ROSALDO, M.
1972 Metaphors and folk classification. Southwestern Journal of Anthropology 28:83.

ROSEN, G.
1973 Health, history and the social sciences. Social Science and Medicine 7:233.

ROSENBERG, C.
1969 The medical profession, medical practice, and the history of medicine. In Modern Methods in the History of Medicine, E. Clarke, ed. London: Athlone Press.

RUBINGTON, E. and M. WEINBERG, eds.
1969 Deviance: The Interactionist Perspective. New York: Macmillan.

SAMORA, J., L. SAUNDERS, and R. LARSON
1962 Knowledge about specific diseases in four selected samples. Journal of Health and Human Behavior 3:176.

SARGENT, M.
1971 A cross-cultural study of attitudes and behavior toward alcohol and drugs. British Journal of Sociology 22:83.

SAUNDERS, L.
1954 Cultural Differences and Medical Care. New York: Russell Sage Foundation.

SCHMALE, A., et al
1970 Current concepts of psychosomatic medicine. In Modern Trends in Psychosomatic Medicine II., O. Hill, ed. New York: Appleton-Century-Crofts.

SCOFIELD, A. and C. W. SUN
1960 A comparative study of the different effect upon personality of Chinese and American training practice. Journal of Social Psychology 52:221.

SHAPIRO, A.
1959 The placebo effect in the history of medical treatment. American Journal of Psychiatry 116:298.

SIEGLER, M. and H. OSMOND
1966 Models of madness. British Journal of Psychiatry 112:1193.
1973 The "sick role" revisited. Hastings Center Studies 1:41.

SIGERIST, H.
1951 A History of Medicine, Vol. I: Primitive and Archaic Medicine. London: Oxford University Press.

SIVIN, N.
1972 Folk medicine in traditional China. Mimeographed paper.

SNOW, C. P.
1973 Human care. Journal of the American Medical Association 225:617.

SNOW, L.
1974 Folk medical beliefs and their implications for care of patients. Annals of Internal Medicine 81:82-96.

SPEIGEL, J.
1964 Cultural variations in attitudes toward death and disease. In The Threat of Impending Disaster, G. Grosser, et al, eds., Cambridge: M.I.T. Press.

SPIRO, M.
   1967   Burmese Super-naturalism: A Study in the Explanation and Reduction of Suffering. Englewood Cliffs, New Jersey: Prentice-Hall.

SPRADLEY, J. and M. PHILLIPS
   1972   Culture and stress. American Anthropologist 74:518.

STIMSON, G.
   1974   Obeying doctor's orders: A view from the other side. Social Science and Medicine 8:97-104.

SUCHMAN, E.
   1965   Social patterns of illness and medical care. Journal of Health and Human Behavior 6:2.

TAMBIAH, S.
   1968   The magical power of words. Man 3:175.

TEICHNER, W.
   1968   Interaction of behavioral and physiological stress reactions. Psychological Review 75:281.

TEMKIN, O.
   1968   Comparative study in the history of medicine. Bulletin of the History of Medicine 42:362.

THOMAS, K.
   1971   Religion and the Decline of Magic. London: Weidenfeld and Nicholson.

TOPLEY, M.
   1953   Paper charms and prayer sheets as adjuncts to Chinese worship. Journal of the Malayan Branch of the Royal Asiatic Society 26:63.
   1970   Chinese traditional ideas and the treatment of disease. Man 5:421.

TSENG, W. S.
   1974a Folk psychotherapy in Taiwan. In Culture and Mental Health in Asia and the Pacific, Volume IV., W. Lebra, ed. Honolulu: University of Hawaii Press, in press.
   1974b Psychiatric Study of Shamanism in Taiwan. Forthcoming in Archives of General Psychiatry.

TSENG, W. S. and J. HSU
   1969   Chinese culture, personality formation and mental illness. International Journal of Social Psychiatry 16:5.

TURNER, V.
   1967   The Forest of Symbols. Ithaca: Cornell University Press.
   1969   The Ritual Process. Chicago: University of Chicago Press.

TWADDLE, A.
1974 The concept of health status. Social Science and Medicine 8:29.

WAITZKIN, H. and J. STOECKLE
1972 The communication of information about illness. Advances in Psychosomatic Medicine 8:180.

WALSER, H. and H. KOELBING, eds.
1971 Erwin Ackerknecht: Medicine and Ethnology. Bern: Huber.

WEISMAN, A.
1972 On Dying and Denying. New York: Behavioral Publications.

WERNER, H. and B. KAPLAN
1967 Symbol Formation. New York: Wiley.

WHITE, K., J. MURNAGHAM, and G. GAUS
1972 Technology and health care. New England Journal of Medicine 287:1223.

WHYBROW, P.
1972 The use and abuse of the medical model as a conceptual frame in psychiatry. Psychiatry in Medicine 3:333.

WILLIAMS, J.
1971 Disease as deviance. Social Science and Medicine 5:219.

WITTKOWER, E. and G. DUBREUIL
1973 Psychocultural stress in relation to mental illness. Social Science and Medicine 7:691.

WOLFF, R.
1965 Modern medicine and traditional culture: Confrontations on the Malay Peninsula. Human Organization 24:201 p. 339.

YALMAN, N.
1964 The structure of Sinhalese healing rituals. Journal of Asian Studies 23:115.

YAP, P.
1952 Mental diseases peculiar to certain cultures: A survey of comparative psychiatry. Journal of Mental Science 407:313.

1967 Ideas of mental health and disorder in Hongkong and their practical influence. In M. Topley, ed.: Some Traditional Chinese Ideas and Conceptions in Hongkong Social Life Today. Hongkong: Hongkong Branch, Royal Asiatic Society.

ZBOROWSKI, M.
1952 Cultural components in responses to pain. Journal of Social Issues 8:16.

ZOLA, I.
1966 Culture and symptoms. American Sociological Review 31:615.

1972a Medicine as an institution of social control. Sociological Review 20:487.

1972b Studying the decision to see a doctor: Review, critique, corrective. *In* Advances in Psychosomatic Medicine, A. Lipowshi, ed. Basel: Karger.

1973 Pathways to the Doctor—From Person to Patient. Social Science and Medicine 7:677.

CHAPTER 22

COMPARATIVE STUDIES IN SCIENCE AND MEDICINE: PROBLEMS AND PERSPECTIVES

EVERETT MENDELSOHN

There is a story that I first heard from a colleague whose father was a missionary in China. During the course of his attempts to bring modernization to a section of China, the father set up a slide projector and screen as part of an attempt to inculcate basic rules of public health. He wanted the household servants to take care against flies and the illnesses that they might bring and he projected on the screen a picture of a common housefly which came out, of course, about human size, or slightly larger. When the session was all over and he had made his point about how dangerous these flies were, the cook in the house said, "I'm sure that in your society where flies are that large they really are dangerous, but here ours are very small." There is something about the things we bring with us in our conceptions of what is important and what scale means that affects our ability to understand what others mean and what we mean. In talking at the conference about comparisons I noticed at least three major axes which were in use. We talked about change or difference across time, the historical comparison; we talked about diffferences across social, cultural and national boundaries; and we talked about social class or other group lines within a given culture or society. Other axes were used, but these certainly loomed large. How shall we handle them? One thing is to be careful of what it is we are bringing to our own analyses. When I thought of why I was asked to take part in the conference session, even though I am not a sinologist and had not focused my studies on Chinese science or medicine—I realized that I had a long history of interest in the biomedical sciences and in science as a social activity. It seemed to me that I might focus on some of the problems and some of the prospects for further study that seem important to someone like myself looking at the history of medicine and science as the study of both cognitive systems and social systems.

What do we bring to our analysis of medicine, science and technology? Have we excluded the analytical techniques of science itself from the framework of our analysis and assumed it as a "given" against which the "sciences" and "medical doctrines and practices" of other cultures are to be measured? If we can avert the assumption of what mathematical or scientific or medical knowledge is, and instead compare under different socioeconomic and cultural conditions how humans have constructed different styles of thought and kinds of explanations and modes of operations and techniques, we can start the problem right. The task, however, turns out not to be simple. One of the underlying sets of disagreements that emerges in discussions of the sort we had in this symposium is the problem of science and rationality (Wilson 1970). Let me turn briefly to 10 different points which provide a number of ways of dealing, albeit indirectly, with science and rationality. The generally-accepted assumption is that we measure the success of some activity against a scientific approach or something which we call rational.

What shall we do with science and rationality? One suggestion is to dethrone it. That is, ask ourselves if we can examine science or a rational system as something that is actually strange to us; treat it as some belief system which we are stumbling upon and which somehow we can come to understand. If we were to examine rationality not only as some sort of cognitive category but as something that is socially constructed and therefore open to sociological inquiry, I think we will have put it in a place where it, among other things, can serve as a cognitive category which is used in some cases, is efficacious in some cases, while in others it is obviously without use. The construction of any body of knowledge, I would suggest, is inextricably linked to the interests of those who produce it, who maintain it, and who practice it. Knowledge is directly tied to the way people live and what it is that they are using that knowledge for. And use here can be everything from a sacred use to a very profane use. If we then look at science or at rationality as socially constructed, what kinds of questions might be asked? As a historian I have looked hard at science in the European contexts. It has often been set aside as something special and which has transnational characteristics. I would point out, to the contrary, that science, as we know it, was created in time, in place, and in context (Merton 1970; Ravitz 1972). What elements were involved?

If we were to transport ourselves back to the year 1600 it would have been very difficult for us to know what science would have looked like by the end of that century—the year 1700. We could not have told whether the images that William Gilbert projected of knowing nature solely through experience and only dealing with the things known through experience would prevail, or whether the image proposed by Giordano Bruno, who wanted to include in a single system of explanation everything from miracles through the motion of natural bodies, would be victorious. When we examine the history of this period—the late sixteenth and early seventeenth centuries—we can see a period of instability in the secular realm and in the sacred realm. These were the years that followed hard upon the Reformation and major wars in Europe; and also included the Cromwellian wars and civil wars in England. This is part of the background of the Scientific Revolution. Who were the revolutionaries? When one looks hard at the European scene, the revolutionaries themselves were a very mixed group. They were Hermetic philosophers; they were experimental philosophers; they included Rosicrucians and Baconians, alchemists, mystics and magicians. While on first appearance they are a strange group, taken together there turn out to be several things they believed in common. They were rebelling against traditional authority at the cognitive level, and at the institutional level where the intellect was concerned. They all were choosing to define new methods. It is no accident that Bacon called his major work the *Novum Organum*. They were directly contradicting the old Aristotelian or authoritarian pattern that was then seen to control university learning. Method was the key to the kind of changes that people wanted to develop. Together with new methods they sought new educational forms. Each of these groups had plans for new universities or schools and offered a variety of new educational forms. The new methods they proposed had an important component in common: they were to be experiential. Experience was one thing which each of these revolutionary groups wanted to see raised in importance. These people had a fundamental social reason to back experience. They were marginal in power and authority in their society. Authority at the cognitive level and the sacred level rested primarily in the church and with the scholastic philosophers. If they were able to replace the Word, the Book, or the Crown with the experience as the arbiter of truth, they had a new chance for gaining authority. Truth would be available to anyone who could become literate, who could take part in observing and that is exactly where these groups wanted to go; they wanted in. They wanted to share the power, authority, and wealth of their time. And they were defining a new method which let them have it. They proposed a series of counter concepts; they proposed knowing nature and controlling nature in new ways. Control was an important new element (Leiss 1972). The assumption stated by Francis Bacon and many others was that we sought to understand nature in order to control it, to gain human dominion over things. They were in their own way a counter culture; they existed on the fringes of the university and on the fringes of the Church. They posed a challenge to the established Church and to the established order or authority of their day. Galileo was not condemned solely because of his ideas about the notions of the bodies in the heaven. Galileo was condemned because of what the new ways of knowing implied and what they did to the position of previously authoritative statements about nature.

Science was being made by marginal men. It turns out when you look at them that they are the same individuals who were a part of the emerging bourgeoisie, the same individuals who Michael Walzer (1965) identified as the radical Protestants, the people existing on the fringes of Protestantism; they were dissenting religionists. What did they hope to do? They wanted social space; they wanted to find their way into society, not at the sufferance of authority. During a period of great social instability they could exist and the early seventeenth century certainly represented just this condition. In England in the 1640's and 1650's, the Rosicrucian and Hermetic philosophers published more works than at any other time. They claimed that it was easier to get things published in England while things were in such turmoil. There was a plurality of views possible in the period of political and social instability and that plurality might or might not last. They rushed to make use of it. But they existed at the sufferance of somebody else's authority, and with the restoration of that authority in England in 1660, the Crown and the Church being restablished, the new members of the Royal Society took a hard look at what they could and could not do. Similarly, as the counter-reformation bore down hard on scientists on the Continent, they too looked at what they could and could not do. What emerged is what the historians called the positivist compromise. Boundaries were drawn around what we now call science—boundaries which prior to that time had not been sharply defined in anyone's mind. The new scientists were responding to the Church; they were responding to the State. When the Royal Society of London drew up their charter, they said "This Society will eschew all discussion of religion, rhetoric, metaphysics, morality, and politics" (cf Purver 1967). They agreed not to deal with the subjective, the normative, and the irrational. They claimed that they would deal with certain knowledge, things which could be known through experience.

The experimental philosophies put forward to understand and command nature and to improve the common weal were powerful. In terms of outlining a way of understanding and organizing human reaction and relation to nature, the experimental philosophy turned out to have enormous efficacy. It had already been demonstrated among such groups as the practical mathematicians, the pharmacists, the architects, and the engineers. This whole subculture had a practical sense of science in the early sixteenth and seventeenth centuries and saw its efficacy burst forward finally in these philosophic tests. Science became institutionalized at a period when it sharply circumscribed the range of phenomena and types of knowledge that it would deal with. It became inextricably linked to the industrial revolution and to the nascent capitalism. What better philosophy of nature could be adopted than one which claims to command nature, but is non-normative, not compelled to ask moral questions. In the years since, we have watched science emerge as the new orthodox way of knowing. Not that it drove all other forms of knowing out of existence, but it drove them from any claim of orthodoxy. While organized science and medicine skirmished with less "orthodox" practices and theories at its boundaries, it insisted on drawing the lines and reading out of the academies and denying licenses to the deviant practitioners. Through their efforts something like an orthodox epistemology arose. We know that there are more readers of astrological columns in the daily newspapers than the astronomical ones. But we also know no astrologist will ever get an appointment in the science faculty of the university; nor will he ever be elected to one of the academies of science or other learned bodies.

Medicine was directly affected by this new outlook in science. Not that it immediately became scientific medicine, but the boundaries were drawn more closely. Why? It turns out that when you look at most of the people who became the practicing scientists, they had entered it through medicine, and many of them earned their livelihood by practicing medicine. What happened then? An increased rationality became linked to therapeutic empiricism. By the late nineteenth century scientific medicine developed, bringing into medicine the system of experimentation as it had earlier developed in science. The new outlook was not necessarily aimed at the health and betterment of the condition of the single patient, but rather at dealing with a whole class of diseases.

Medicine had had an alternative epistemology from the epistemology of science. A physician would not have been heard saying, "I am searching for this new knowledge for the sake of the knowledge itself." In fact, to this day I expect physicians generally would not find themselves in that position. Medical scientists, on the other hand, might, and this is a tension that exists in medicine today. Throughout the West there is little doubt that the impact of science on medicine has been to create an alternative epistemology more closely allied to that of science: not a therapy-oriented medicine, but a science-oriented medicine. And it is this that I think creates confusion when we look at scientific medicine or Western medicine as it interacts with other cultures. There are several parts or traditions of Western medicine interacting, and I think we have to separate them clearly. The point that I believe must be stressed is that science and medicine have not been with us from the beginning in unchanged form. They have undergone the changes of institutionalization, professionalization, and enormous success. Science and medicine will not remain unchanged into the future. They are not constants. They must be among the objects of anthropological and sociological studies, not constants to bring to anthropological and sociological studies.

Having digressed at great length on these facets of the social organization of science, let us turn to the second point—the question of expert or esoteric knowledge and technique. This is one of the areas that interests me particularly in light of the comparative discussions in which we are engaged. Who holds the knowledge and who generates it? Do they differ from those who use the knowledge or are affected by it? It is a long-term problem that transcends science and obviously occurs in other fields as well. The question that emerges when we look at science and medicine is what is the nature of the gap between those who hold expert or esoteric knowledge and those who are affected by it or use it? Is there a difference in their way of perceiving their knowledge and handling it? If there is a difference (and I would contend there almost always is), is there a feedback loop? Do the users, those affected by it, in any way affect the nature of the new knowledge to be generated? If they don't, what is the focus of the new knowledge? What is the social locus of the knowledge and technique that we call medical or scientific? Are there differences in social distance, or cognitive distance, between the generators and holders of special knowledge and those who are affected by it or use it?

Let me turn directly now to the third point—activities at the margins and boundaries of science and medicine. As I look at Western medicine and science (those developed in the European culture area) there is an orthodox core more-or-less clearly identified, albeit it varies in time and across history. It has been institutionalized and professionalized. It has had an enormous increase in its authority as both formal and informal means of ordering its practice, ordering its use. It has created in many ways a knowledge elite with limited access. There are educational and class hurdles to entering that knowledge elite. At the boundaries of this organized and institutionalized group of professional practitioners of either science or medicine there seems to be a lot of other activity at any given point in human history. Recent years have seen an increase in the numbers of devotees and followers of activities at the boundaries as compared with those committed to activities at the core. The orthodox may have power, but may not have followers. One of the interesting characteristics that I found while looking at what have been derogatorily called pseudo sciences or popular medicine, quack medicine in Western societies, is that they often have the characteristics of social movements, or political movements. This is in marked contrast to the clearly institutionalized or professionalized organizational form of orthodox knowledge. I would love to see some further study of this kind of difference. Why is it that when you exist on the fringes you seem to take part in political movements or social movements, whereas when you are a part of the core you have organized your activities in a different way and you seem to ask for different canons of proof and often even turn toward different problems? Further, it appears that the heterodox practitioners relate to the recipients of the knowledge in a different manner.

This relates directly to a fourth point—the audiences, the public and the clients of both science and medicine. What forms of legitimation and support are developed, where do they come from and how do we locate them? There was a lot of informal discussion on this topic, but I would like to see it examined more directly on a comparative basis. We might begin by examining why we can have in some cultures or societies plural systems of medical practice seemingly equal or at least non-oppressive of one another, whereas in other cultures we cannot. What is the difference? What do the social mechanisms of it look like? I think this is a question which will lead us to a better understanding of the experience in the PRC.

Point five—pop culture, as I would call it. We know that our children learn much more out of school than they do within the classroom. Most of their images of society are gained at the corner drug store, from the television, from comic books, from their friends, and from a variety of non-formal educational activities. What kinds of images are developed in different cultures and societies? What kinds of images are created of scientists or those in medicine? How do they compare? How does the healer compare to other people within a given culture? And most important of all, what kinds of expectations are created? What does the pop culture create by way of expectations on the part of those who live within a society in its children's games, for example? Everyone of us knows a child who plays doctor at one time or another. Does a game like that exist elsewhere? Does someone in a Taiwanese village play healer? How does the game work? It would be interesting to see what the mode of setting up the expectations looks like. Are they similar or not? These to my mind are part of the tacit clues which are passed on in any society or culture as the way we recognize and then later organize our responses to the organized forms and informal forms of knowing nature and using healing.

Sixth point—what I would call the architecture of science and medicine. Look at it. There we were in a center for medical education, and we sat for 3 days in a room and never looked out of a window. What does it tell us about the nature of an activity, when it is physically practiced in a setting which clearly is an exclusive one? What does the architecture tell us about where in a society different forms of knowledge exist? Think back to the ancient European universities or try Harvard as a latter-day place on this continent. Without exception you will find that science is practiced on the periphery. Post-1945, the science buildings were the largest and most expensively furnished. Take the examination of the architecture of science and medicine one step further—where is it practiced? Is it practiced in a market place? Is it practiced in a church? Is it practiced in a university, in a hospital, in a laboratory, in a village hut? I think these give us some indication of the manner in which the physical structures tell us something about access to the knowledge and technique, tell us about the exclusiveness or inclusiveness of the activity itself.

Seven—the lure of development models. They came up over and over again in our discussions, sometimes formally, sometimes we inadvertently slipped into them. Here I think we can blame Karl Marx to begin with, and perhaps Walt Rostow in the second spot. There seems to be a continuing assumption that there are stages of growth, take-off points, and assumed directions in which we will go. The assumption that I heard being made was that traditional medicine will go through a series of forms and end up where we are today. This seems to be a model full of justification of where we are today. By contrast, a true evolutionary model does not have a predictable outcome. All cultures and societies go through some sort of change whether we call them evolutionary or not. We have too easily slipped into taking a developmental model as a guide, seeming to know the final point almost as we start. I do not think it is helpful.

Eight—a question I would love to learn more about but will just allude to is the role of literacy. It has been brought up briefly in our discussions. Jack Goody (1963) makes the point that there is something like a cultural homeostasis in oral cultures and that the achievement of literacy allows for greater change and innovation. In examining scientific or medical systems it would seem important to compare the changes that literacy has brought to their development in different cultures. Are there methods of change built into some systems of knowledge and not others? As we look at comparisons I think it is important for us to recognize whether or not a dynamic for change exists or whether by bringing the assumption of change we are basically altering the cultural traditions.

Nine—I will deal very briefly with the problem of transfer and exchange. It seems to me that a basic problem of dealing with Western science and medicine in relation to non-Western societies has been the assumption that we are looking at a one-way system of "impact." Yet, everything I know about the history of human cultures suggests to me that over any significant time-span the impact is not unidirectional. For example, will Western or scientific medicine emerge unchanged from its contact with other culture systems? I cannot believe that will be the case. In our research are we even looking for those changes or are we looking only at results expected from impact? I think that this is a question which we have to retool ourselves to ask in an alternative fashion.

Finally, point ten. In an earlier paper I asked a question about the makeup of the practitioners of science and medicine (Mendelsohn 1973). I noted that science, as we know it now, is done by white males who, by the nature of the activity, are middle class. The question I asked is, would the activity look the same if it were being done by the poor, the black, the females in our society? The answer I hear from the particular studies at the anthropological level is obviously not. How do we bridge this gap? The assumption the scientist makes is that anyone coming in to look at science will bend themselves to fit its mode and its epistemology. Yet everything I have heard in the anthropological discussions and seen in the literature I read is that there are competing epistemologies (Horton and Finnegan 1973). If our activity is socially constructed by white males of the middle class and it provides the guidelines of research, how can we possibly hope to understand cross-cultural comparisons and understand systems which have been designed by entirely different segments of the populations?

Comparative studies of science and medicine are certainly important for what they may tell us of these activities in other cultures (Thackery and Mendelsohn 1974). But these studies may be even more important in that they force us to re-examine our own research methods to enable the researcher to focus on those methods themselves as objects of anthropological and sociological scrutiny.*

---

*For reports of the conference discussions Mendelsohn refers to, see Chapters (17), (18), (27), (33), (42), (48) in *Medicine in Chinese Cultures* (A. Kleinman et al, eds. Bethesda, Md.: Fogarty International Center, N.I.H., 1975).

REFERENCES

GOODY, J. and I. WATT
1963 The consequences of literacy. Comparative Studies in Society and History, 5: 304.

HORTON, R. and R. FINNEGAN, eds.
1973 Modes of Thought: Essays on Thinking in Western and Non-Western Societies. London: Faber.

LEISS, W.
1972 The Domination of Nature. New York: G. Braziller.

MENDELSOHN, E.
1973 A human reconstruction of science. Boston University Journal, 21: 45–52.

MERTON, R.
1970 Science, Technology and Society in Seventeenth-Century England. New York: H. Fertig.

PURVER, M.
1967 The Royal Society: Concept and Creation. London: Routledge.

RAVITZ, J.
1972 Scientific Knowledge and its Social Problems. London: Oxford University Press.

THACKERY, A. and E. MENDELSOHN, eds.
1974 Science and Values: Patterns of Tradition and Change. New York: Humanities Press.

WALZER, M.
1965 The Revolution of the Saints: A Study in the Origins of Radical Politics. Cambridge: Harvard University Press.

WILSON, B., ed.
1970 Rationality. New York: Harper and Row.

INDEX

A

Acupuncture
  acceptance in Hongkong, 135
  anesthesia by, 115, 302
  in Hongkong, 115, 303, 306
  instruction in Malaysia, 164
  Kwun Tong, in, 300
  "no demand for it" in Taiwan
    market town, 42
  stress syndrome, and the, 95
  Taiwan, practitioners rendering, 281
  use in Japan, 267
  Western demand for, 235
Adaptive functions of medical systems,
  table of, 403
Adjectives applied to medical systems,
  table of, 403
Ahtelan hsaya (Exorcists, Burmese),
  223
Air or wind (*lom*), 198, 199
Alcoholic beverages considered heating, 72–73
Alcoholism, not prevalent in Taiwan,
  323–324
All-India Ayurvedic Congress, 245
Almanac, Chinese (*Tung Seng*), 160
American culture and study of health-
  care explanatory models, 422
American visitors to China, short-term,
  383
Amnesia diagnosed as soul loss, 79
Amulets
  used in Burmese preventive medicine,
    221
  worn by baby in Malaysia, 159
Analytical dichotomy between tradi-
  tional and modern medicine, 408
Ancestral spirits
  in Thailand, 191
  obligations to, 207
Angelica sinensis, 160
Animal sacrifices and spirit-caused ill-
  ness, 192, 193
Animistic medical system, early, in
  Japan, 266
Anthropological study of medical sys-
  tems, comparative, 393–404
Antiseptics germ-killing theory, accept-
  ance of in Taiwan village, 107
Arabic medicine
  See also Yumani medicine and the
    Classical Western tradition, 428

Arabic-Persian medicine in Malaysia,
  155
Architecture of science and medicine,
  the, 451
Artemisia and sweet flag in Chinese folk
  medicine, 22
Aryan Medical School, Bombay, 244
Asian medical systems, Western image
  of, 236
Astrology, 266
Attitudes of patient and practitioner in
  Chinese setting, modern, 275–287
Aulan hsaya (Master witches, Burmese), 219
Ayurveda, 253–262
  "cultural diseases" in, 253, 257, 258
  emulating Western medical model,
    254
  Five Elements, and the, 256, 258
  professionalized, 254
  what is the future of?, 256
Ayurvedic medicine
  a major non-Western form of medi-
    cine, 408, 409
  available in Malaysia, 151, 155, 166
  in India, 238
Ayurvedic texts, courses based on, 245

B

Bamboo stick, divination (*chouchien*),
  314
Bandar (urban, Malay), 144
Beer in Chinese dietetics, 74
Behavior
  beliefs and, 85
  Burmese, and psychopathology, 228
  cognitive systems, and associated,
    396
  cultural analysis of, 394
  health consequences of, 394
  illness, 417, 418
  individual, in cross-cultural analyses,
    407
  medical, Peninsular Malaysia, in, 144
  tribal, in Thailand, 208
  personal health, 156
  social, illness and, 185
Behavioral science perspectives in the
  study of medical systems, 408
Beliefs
  about food, 75–76

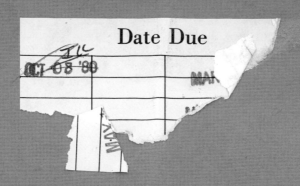